COMMON MEDICAL DIAGNOSES: AN ALGORITHMIC APPROACH

SECOND EDITION

Patrice M. Healey, M.D.
Assistant Clinical Professor of Medicine
UCLA School of Medicine
Los Angeles, California

Edwin J. Jacobson, M.D.
Clinical Professor of Medicine
UCLA School of Medicine
Los Angeles, California

D1317775

W.B. SAUNDERS COMPANY
A Division of Harcourt Brace & Company
Philadelphia ■ London ■ Toronto ■ Montreal ■ Sydney ■ Tokyo

W.B. SAUNDERS COMPANY
A Division of
Harcourt Brace & Company

The Curtis Center
Independence Square West
Philadelphia, Pennsylvania 19106

Library of Congress Cataloging-in-Publication Data

Healey, Patrice M.

   Common medical diagnoses : an algorithmic approach / Patrice M.
Healey, Edwin J. Jacobson.—2nd ed.

     p.   cm.

Includes index.

ISBN 0–7216–5401–0

1. Medical protocols.   2. Diagnosis, Differential.   I. Jacobson,
  Edwin J.   II. Title.
  [DNLM: 1. Algorithms.   2. Decision Support Techniques.
  3. Diagnosis.   WB 141 H434c 1994]

RC64.H43 1994

616.07′5—dc20

DNLM/DLC   93–38502

Common Medical Diagnoses: An Algorithmic Approach, Second Edition   ISBN 0–7216–5401–0

Printed in the United States of America

Last digit is the print number: 9   8   7   6   5   4   3   2

For Martha, Emily, and Bob

Foreword

According to William Osler, to study medicine without reading books is like navigating without maps; however, trying to become a physician without seeing patients is never to go to sea at all.

In the light of what they have read, thoughtful students and physicians learn from their patients, and what they learn from patients in turn enhances what it is possible for them to learn from reading. Access to the experience of others and one's own experience combine synergistically in the acquisition of clinical wisdom.

In practice, interpretation of the history and physical examination is often commingled with the weighing of other diagnostic clues from laboratories and special procedures. The diagnostician may at many stages in the analysis of a patient's illness shorten the distance from complaint to diagnosis—and render the trip less expensive—by finding out before ordering it how helpful a particular test or procedure has generally proved to be. The doctor's bedside findings lead to a fork in the road. At this point for this patient, which pathway is better?

Burgeoning techniques, which when used wisely greatly improve diagnostic accuracy, can also make the choice of pathways more complicated or unnecessarily expensive. Even to know where to look or whom to consult for help requires not only skillful gathering of data but also logical use of them.

Doctors Healey and Jacobson have approached the diagnostic process by considering such common clinical problems as headache and fever through algorithms. The word algorithm, derived from the name of a ninth century Arabic mathematician, means step-by-step, logical problem-solving.

Algorithms prepared in advance cannot infallibly be applicable to all patients, who vary enormously. In a sense every patient requires step-by-step logical problem-solving for his or her specific problem(s). Algorithms can, however, help the physician to develop logical steps in differential diagnosis by indicating in stepwise fashion frequently encountered bifurcations in the reasoning process and how, generally, to choose the best route.

An additional benefit of this work is that the algorithms are cross-referenced to two medical textbooks. Thus this book can enhance for students of all ages the circle of learning that proceeds for a lifetime from patients to medical literature and back to patients again.

SHERMAN M. MELLINKOFF, M.D.
Professor of Medicine
UCLA School of Medicine
Former Dean, UCLA School of
Medicine, 1962–1986
Los Angeles, California

Preface

The first edition of *Common Medical Diagnoses: An Algorithmic Approach* was written with the student and house officer in mind, but we found the book to be extremely well received by the experienced clinician as well.

In preparing the second edition of *Common Medical Diagnoses,* we undertook an extensive review of the recent literature in order to incorporate into the algorithms changes in technology and new testing procedures so that the algorithms reflect the technological advances in the diagnosis of medical problems. Four new algorithms have also been added.

As with the first edition, we have classified common clinical problems as they present to us in everyday practice: as signs, symptoms, and laboratory abnormalities. Although an algorithm cannot take into account the circumstances of the individual patient, these decision trees suggest a logical, cost-effective approach to diagnosis. Certainly there are many ways to approach a clinical problem; these algorithms are but one approach. The algorithms provide a directed approach to breaking down large lists of differential diagnoses into smaller, more manageable lists, through clinical examination and the judicious use of diagnostic testing. Algorithms presume familiarity with clinical medicine and the ability of the user to make intelligent choices in approaching a particular problem.

As with the first edition, although many of the algorithms suggest a diagnostic test at the outset, it is presumed that a thorough history and physical examination have been performed prior to any diagnostic testing. The comments provide clinical insights and clarification of the algorithms but are by no means complete reviews of each diagnostic category. All of the algorithms are directed toward diagnosis only; treatment is never addressed unless treatment is used as a diagnostic test. Each algorithm is cross-referenced to the latest editions of the major textbooks of medicine, *Cecil Textbook of Medicine,* 19th Edition, Wyngaarden JB, Smith LH, and Bennett K (eds.), Philadelphia, WB Saunders, 1992; and *Harrison's Principles of Internal Medicine,* 12th Edition, Braunwald E (ed.), New York, McGraw-Hill, 1990.

We anticipate that the second edition will be as useful to and as well-received by students of medicine as the first edition was.

PMH
EJJ

Acknowledgments

Many people have contributed to the writing of this book. The authors would like to thank Doctors Saleh Saleh, Franklin Murphy, Allen Nissenson, Jan Tillisch, Paul Bellamy, John Child, James Roach, Michael Rosove, Sheldon Jordan, Marvin Derezin, Edwin Amos, Charles Frankel, Kenneth Kalunian, Gary Lazar, John Glaspy, Richard P. Kaplan, Larry Ford, Inder Chopra, Jaime Moriguchi, Gayle Randall, and Martin Pops for their help in reviewing the manuscript. John Dyson, Senior Editor at W. B. Saunders, who guided us through the first edition, has retired. We thank Ray Kersey, who has replaced John Dyson as Editor, for his patience and skill in guiding us through this second edition.

PMH
EJJ

Contents

COMMON MEDICAL DIAGNOSES: AN ALGORITHMIC APPROACH

1 ▪ Generalized Disorders

Signs and symptoms:	Weight loss
Fatigue	Weight gain
Fever of unknown origin	

Fatigue

1 Fatigue is one of the most common physical complaints. It is the chief complaint in as many as 55 per cent of visits to primary care physicians. Almost everyone feels fatigue at some time during his or her life. The causes of the fatigue usually are stress, overactivity, poor physical conditioning, or inadequate sleep. At times, however, fatigue may be severe. When fatigue lasts more than a few days, or when fatigue affects the normal activities of daily life, a more serious underlying disorder may be present, and a thorough evaluation is necessary.

2 Drugs may cause fatigue as a direct effect, or as an indirect effect by altering normal sleep patterns or metabolism. Drugs most commonly associated with fatigue include sedatives and hypnotics, tranquilizers, some antihistamines, most analgesics, tetracyclines, colchicine, steroids, birth control pills, centrally acting antihypertensives, many beta-blockers, and some of the nonsteroidal anti-inflammatory drugs. Digitalis toxicity is a common cause of fatigue and should be evaluated in any patient taking the drug. Many hypnotics, tranquilizers, and antidepressants may interfere with normal rapid eye movement (REM) sleep. The resultant abnormal sleep pattern is a common cause of fatigue even though the number of hours slept may be normal.

3 The medical history and physical examination provide clues for many of the causes of fatigue. Most often, fatigue of an organic etiology is worse in the evenings and is partially relieved by sleep. Psychogenic fatigue, on the other hand, usually has the opposite pattern. Many times, however, no specific cause can be determined on examination. Further evaluation, including the use of laboratory tests, radiographic examinations, various imaging techniques, and an extensive psychological profile, may be necessary in order to determine the cause of the fatigue.

4 Fatigue is often associated with infections. Acute bacterial infections are usually obvious from the medical history and physical examination. Diagnosing chronic infections may require a more extensive evaluation. The evaluation may require cultures of blood, other body fluids, and secretions for bacteria, fungus, and acid-fast organisms. Radiographic examinations of the lungs and sites of bone pain may be helpful. Stool examination for parasites should be performed for individuals with an appropriate history or a change in bowel habits. Other imaging techniques such as bone scan, computed tomography (CT), or magnetic resonance imaging (MRI) may also be useful in appropriate settings.

5 Fatigue is often a sign of an advanced or end-stage malignancy. Abnormalities on the physical examination or historical clues as well as a statistical likelihood should direct the evaluation for occult malignancy. Leukemias and lymphomas are the malignancies most often associated with fatigue, although fatigue may accompany any cancer.

6 Any nutritional deficiency may cause fatigue. The most common deficiencies include protein, calories, and certain vitamins. Although malnutrition is not thought of commonly in industrialized nations, fad diets, malabsorption syndromes, and eating disorders may all contribute to significant nutritional deficiencies.

7 Depression is probably the most common cause of chronic fatigue. In classic depression, fatigue is often accompanied by mood changes, anorexia, and sleep disturbances. Depression can present in more subtle ways and should always be suspected when no obvious cause for the fatigue can be found, especially in elderly persons.

8 Chronic viral infections are controversial causes of fatigue. After initial infection, many viruses remain in latent states within various tissues of the body. The most common of these viruses are the herpesvirus, Epstein-Barr virus, and cytomegalovirus. Any of these viruses may become reactivated and cause serious disease in the immunocompromised host. Several of these viruses, most notably the Epstein-Barr virus, have been implicated in patients with a variety of systemic complaints, including fatigue. There is little firm evidence, however, linking chronic viral diseases with fatigue in the immunocompetent patient.

9 Chronic fatigue syndrome is the name given to a symptom complex consisting of chronic severe fatigue, mild systemic complaints such as pharyngitis, and occasional myalgias. The illness usually affects women between 20 and 45 years of age. It is frequently associated with an active, high-stress lifestyle. Although chronic viral diseases have, in the past, been thought to play a role in the illness, it now appears that some combination of stress, a form of chemical depression, and possibly allergy may be the cause of the fatigue and many of its associated symptoms.

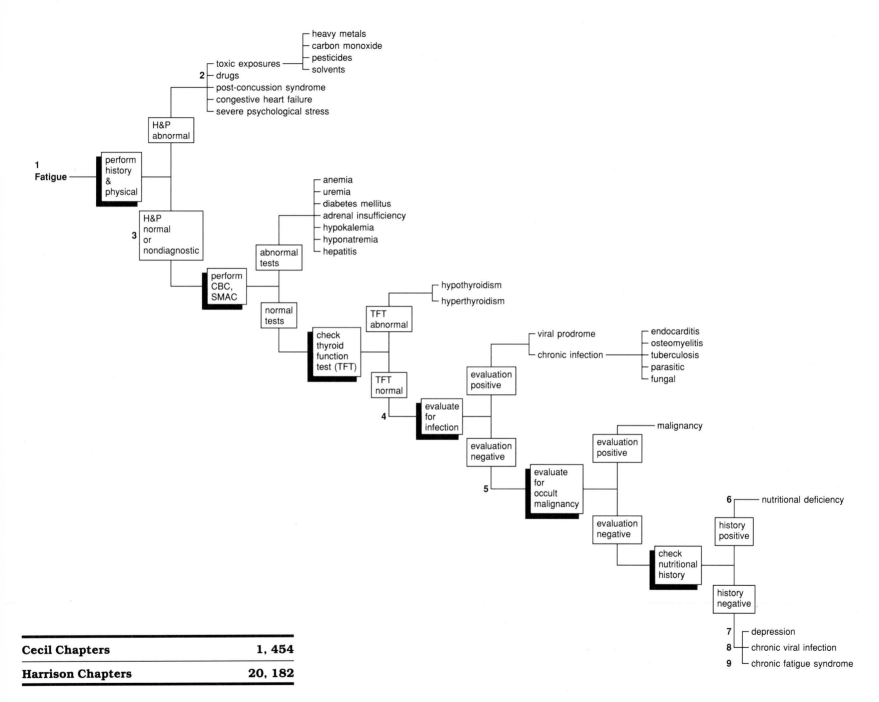

1
Fatigue

perform history & physical

H&P abnormal

2
├ toxic exposures ─┬ heavy metals
│   ├ carbon monoxide
│   ├ pesticides
│   └ solvents
├ drugs
├ post-concussion syndrome
├ congestive heart failure
└ severe psychological stress

3
H&P normal or nondiagnostic

perform CBC, SMAC

abnormal tests
├ anemia
├ uremia
├ diabetes mellitus
├ adrenal insufficiency
├ hypokalemia
├ hyponatremia
└ hepatitis

normal tests

check thyroid function test (TFT)

TFT abnormal
├ hypothyroidism
└ hyperthyroidism

TFT normal

4
evaluate for infection

evaluation positive
├ viral prodrome
└ chronic infection ─┬ endocarditis
                     ├ osteomyelitis
                     ├ tuberculosis
                     ├ parasitic
                     └ fungal

evaluation negative

5
evaluate for occult malignancy

evaluation positive ── malignancy

evaluation negative

check nutritional history

6
history positive ── nutritional deficiency

history negative

7 ─ depression
8 ─ chronic viral infection
9 ─ chronic fatigue syndrome

Cecil Chapters	1, 454
Harrison Chapters	20, 182

Generalized Disorders—Fatigue   3

Fever of Unknown Origin

1 The body's temperature regulation is an excellent indicator of general health. Although "normal" temperature may vary from person to person, deviation from an individual's normal pattern is usually an indication of disease. Heavy meals, strenuous exercise, ovulation, and menstruation may cause significant increases in body temperature, but these increases are short-lived and fit a predictable pattern. In general, an oral temperature over 99°F or a rectal temperature over 100°F is defined as fever. Fevers that last less than 1 week are virtually always associated with some form of infection. Fevers that last longer than 1 week are usually associated with serious disease. If fever lasts more than 3 weeks with daily temperature elevations to greater than 101°F and no diagnosis is readily apparent from routine history and physical examination, the fever is classified as fever of unknown origin (FUO). In 90 per cent of cases, FUOs are associated with serious infections, malignancies, and collagen vascular diseases. An extensive evaluation may be necessary in order to reach a diagnosis. Many approaches have been devised to evaluate FUOs. This algorithm represents only one such approach.

2 Cultures of blood, bodily secretions, the throat, or other abnormal-appearing areas of the body are the cornerstone of the evaluation of FUO. In addition to routine culture for bacteria, special methods for fungal and acid-fast culture should always be performed on appropriate fluids or tissues. The selection of the proper culture media and collection methods is essential. In most large series, 30 to 35 per cent of FUOs are due to previously undiagnosed infection.

3 Endocarditis should always be suspected in the patient with FUO. Individuals with underlying cardiac valvular abnormalities, especially those who have recently undergone procedures associated with bacteremia, such as dental, abdominal, gynecologic, or urinary tract surgery, are particularly susceptible to endocarditis. Intravenous drug users are also susceptible to endocarditis, many times with infection involving the right side of the heart. The bacteremia associated with endocarditis may be intermittent, and several blood cultures may be necessary to detect the organism. Most studies have shown that six sets of blood cultures are necessary to detect 90 per cent or more of patients with endocarditis. Fungal blood cultures should always be performed in immunocompromised patients and intravenous drug users.

4 Tuberculosis is one of the most common causes of FUO, accounting for 5 to 15 per cent of all cases. Prolonged fever is usually caused by extrapulmonary spread of the disease. Disseminated tuberculosis is more common in blacks than in whites. The most common extrapulmonary sites of infection are the liver, bone marrow, and kidney.

5 Lymphomas are the malignancies most commonly associated with fever. These tumors account for as many as 20 per cent of FUOs. Non-Hodgkin's lymphomas are more likely to be associated with fever. Other systemic symptoms usually accompany fever in these patients. These symptoms include weight loss, anorexia, and night sweats. These systemic symptoms constitute the B category when grading or staging various lymphomas. B-type symptoms are associated with shorter survival.

6 Several methods are available for detecting antibody to the human immunodeficiency virus (HIV) in blood. The most common method is the enzyme-linked immunosorbent assay (ELISA). Although the test is very sensitive, there is a 10 to 15 per cent false-positive rate. A test, most commonly the Western blot, should be performed to confirm exposure to HIV. Detection of HIV antibody is only an indication of exposure to the virus, but it is thought that the majority of persons exposed will progress to the full-blown acquired immunodeficiency syndrome (AIDS).

7 Fever is a common form of allergic reaction to many drugs. The mechanism of the fever may be related to the classic serum sickness reaction or may be an immune-mediated form of vasculitis. Most of the antibiotics can cause allergic-type fever. Other drugs associated with drug fever include allopurinol, captopril, heparin, hydralazine, hydantoins, methyldopa, procainamide, propylthiouracil, quinine, and quinidine.

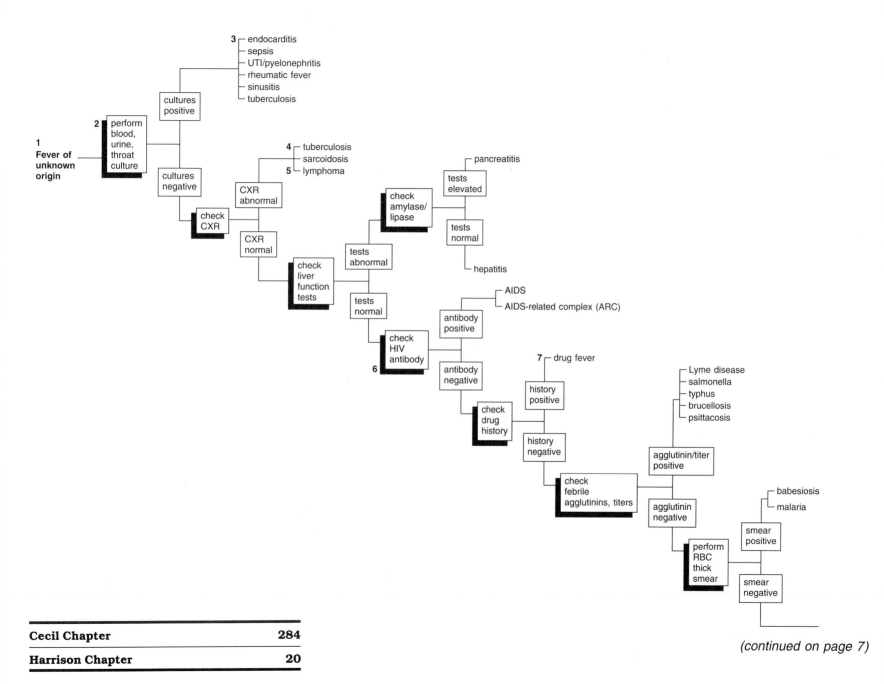

1
Fever of unknown origin

2 perform blood, urine, throat culture

cultures positive

3 endocarditis
sepsis
UTI/pyelonephritis
rheumatic fever
sinusitis
tuberculosis

cultures negative

check CXR

CXR abnormal

4 tuberculosis
sarcoidosis
5 lymphoma

CXR normal

check liver function tests

tests abnormal

check amylase/lipase

tests elevated

pancreatitis

tests normal

hepatitis

tests normal

check HIV antibody **6**

antibody positive

AIDS
AIDS-related complex (ARC)

antibody negative

check drug history

history positive

7 drug fever

history negative

check febrile agglutinins, titers

agglutinin/titer positive

Lyme disease
salmonella
typhus
brucellosis
psittacosis

agglutinin negative

perform RBC thick smear

smear positive

babesiosis
malaria

smear negative

(continued on page 7)

Cecil Chapter	**284**
Harrison Chapter	**20**

Fever of Unknown Origin
(Continued)

8 Metastatic carcinoma of the lung, pancreas, and stomach is frequently associated with fever. Liver metastases are usually present before fever becomes a prominent feature of the disease.

9 Cardiac myxomas are rare primary tumors of the heart. Myxomas most commonly occur in the left atrium. Myxomas occur most frequently in women and usually present in the middle decades of life. Fever, malaise, arthralgias, and an elevated sedimentation rate are frequently associated with myxomas, and the presentation can easily be confused with any chronic infection. Clues to the diagnosis include paroxysmal positional congestive heart failure and systemic or pulmonary embolization.

10 Nonlupus vasculitis is a common cause of FUOs, accounting for approximately 10 per cent of cases. This form of vasculitis is also associated with other constitutional symptoms, including intense myalgias, arthralgias, and occasionally rashes. Some of the highest fevers occur in patients with this syndrome.

11 Familial Mediterranean fever is a rare inherited disease. Persons of Middle Eastern and southern European ancestry have the highest incidence of the disease. Familial Mediterranean fever is characterized by recurrent episodes of fever, peritonitis, arthralgias, arthritis, elevated sedimentation rate, and occasionally pleuritis. The episodes are self-limited, but amyloidosis is a frequent late complication.

12 Among the solid localized tumors, hypernephromas have the highest incidence of associated fever.

13 Viral cultures are often difficult, time-consuming, and expensive. The highest yield comes from cultures of urine, pharyngeal secretions, and the buffy coat of the blood. A more practical approach is the measurement of viral and *Toxoplasma* antibody titers. The presence of elevated IgM antibody titer or a four-fold or more increase in IgG antibody titers is presumptive evidence of active infection.

14 As many as 10 per cent of FUOs may go undiagnosed after extensive evaluation. About half of these will eventually be diagnosed, usually with some form of malignancy. The remainder will continue undiagnosed, with fever in about half of this group remitting spontaneously and the other half responding to antipyretics and anti-inflammatory drugs.

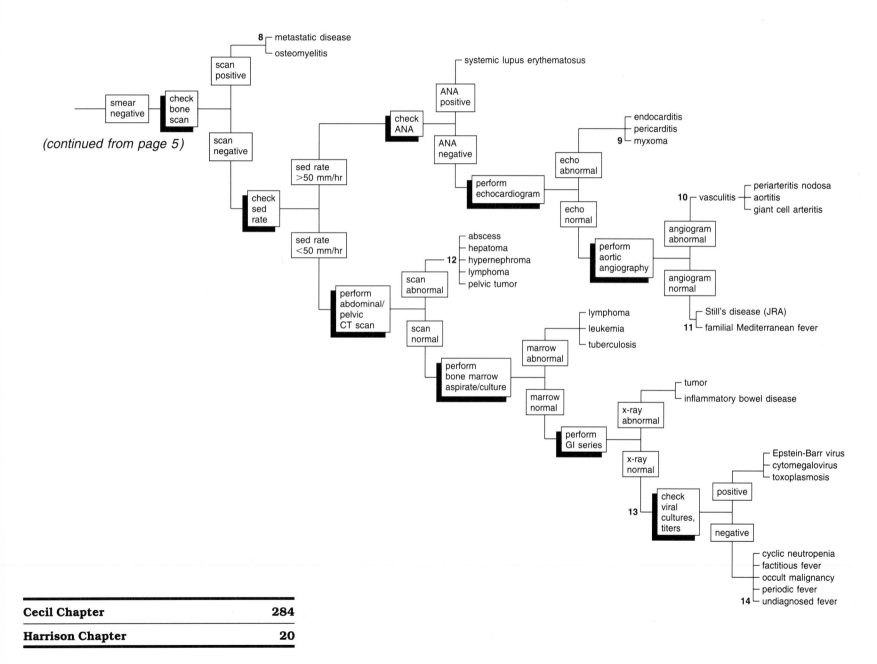

(continued from page 5)

8 ─ metastatic disease
     └ osteomyelitis

9 ─ endocarditis
     ├ pericarditis
     └ myxoma

10 ─ vasculitis ─ periarteritis nodosa
                    ├ aortitis
                    └ giant cell arteritis

11 ─ Still's disease (JRA)
      └ familial Mediterranean fever

12 ─ abscess
      ├ hepatoma
      ├ hypernephroma
      ├ lymphoma
      └ pelvic tumor

13 check viral cultures, titers
positive ─ Epstein-Barr virus
         ├ cytomegalovirus
         └ toxoplasmosis

negative ─ cyclic neutropenia
         ├ factitious fever
         ├ occult malignancy
         ├ periodic fever
14   └ undiagnosed fever

Cecil Chapter	**284**
Harrison Chapter	**20**

Weight Loss

1 Involuntary weight loss is one of the most ominous signs in medicine. The weight loss is usually a sign of a serious underlying physical or psychological disorder. True weight loss is usually defined as a 5 per cent or greater reduction in the patient's usual weight over a period of 6 months or less. More rapid weight loss, especially if it is accompanied by other systemic symptoms such as fatigue or fevers, is usually associated with more serious underlying conditions. Many patients do not complain of weight loss unless it is extremely rapid. Most often the physician detects the weight loss during routine examination. The diagnosis of true weight loss must be made on the basis of actual weight measurements rather than on historical data such as a change in clothing size or fit.

2 Weight loss may be caused by a deficiency of intake or absorption of sufficient calories to meet metabolic needs. Increased metabolic demands may also cause this caloric imbalance in spite of normal food intake. There are numerous formulas that allow for an accurate estimation of normal basal caloric needs. These formulas may be modified to account for any unusual expenditure of calories as a result of increased activity or increased metabolic needs. A reliable rule states that a 1-pound weight reduction will occur for each 3500-kcal deficit. Keeping a careful dietary history, including diet logs and formal calorie counts, is essential to determine whether the cause of the weight loss is decreased intake of calories rather than decreased absorption or increased metabolic demands.

3 More than 50 per cent of cases of inflammatory bowel disease are associated with weight loss. Weight loss is more common with Crohn's disease than with ulcerative colitis because involvement of the small bowel is usually more extensive. The weight loss may be secondary to decreased absorption of calories as well as to a rapid transit time of food in the intestine. Physical symptoms such as pain and early satiety may contribute to decreased intake of food and subsequent weight loss.

4 Celiac disease (nontropical sprue) is the result of gluten-associated inflammation of the epithelium of the small bowel. The inflammation results in malabsorption of nutrients and calories. The disease occurs in approximately 0.5 per cent of the general population. There is a strong family history in 20 per cent of patients with celiac disease. The disease is associated with weight loss, steatorrhea, anemia, cramps, and diarrhea. Severe vitamin and calcium deficiencies may occur. A classic pattern may be seen on small bowel barium studies, but the definitive diagnosis is made by small bowel biopsy. A gluten-free diet will result in resolution of the abnormalities.

5 The abdominal CT scan may be useful in diagnosing obstruction of the lymphatic drainage of the bowel and mesentery. Weight loss is caused by decreased absorption of food owing to edema of the intestinal wall. The etiology of the lymphatic obstruction, however, usually requires tissue samples and cultures obtained at laparotomy.

6 Several resins are used in the treatment of hyperlipidemia and hyperkalemia, including cholestyramine and sodium polystyrene sulfonate. These drugs may bind nutrients in the intestine if taken immediately prior to or after meals.

7 Several drugs can cause weight loss as a result of anorexia, nausea and vomiting, or changes in absorption in the intestine. These drugs include digitalis, anti-arrhythmics, diuretics, opiates, some antibiotics, some nonsteroidal anti-inflammatory drugs, hypoglycemic agents, cytotoxics, sucralfate, and several antihistamines.

8 Anorexia and weight loss are common with severe chronic congestive heart failure. The anorexia is secondary to fatigue, depression, and dyspnea. Increased metabolism may also play a role in the weight loss owing to the increased work of breathing. The actual weight loss may at times be masked by fluid retention but will be uncovered when the patient is made euvolemic during treatment.

9 Chronic infection is a common cause of weight loss. Granulomatous disease, deep fungal infections, intestinal and hepatic parasites, and subacute bacterial endocarditis are the most common infections associated with significant weight loss.

10 Weight loss and anorexia may be prominent components of many of the collagen vascular diseases. The collagen vascular diseases most commonly associated with weight loss include systemic lupus erythematosus, polyarteritis nodosa, rheumatoid arthritis, polymyositis, scleroderma, ankylosing spondylitis, polymyalgia rheumatica, and temporal arteritis.

11 As much as 15 to 20 per cent of total body weight may be lost during the course of AIDS. The etiology of this weight loss is multifactorial. Infections involving the mouth, teeth, esophagus, and intestine are common. The most common organisms include *Candida,* herpes simplex, *Cryptosporidia,* Campylobacter, and *Entamoeba histolytica.* Kaposi's sarcoma and AIDS-related lymphoma may involve the gastrointestinal tract. Decreased appetite may also arise from depression or as a part of AIDS encephalopathy.

12 Eating disorders are being diagnosed with increased frequency. Anorexia nervosa and bulimia are the most common of these disorders. Although any severe psychological illness can cause weight loss, a greater than 25 per cent weight loss secondary to decreased intake alone is classified as anorexia nervosa. The prevalence of this disorder may be as high as 1 in 200 in the general population, with a female predominance of 30 to 1. The disease is more common in Western society, where slimness is a cultural goal. Other, more severe, underlying psychological factors may play an important role in the etiology of the illness. Bulimia, the syndrome of eating and purging for the purpose of losing or maintaining weight, may be a separate disorder or can be associated with anorexia nervosa. Both of these disorders can lead to endocrine abnormalities, especially amenorrhea, and can ultimately lead to serious physical complications as a result of starvation and electrolyte imbalances.

13 Social stresses including poverty and physical or mental infirmity, as well as inadequate knowledge of proper nutrition and inadequate access to food, may lead to weight loss. This condition is probably much more widespread, even in developed countries, than is commonly thought.

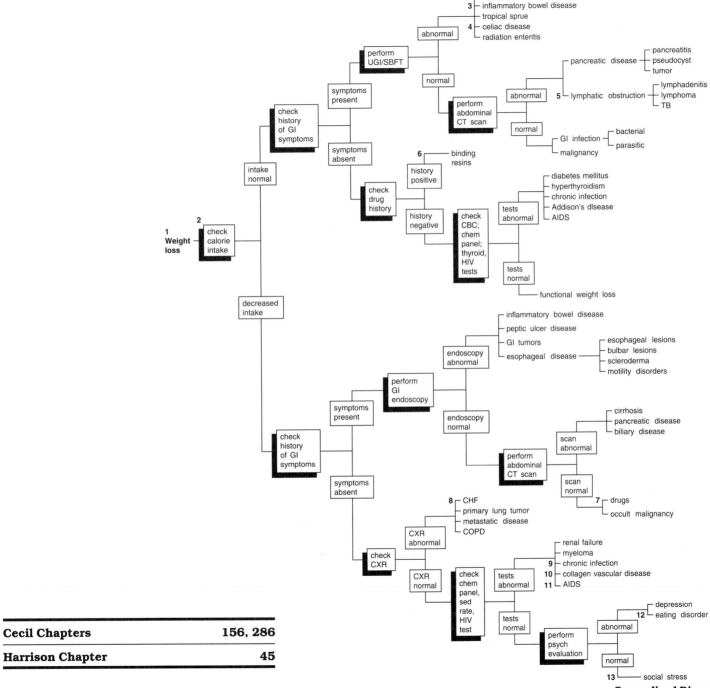

1 Weight loss — **2** check calorie intake

intake normal

check history of GI symptoms

symptoms present — **perform UGI/SBFT**

abnormal
- **3** GI tumor
- inflammatory bowel disease
- tropical sprue
- **4** celiac disease
- radiation enteritis

normal — **perform abdominal CT scan**

abnormal
- pancreatic disease
  - pancreatitis
  - pseudocyst
  - tumor
- **5** lymphatic obstruction
  - lymphadenitis
  - lymphoma
  - TB

normal
- GI infection
  - bacterial
  - parasitic
- malignancy

symptoms absent — **check drug history**

history positive — **6** binding resins

history negative — **check CBC; chem panel; thyroid, HIV tests**

tests abnormal
- diabetes mellitus
- hyperthyroidism
- chronic infection
- Addison's disease
- AIDS

tests normal — functional weight loss

decreased intake

check history of GI symptoms

symptoms present — **perform GI endoscopy**

endoscopy abnormal
- inflammatory bowel disease
- peptic ulcer disease
- GI tumors
- esophageal disease
  - esophageal lesions
  - bulbar lesions
  - scleroderma
  - motility disorders

endoscopy normal — **perform abdominal CT scan**

scan abnormal
- cirrhosis
- pancreatic disease
- biliary disease

scan normal — **7** drugs / occult malignancy

symptoms absent — **check CXR**

CXR abnormal
- **8** CHF
- primary lung tumor
- metastatic disease
- COPD

CXR normal — **check chem panel, sed rate, HIV test**

tests abnormal
- renal failure
- myeloma
- **9** chronic infection
- **10** collagen vascular disease
- **11** AIDS

tests normal — **perform psych evaluation**

abnormal
- depression
- **12** eating disorder

normal — **13** social stress

Cecil Chapters	156, 286
Harrison Chapter	45

Generalized Disorders—Weight Loss

9

Weight Gain

1 The causes of weight gain may include physical, psychological, and socioeconomic factors. Six to 15 per cent of children and adolescents are overweight. Approximately 25 per cent of men and 30 per cent of women are overweight. There is also an inverse relationship between socioeconomic status and the prevalence of obesity. Genetic factors, such as fat type and distribution, may play important roles in the way weight is gained and lost. By far, the most common etiology for weight gain is excessive caloric intake. Drug-induced changes in appetite or metabolism are also common. Only rarely can a physical cause such as an endocrine imbalance be found.

2 Excessive caloric intake is the most common cause of weight gain. Many patients may be reluctant to discuss their dietary habits or may not realize how the quantity and type of food they are eating affect their weight. An effective tool for dietary evaluation is a log kept by the patient and then analyzed for total calories consumed. This calorie count, when combined with an estimate or measurement of metabolic rate, can give a good assessment of the possible contribution of diet to the patient's weight gain.

3 Several classes of drugs are associated with weight gain. Their mechanisms are usually not well understood, but these medications may affect both appetite and metabolism. The dosage and the route of administration may also have an effect. Generally, the more sedating the drug, the greater the potential for weight gain.

4 The cessation of smoking is usually associated with a modest weight gain, averaging 10 pounds. Stopping nicotine decreases the patient's resting metabolic rate. There may also be a concomitant increase in caloric intake. This effect usually lasts no longer than 2 months.

5 Psychiatric disorders must be considered in the evaluation of weight gain. Many neuroses and some forms of depression may involve overeating. Among the more severe disorders, bulimia nervosa is most commonly associated with weight gain. This disorder is associated with binge eating alternating with caloric restriction. Bulimia nervosa should be distinguished from other variants, in which purging usually leads to weight loss. Bulimia nervosa is more common than previously thought; it may affect 10 per cent of women and 1 to 2 per cent of men in the United States.

6 Routine blood chemistries may reveal clues to several causes of weight gain. A high incidence of rapid weight gain and obesity has been found associated with the onset of non–insulin-dependent diabetes. Other abnormalities in electrolytes such as potassium and total CO_2 may be found in the pituitary cause of Cushing's disease or the adrenal cause of Cushing's syndrome. If either of these disorders is suspected, a serum cortisol is the single most useful confirmatory test. Should the serum cortisol be elevated, then a dexamethasone suppression test may be used to further define the disorder.

7 Although commonly suspected in weight gain, hypothyroidism is rarely a cause. Even with the severe deficiency in thyroid hormone seen in myxedema, the majority of the weight gain is secondary to fluid retention. Occasionally, weight gain may occur when excess artificial hormone is withdrawn.

BIBLIOGRAPHY

Jacobson E: Chronic mononucleosis—it almost never happens. Postgrad Med 83:56–65, 1988.

Louis AA (ed): Handbook of Difficult Diagnoses. New York, Churchill Livingstone, 1990.

Norton J: Gastrointestinal Disorders. 2nd ed. Chicago, Year Book Medical Publishers, 1981.

Sugarman JR: Evaluation of fatigue in family practice. J Fam Pract 19:643–647, 1984.

Taylor RB: Difficult Diagnosis. Philadelphia, W. B. Saunders Company, 1985.

Wyngaarden JB, Smith LH Jr (eds): Cecil Textbook of Medicine. 19th ed. Philadelphia, W. B. Saunders Company, 1992.

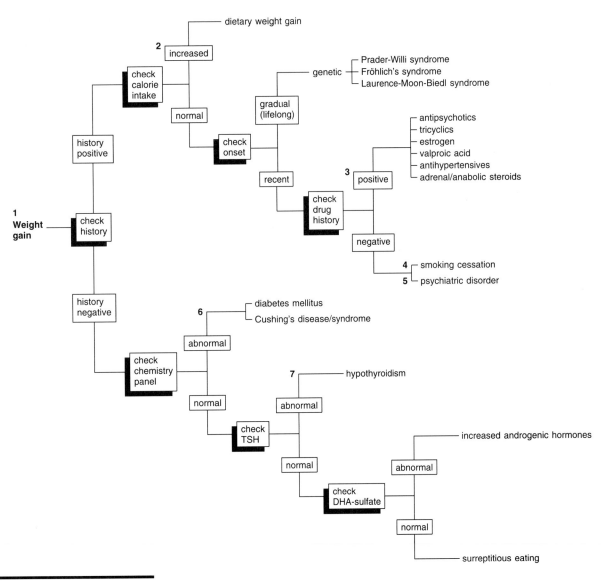

dietary weight gain

2 increased

check calorie intake

normal

genetic — Prader-Willi syndrome
— Fröhlich's syndrome
— Laurence-Moon-Biedl syndrome

gradual (lifelong)

check onset

antipsychotics
tricyclics
estrogen
valproic acid
antihypertensives
adrenal/anabolic steroids

recent

3 positive

history positive

check drug history

negative

1 **Weight gain**

check history

4 ┌ smoking cessation
5 └ psychiatric disorder

history negative

diabetes mellitus
Cushing's disease/syndrome

6 abnormal

check chemistry panel

hypothyroidism

7 abnormal

normal

check TSH

increased androgenic hormones

normal

abnormal

check DHA-sulfate

normal

surreptitious eating

Cecil Chapters	1, 454
Harrison Chapters	20, 182

2 ▪ Respiratory Disorders

Signs and symptoms:
Cough
Dyspnea
Hemoptysis
Cyanosis

Labs:
Pleural effusion
Hypercarbia

Cough

1 Cough is the most common respiratory symptom. Cough is normally a protective mechanism for clearing the airway of secretions, foreign material, or irritants. The cough is initiated by mechanical stimulation of the irritant receptors in the nose, ears, esophagus, larynx, trachea, and larger bronchi, as well as the pleura, pericardium, and diaphragm. The stimulation is carried via the afferent fibers of the vagus nerve to the "cough center" in the lower medulla and the upper pons. The reflex arc is completed via the efferent fibers of the vagus nerve and the spinal nerves C2 and C3 to the muscles of the diaphragm, chest wall, and abdomen. It is the contraction of these muscles followed by the sudden opening of the glottis that creates the cough. Air flows exceeding 500 miles per hour have been documented during cough.

2 The forced expiratory volume in 1 second (FEV_1), the peak flow, and the vital capacity are the most useful pulmonary function tests to determine the presence of an obstructive pulmonary defect. The most common causes of obstructive pulmonary function test abnormalities are intrinsic airway hyperreactivity as seen in asthma and extrinsic airway obstruction secondary to compression from lymph nodes, masses, or aneurysms.

3 Cigarette smoking is the most common cause of chronic cough. The cough does not necessarily occur when the patient is actually smoking but is usually more severe in the early morning. The cough is usually not productive unless accompanied by bronchitis. Some studies have shown that complete cessation of the cough may occur as soon as one month after smoking has been stopped.

4 Common air pollutants such as sulfur dioxide, nitrogen dioxide, and ozone are frequent causes of cough. Many industrial and agricultural exposures can cause an acute or chronic cough. Symptoms may appear minutes to years after the exposure. A cough that initially begins after work or at night is a clue to exposure to airway irritants.

5 Psychogenic cough is a diagnosis of exclusion. The cough is most common in adolescents with concomitant emotional disorders. The cough does not produce sputum, usually does not occur at night, and is not affected by commonly used cough suppressants.

6 Lung biopsies may be performed by the transbronchial or the transthoracic method depending on the location of the lesion or area to be sampled. When the diagnosis is not evident or a large amount of lung tissue is required, open lung biopsy may be necessary.

7 Cough occurs more commonly with bronchogenic carcinoma than with metastatic disease. Seventy to 90 per cent of patients with bronchogenic carcinoma have cough as a prominent symptom. Isolated cough, even in the absence of radiographic findings, may be the first symptom of bronchogenic carcinoma in a patient at risk. Sputum cytology or bronchial washings may be of help in making the diagnosis in this setting.

8 Cough is common in patients with interstitial lung disease. The cough is probably caused by changes in the airways with activation of stretch receptors as a result of the increase in fibrous tissue within the lung. The cough in this setting is usually increased by deep breathing.

9 Recurrent aspiration is usually seen in elderly patients and patients with central nervous system or swallowing disorders. The cough may be provoked by either solids or liquids or may occur during sleep. Chronic aspiration with resulting lipoid pneumonitis is commonly seen in patients who use mineral oil as a nighttime laxative.

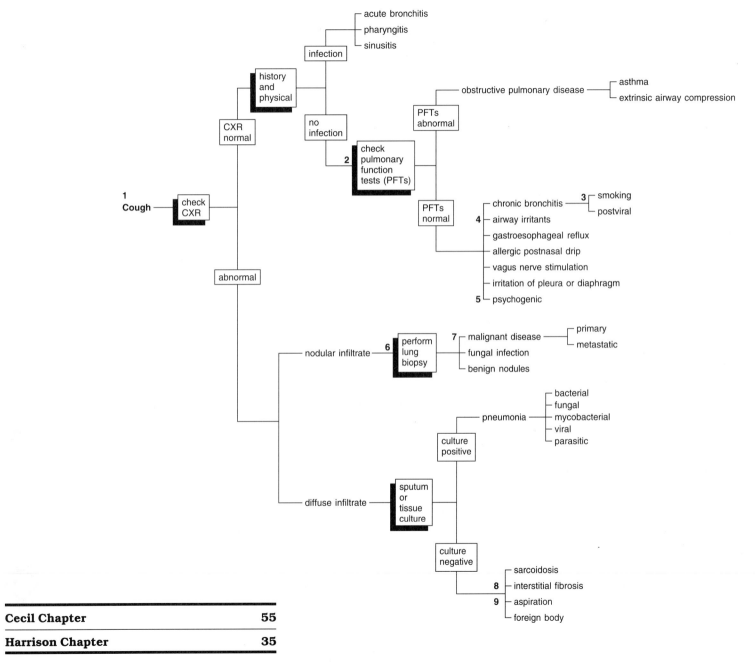

acute bronchitis
pharyngitis
sinusitis

infection

history
and
physical

obstructive pulmonary disease
asthma
extrinsic airway compression

PFTs
abnormal

CXR
normal

no
infection

2 check
pulmonary
function
tests (PFTs)

PFTs
normal

chronic bronchitis **3** smoking
postviral

4 airway irritants
gastroesophageal reflux
allergic postnasal drip
vagus nerve stimulation
irritation of pleura or diaphragm
5 psychogenic

1
Cough — check
CXR

abnormal

nodular infiltrate **6** perform
lung
biopsy

7 malignant disease
primary
metastatic

fungal infection
benign nodules

pneumonia
bacterial
fungal
mycobacterial
viral
parasitic

culture
positive

diffuse infiltrate sputum
or
tissue
culture

culture
negative

sarcoidosis
8 interstitial fibrosis
9 aspiration
foreign body

Cecil Chapter	55
Harrison Chapter	35

Dyspnea

1 Dyspnea is one of the most common symptoms for which patients seek medical attention. The various forms of dyspnea may provide important diagnostic clues. Orthopnea, or dyspnea in the supine position, along with paroxysmal nocturnal dyspnea, is usually associated with pulmonary venous congestion. Platypnea, or dyspnea on sitting upright, is usually associated with intracardiac or intrapulmonary shunts and neuromuscular disorders of the chest wall muscles. Trepopnea, or dyspnea in the lateral decubitus position, is usually associated with congestive heart failure. Even if the patient does not or cannot complain of the condition, dyspnea can be suspected when other signs such as gasping, intercostal muscle retraction, audible wheezing, or flaring nostrils are present.

2 Spirometry should include the FEV_1, the maximum voluntary ventilation (MVV), the forced vital capacity (FVC), total lung capacity (TLC), and the diffusion of carbon monoxide (D_{CO}). An FEV_1 and an MVV of 25 to 40 per cent of the predicted level are associated with moderate to severe dyspnea. An FEV_1 and an MVV of 15 per cent or less are associated with dyspnea at rest. FEV_1/FVC ratios of less than 70 per cent are found with obstructive airway diseases. If the FEV_1/FVC ratio is greater than 70 per cent, a restrictive defect should be sought using additional tests such as the TLC and the D_{CO}. Pulmonary function testing may also be useful in diagnosing dyspnea associated with some abnormal chest radiographic findings.

3 Direct measurement of the oxygen saturation by oximetry is necessary to determine the true saturation of the hemoglobin. The value reported with most routine blood gas measurements is a calculated value derived from the oxygen partial pressure (P_{O_2}), the pH, and the body temperature. This calculated value will not reflect the true saturation in the presence of carbon monoxide or abnormal hemoglobins.

4 When the etiology of the dyspnea is not evident after standard pulmonary function tests (PFTs) and the resting arterial P_{O_2} is normal, exercise pulmonary function testing may be useful. The object of the test is to determine the ability of the oxygen transport system (heart, lungs, and respiratory muscles) to supply the necessary increase in oxygen delivery to the tissues during exercise. The test may also induce bronchospasm not evident at rest. Usually a bicycle ergometer or a treadmill is used to increase physical activity in a controlled manner. Minute ventilation (V_E), oxygen consumption (V_{O_2}), and carbon dioxide production (V_{CO_2}), as well as heart rate (HR) and traditional spirometry, are measured during the test.

5 Disorders that limit the heart from increasing cardiac output when needed include certain valvular abnormalities, decreased myocardial mass or contractility, and pericardial disease causing restriction of diastolic filling. The exercise PFT abnormalities most commonly seen with fixed cardiac output syndromes include failure of the V_{O_2} to increase at the start of exercise, or a low V_{O_2}/HR. Both of these findings are due to a decreased stroke volume.

6 Psychogenic dyspnea and hyperventilation are often associated with various anxiety neuroses. The dyspnea is intermittent, does not accompany all forms of physical exertion, and usually occurs in patients under 40 years of age. The dyspnea may be accompanied by dizziness, giddiness, difficulty with concentration, palpitations, and fatigue. Both standard and exercise PFTs are normal.

7 Although cardiac catheterization remains the "gold standard" in diagnosing intracardiac shunts and pulmonary hypertension, several less invasive tests are available and may be helpful. These tests include "bubble" echocardiography for the determination of intracardiac shunts and lung perfusion scans with differential counting over the brain and kidney to detect particles shunted through dilated pulmonary vessels.

8 Pulmonary hypertension may be a primary disorder of unclear etiology or the result of multiple pulmonary emboli. Other evidence of right-sided cardiac failure may be present, including accentuation of the second heart sound, fixed splitting of the second heart sound, or a right ventricular heave. The diagnosis is confirmed by right-sided cardiac catheterization.

9 Large airway obstruction may be either internal or external to the trachea or main stem bronchi. The most common forms of external compression come from neoplasms within the neck or mediastinum or large goiters. Internal obstruction may also be caused by neoplasms, but foreign bodies must always be considered.

10 Respiratory muscle weakness may result from dysfunction of the motor nerves, the neuromuscular junction, or the muscle cells themselves. For a more complete explanation of respiratory muscle weakness, refer to the hypercarbia algorithm (see page 22).

11 Pneumothorax may occur spontaneously or as a result of trauma. Spontaneous pneumothorax occurs most commonly in patients with cystic fibrosis or in young adults idiopathically, but it may also occur with *Staphylococcus aureus* pneumonia, chronic obstructive pulmonary disease, pulmonary tuberculosis, asthma, interstitial lung disease (such as sarcoidosis), malignancy, endometriosis, and Marfan's syndrome.

12 Interstitial lung disease presents as a diffuse pulmonary parenchymal process without airway obstruction. Idiopathic pulmonary fibrosis, rheumatoid lung disease, sarcoidosis, and various pneumoconioses are the most common interstitial lung diseases. Exertional dyspnea is invariably present and usually occurs before any changes on spirometry are noted. Chest radiographic findings may initially be subtle, but with time, radiographic changes in the parenchyma, as well as volume loss, will become evident.

13 Progressive exertional dyspnea is a common presentation of cardiovascular disease. The echocardiogram and radiographic changes in cardiac size and shape will help to define whether the abnormality is valvular, myocardial, or pericardial in origin. Cardiac catheterization may be necessary to confirm the diagnosis.

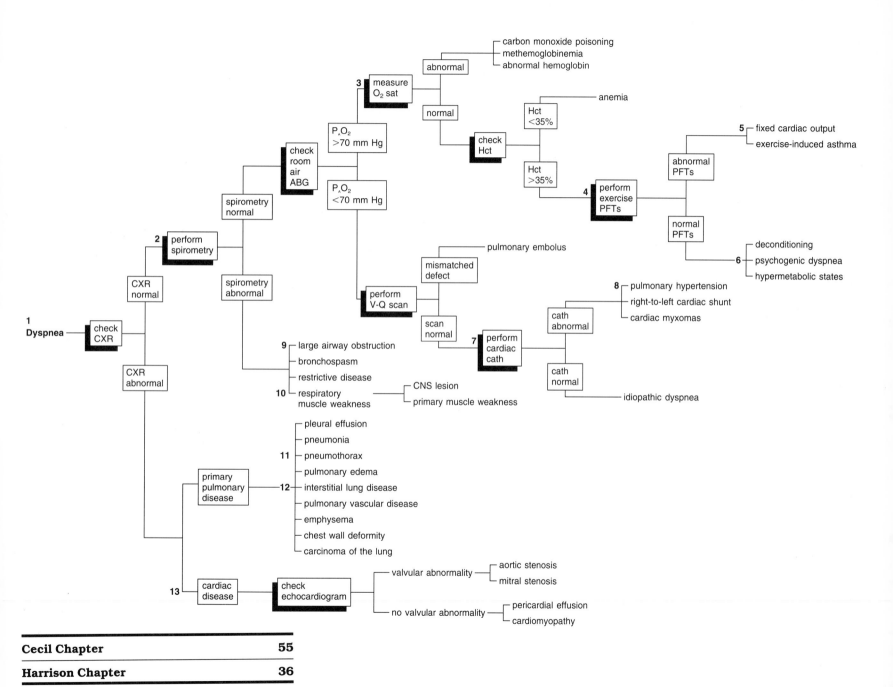

1 **Dyspnea** — check CXR

CXR normal

2 perform spirometry

spirometry normal — check room air ABG

P_AO_2 >70 mm Hg

3 measure O_2 sat

abnormal
- carbon monoxide poisoning
- methemoglobinemia
- abnormal hemoglobin

normal — check Hct

Hct <35% — anemia

Hct >35%

4 perform exercise PFTs

abnormal PFTs
- 5 — fixed cardiac output
- exercise-induced asthma

normal PFTs
- 6 — deconditioning
- psychogenic dyspnea
- hypermetabolic states

P_AO_2 <70 mm Hg

perform V-Q scan

mismatched defect — pulmonary embolus

scan normal

7 perform cardiac cath

cath abnormal
- 8 — pulmonary hypertension
- right-to-left cardiac shunt
- cardiac myxomas

cath normal — idiopathic dyspnea

spirometry abnormal
- 9 — large airway obstruction
- bronchospasm
- restrictive disease
- 10 — respiratory muscle weakness
  - CNS lesion
  - primary muscle weakness

CXR abnormal

primary pulmonary disease
- 11 — pleural effusion
- pneumonia
- pneumothorax
- pulmonary edema
- 12 — interstitial lung disease
- pulmonary vascular disease
- emphysema
- chest wall deformity
- carcinoma of the lung

13 cardiac disease — check echocardiogram

valvular abnormality
- aortic stenosis
- mitral stenosis

no valvular abnormality
- pericardial effusion
- cardiomyopathy

Cecil Chapter	55
Harrison Chapter	36

Hemoptysis

1 Hemoptysis is the expectoration of blood arising from the respiratory tract. The quantity of blood may range from streaking of the sputum to a massive hemorrhage. Hemoptysis of greater than 100 ml/24 hr is considered potentially life-threatening. Expectorated blood does not always arise from the respiratory tract. Hemoptysis must be distinguished from epistaxis, oral or laryngeal bleeding, and hematemesis. A careful head and neck examination is always necessary as part of the evaluation of hemoptysis. The usually bright red color and alkaline pH of respiratory tract bleeding may help distinguish hemoptysis from hematemesis.

2 The history and physical examination may be useful in both the diagnosis and localization of the bleeding. Trauma to the lungs or thorax is a common cause of hemoptysis. The most common traumatic causes of hemoptysis are pulmonary contusion from blunt trauma such as impact with a steering wheel, rib fracture, and inhalation of toxic fumes. Even when the history and physical examination fail to pinpoint the exact diagnosis, findings like fever, cough, weight loss, cardiac murmurs, adenopathy, and clubbing may give useful clues. Patients may often be able to localize the site of the bleeding to one lung or the other by feeling the sensation of fluid in the bronchi. The physical finding of isolated rhonchi or wheezes may further narrow the search for the site of the bleeding.

3 The chest radiograph is the most useful diagnostic test in the evaluation of hemoptysis. Primary diseases of the respiratory tract such as infiltrates or nodules will be evident. Aids to the diagnosis of hemoptysis secondary to nonpulmonary organ dysfunction may be found on the radiograph. Cardiomegaly, Kerley's lines, and hilar adenopathy may be useful in determining the cause of the hemoptysis. It should be noted, however, that an abnormality on the chest radiograph does not always indicate the site of the bleeding. Old inflammatory changes may coexist with a radiologically undetectable tumor. Bleeding from any area of the lung may spread throughout the pulmonary tree, giving the false impression of diffuse disease on radiography. In addition, some studies have shown that up to 50 per cent of patients with hemoptysis may initially have normal chest radiographs.

4 Most primary lung neoplasms are malignant. In smokers over the age of 40, 90 per cent of these lesions are bronchogenic carcinomas. Hemoptysis occurs in more than 50 per cent of patients with lung cancer at some point in the course of their disease. The hemoptysis is caused by erosion of the tumor into the bronchus or by necrosis of bulky fungating tumors. Benign tumors of the lung rarely cause hemoptysis; therefore, other sources of bleeding should be sought if the mass is found to be benign.

5 Most metastatic tumors do not cause hemoptysis. However, osteogenic sarcoma and metastatic choriocarcinoma have been frequently associated with massive hemoptysis and should be suspected in the appropriate clinical setting.

6 Infection is the most common cause of hemoptysis. Acute and chronic bronchitis are the most common respiratory infections causing hemoptysis. Primary bacterial infections of the lungs causing hemoptysis are most commonly due to *Staphylococcus, Klebsiella,* and *Pseudomonas* species. Pneumococcal pneumonia rarely presents with hemoptysis, although the sputum can be rust-colored. Often the infectious agent responsible for the bronchitis cannot be isolated and empiric therapy must be begun.

7 Tuberculosis is a common cause of hemoptysis. The bleeding arises from anastomoses between the bronchial and pulmonary circulations within the tuberculous cavity walls. These lesions are sometimes called Rasmussen's aneurysms. Because the bleeding is not related to the tuberculous infection itself, massive hemoptysis may occur even when distinct cavities are no longer visible.

8 Most pulmonary fungal infections can cause hemoptysis, and bleeding is most commonly associated with a mycetoma or a fungal ball. A mycetoma is usually caused by *Aspergillus fumigatus* growing in an old tuberculous cavity. The bleeding may be caused by the release of certain fungal enzymes and by local irritation.

9 A wide variety of immunologically mediated diseases may cause hemoptysis. The diseases can be broken down into two groups. The first is characterized by antibody-mediated damage to the pulmonary capillary membranes. The capillary damage may occur in an isolated form or in conjunction with renal failure, as in Goodpasture's syndrome. In the second and more common group, pulmonary damage is caused by deposition of antibody or immune complexes in the lung. Lupus pneumonitis, periarteritis nodosa, sarcoidosis, Behçet's syndrome, and Wegener's granulomatosis are examples of this group of diseases.

10 Hemoptysis is seen in 10 to 20 per cent of patients with mitral stenosis. The hemoptysis is most common in young people and tends to occur after exercise. The bleeding is due to the rupture of pulmonary veins and capillaries caused by the markedly elevated left atrial pressure.

11 Hemoptysis may occur in either viral or bacterial bronchitis. Because the inflammatory process is localized to the bronchial tree, the chest x ray will usually be negative. In addition to standard cultures, bronchial brushings and washings should be performed specifically for fungal or opportunistic disease.

12 Twenty-five to 40 per cent of patients with pulmonary embolus and infarction present with hemoptysis. The suspicion of embolus is increased when the other "classic" symptoms of dyspnea, cough, and pleuritic pain are present. The diagnosis of pulmonary embolus should, however, be considered in any patient with a sudden onset of hemoptysis.

13 Even after thorough examination, 5 to 15 per cent of patients have no explanation for their hemoptysis. A significant number of these patients eventually manifest an initially occult disease during careful follow-up.

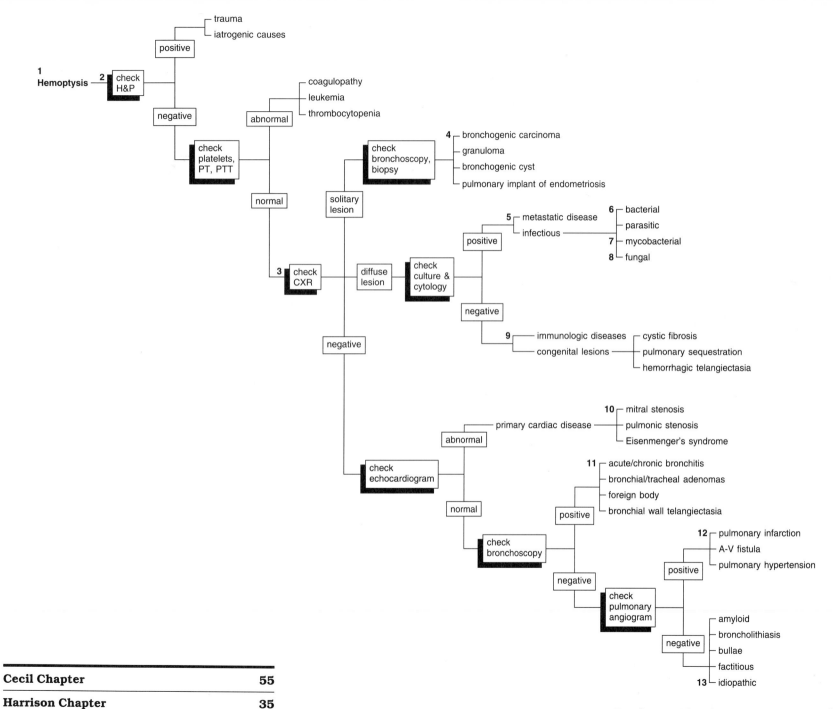

1
Hemoptysis — **2** check H&P

positive
— trauma
— iatrogenic causes

negative — check platelets, PT, PTT

abnormal
— coagulopathy
— leukemia
— thrombocytopenia

normal — **3** check CXR

solitary lesion — check bronchoscopy, biopsy
4 — bronchogenic carcinoma
— granuloma
— bronchogenic cyst
— pulmonary implant of endometriosis

diffuse lesion — check culture & cytology

positive
5 — metastatic disease
— infectious
6 — bacterial
— parasitic
7 — mycobacterial
8 — fungal

negative
9 — immunologic diseases
— congenital lesions
— cystic fibrosis
— pulmonary sequestration
— hemorrhagic telangiectasia

negative — check echocardiogram

abnormal — primary cardiac disease
10 — mitral stenosis
— pulmonic stenosis
— Eisenmenger's syndrome

normal — check bronchoscopy

positive
11 — acute/chronic bronchitis
— bronchial/tracheal adenomas
— foreign body
— bronchial wall telangiectasia

negative — check pulmonary angiogram

positive
12 — pulmonary infarction
— A-V fistula
— pulmonary hypertension

negative
— amyloid
— broncholithiasis
— bullae
— factitious
13 — idiopathic

Cyanosis

1 Cyanosis occurs when the level of unsaturated hemoglobin reaches 5 gm/100 ml of capillary blood. Cyanosis is difficult to detect clinically when serum hemoglobin is less than 7 gm/100 ml. Carboxyhemoglobinemia may be confused with cyanosis owing to the reddish flush seen in this setting. Changes in skin pigmentation, such as the blue coloration seen with argyria or the brownish discoloration in Addison's disease or hemochromatosis, may also be confused with cyanosis.

2 Raynaud's phenomenon is defined as episodes of pallor and cyanosis of the hands and feet, usually in response to cold or stress. When the disorder is primary, it is called Raynaud's disease. The disease is more common in women, with a peak occurrence between 20 and 40 years of age. The etiology is unknown but may involve increased activity of the sympathetic nervous system. The disease has been described in several families. The secondary form of the disorder is seen in association with several groups of diseases. These include (1) occlusive arterial disease such as thromboangiitis obliterans; (2) connective tissue diseases including systemic lupus erythematosus, rheumatoid arthritis, and scleroderma; (3) repeated minor trauma to the digits; (4) neurogenic disorders including thoracic outlet syndrome; (5) chemically induced forms secondary to drugs like ergotamine, beta-blockers, and methysergide, as well as chemicals like polyvinyl chloride; (6) intravascular coagulation of blood elements as seen in cryoglobulinemia and with cold agglutinins; and (7) primary pulmonary hypertension.

3 Cyanosis that is greater in the upper extremities is usually associated with transposition of the great arteries and a preductal coarctation of the aorta. The secondary pulmonary hypertension causes a reversal of blood flow in the ductus, with a resultant increased delivery of oxygenated blood to the legs.

4 The pulmonary hypertension associated with a patent ductus arteriosus may lead to increased cyanosis and clubbing of the feet compared to the left hand and the relatively normal right hand. The "differential cyanosis" is due to the reversal of blood flow through the ductus, which enters the aorta distal to the left subclavian artery.

5 Oxygen saturation must be measured directly by oximetry. The saturation reported on routine blood gas determinations is a calculated value and would therefore not detect abnormal hemoglobins such as carboxyhemoglobin or methemoglobin.

6 Acrocyanosis is a benign condition in which cyanosis is caused by congenital differences in capillary density or transient local changes in capillary flow with resultant increased oxygen extraction by the tissues. Placing a cyanotic extremity in warm water will reverse the cyanosis. There may be some difficulty distinguishing acrocyanosis from Raynaud's disease.

7 The findings on cardiac examination in the setting of cyanotic heart disease will depend on the site of the abnormality, associated lesions, and the duration and severity of the anatomic lesion. The most consistent abnormalities are pathologic murmurs. The electrocardiogram (EKG) and the configuration of the heart on chest radiograph may, at times, be normal.

8 Cyanotic heart disease requires a major right-to-left intracardiac shunt. The shunt may be primary or secondary to increased pulmonary arterial pressure, with reversal of flow through an intracardiac abnormality. The cyanotic heart diseases may be classified by their anatomic location. The great arteries may be involved in patent ductus arteriosus (see No. 4), aorticopulmonary window, or transposition of the great arteries. The atria may be involved via an atrial septal defect, anomalous pulmonary venous drainage, or a patent foramen ovale. Ventricular lesions such as ventricular septal defects, Fallot's tetralogy, and single ventricle may be associated with cyanotic heart disease.

9 Mismatched perfusion defects seen on a ventilation-perfusion (V/Q) scan are specific for pulmonary embolus. The scan may, however, be more difficult to interpret in the presence of other lung abnormalities or when matched defects are seen. The pulmonary arteriogram remains the "gold standard" in the diagnosis or exclusion of pulmonary embolus.

10 The most common causes of cyanosis secondary to abnormal hemoglobin are methemoglobinemia and sulfhemoglobinemia. Methemoglobinemia may be congenital or due to the ingestion of sulfonamides, nitrites, or aniline derivatives in susceptible individuals. Sulfhemoglobinemia may be the result of ingestion of toxic doses of phenacetin or acetanilid or exposure to large amounts of aromatic amino and nitro compounds. Excess hydrogen sulfide produced in the intestine has also been implicated in this disorder. Unlike methemoglobinemia, which is reversible when the cause is discontinued, sulfhemoglobinemia may persist for weeks.

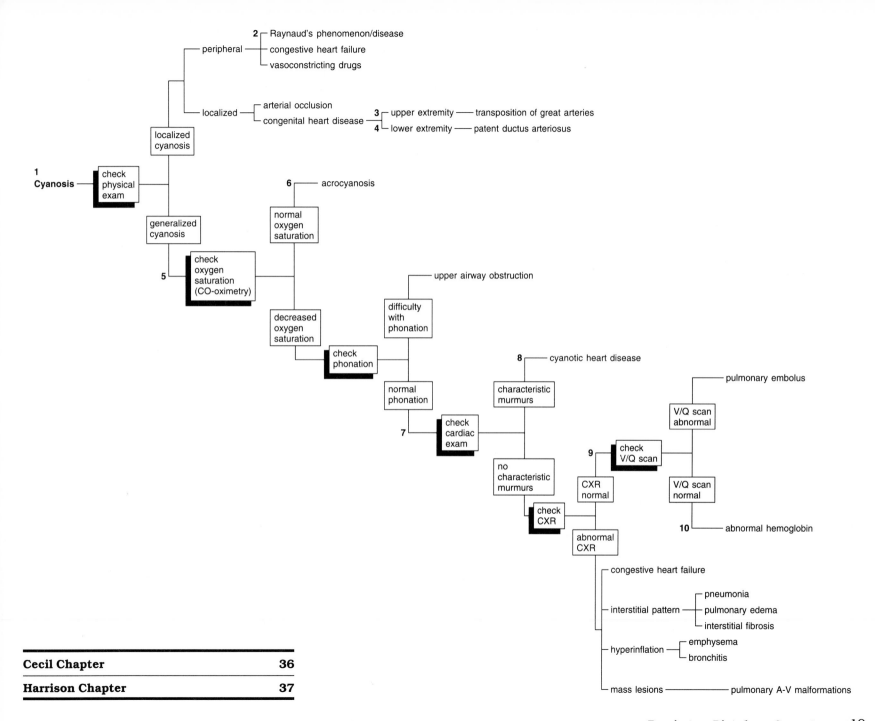

1
Cyanosis

check physical exam

localized cyanosis

peripheral

2 Raynaud's phenomenon/disease
congestive heart failure
vasoconstricting drugs

localized

arterial occlusion
congenital heart disease

3 upper extremity —— transposition of great arteries
4 lower extremity —— patent ductus arteriosus

generalized cyanosis

5 check oxygen saturation (CO-oximetry)

normal oxygen saturation

6 acrocyanosis

decreased oxygen saturation

check phonation

difficulty with phonation

upper airway obstruction

normal phonation

7 check cardiac exam

characteristic murmurs

8 cyanotic heart disease

no characteristic murmurs

check CXR

CXR normal

9 check V/Q scan

V/Q scan abnormal —— pulmonary embolus

V/Q scan normal

10 abnormal hemoglobin

abnormal CXR

congestive heart failure

interstitial pattern

pneumonia
pulmonary edema
interstitial fibrosis

hyperinflation

emphysema
bronchitis

mass lesions —— pulmonary A-V malformations

Pleural Effusion

1 A pleural effusion is an abnormal accumulation of fluid within the pleural space. The fluid may be an ultrafiltrate of the plasma, an inflammatory exudate, chyle, or blood (see No. 3). Effusions of more than 300 ml may be detected on physical examination as decreased fremitus and dullness to percussion. Effusions of greater than 2000 ml may cause severe dyspnea and mediastinal shift. On chest radiographic examination, effusions of less than 300 ml are usually noted on the lateral film only. Effusions of less than 150 ml may be seen only on lateral decubitus films.

2 Pleural effusions will occur in more than half of the patients who develop a pulmonary embolus. Effusions rarely develop, however, unless pulmonary infarction has also occurred. The effusion is usually bloody and occasionally bilateral.

3 Most pleural effusions have traditionally been classified as transudates or exudates based on the protein concentration of the fluid. Greater than 3 gm/100 ml of protein denotes an exudate, whereas less than 3 gm/100 ml indicates a transudate. Recent evidence has demonstrated that the use of this criterion alone leads to an inaccurate classification in more than 10 per cent of cases. A more accurate diagnosis of an exudate may be made when three separate criteria are met: (1) a pleural fluid protein–to–serum protein ratio of 0.5 or greater; (2) a pleural fluid lactate dehydrogenase (LDH)–to–serum LDH ratio of more than 0.6; (3) an absolute pleural fluid LDH greater than 200 U/L. The glucose concentration or the absolute cell count of the fluid is less specific. A glucose concentration of less than 60 mg/dl, however, is usually associated with an exudate.

4 Meigs' syndrome is the triad of ascites, ovarian tumor, and large pleural effusion. The tumor may be malignant or may be a benign fibroma. The effusion is serosanguineous and usually resolves after the removal of the tumor. The mechanism of the effusion is not understood, but Meigs' syndrome should be considered when the source of the effusion is obscure and there is evidence of pelvic disease.

5 Pleural fluid pH is of value in the further differentiation of exudative effusions. With the exception of direct rupture of gastric contents into the pleural space, the pleural fluid pH is determined by both fixed acids and CO_2 content. Damaged pleura decreases CO_2 efflux from the pleural space, causing pH to fall. An exception is the alkaline pH of the pleural fluid at times associated with congestive heart failure and empyema owing to *Proteus mirabilis* infection.

6 Empyema is defined as pus in the pleural space. The empyema develops as a result of infection in the pleural space, or as a complication of pneumonia with spread of the infection into the pleural space. Common pathogens include *Staphylococcus aureus, Streptococcus pneumoniae,* and gram-negative and anaerobic organisms. The empyema usually contains a white blood count of greater than 10,000 cells/mm.[3] A parapneumonic effusion, on the other hand, is an effusion that resembles a true empyema but develops as a result of local inflammation near the site of a pneumonia without direct extension of the infection into the pleural space.

7 Rheumatoid pleuritis develops in approximately 5 per cent of patients with rheumatoid arthritis. The effusion usually occurs in the absence of rheumatoid lung disease. The pH and glucose are low, and rheumatoid factor is usually present. The effusion may persist for weeks following successful treatment of the disease.

8 Pleural fluid cytology is positive in 50 to 75 per cent of patients with malignant processes involving the pleura. False-negative results may be due to the chronicity of the effusion or degeneration of the malignant cells during processing of the sample. A pleural biopsy may be necessary if cytology is negative and there is a strong suspicion of malignancy. Needle biopsy of the pleura and open thoracotomy are the most commonly employed techniques for determining malignancy, but the endoscopic procedure of pleuroscopy in well-trained hands may be useful as well. In the absence of direct pleural involvement, malignancy may cause pleural effusion through lymphatic obstruction, endobronchial obstruction with postobstructive pneumonia, or atelectasis. Under these conditions, pleural fluid cytology will be negative.

9 Metastatic disease, most frequently from carcinoma of the colon or breast, is the most common form of pleural malignancy. However, malignancies arising from virtually any other tissue may involve the pleura. Primary malignancies of the pleura are rare. Mesotheliomas are the most common primary pleural tumors. In older age groups, 30 to 40 per cent of pleural effusions are malignant.

10 Tuberculous effusions may be found even in the absence of other radiographic findings of active tuberculosis. The effusion may represent a pleural reaction to the tuberculous protein. For this reason, smears and cultures of the pleural fluid for acid-fast organisms are rarely positive. Culture of pleural tissue obtained at biopsy, however, yields a positive result in 55 to 80 per cent of cases. Because of the ubiquitous nature of this disease, all specimens of pleural fluid or tissue should be cultured for tuberculosis.

11 Several drugs have been associated with pleural effusions with or without pleural disease. These include nitrofurantoin, dantrolene, methysergide, bromocriptine, procarbazine, and amiodarone. Pleural effusions are usually associated with an eosinophil count of greater than 10 per cent.

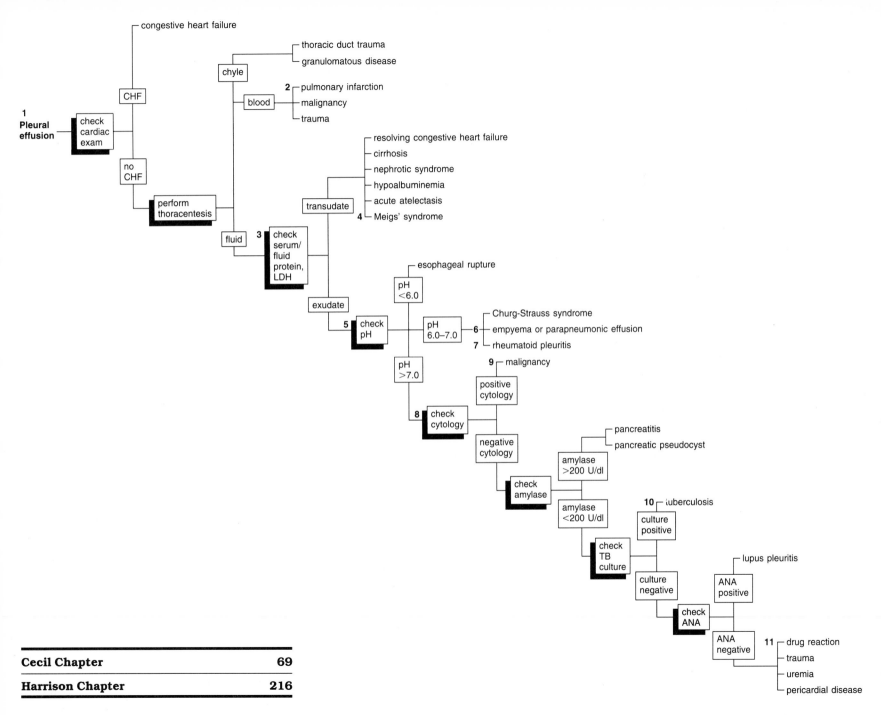

1
Pleural effusion — check cardiac exam

- CHF — congestive heart failure
- no CHF — perform thoracentesis — fluid
  - chyle
    - thoracic duct trauma
    - granulomatous disease
  - blood
    - 2 — pulmonary infarction
    - malignancy
    - trauma
  - 3 check serum/fluid protein, LDH
    - transudate
      - resolving congestive heart failure
      - cirrhosis
      - nephrotic syndrome
      - hypoalbuminemia
      - acute atelectasis
      - 4 — Meigs' syndrome
    - exudate
      - 5 check pH
        - pH <6.0 — esophageal rupture
        - pH 6.0–7.0
          - Churg-Strauss syndrome
          - 6 — empyema or parapneumonic effusion
          - 7 — rheumatoid pleuritis
        - pH >7.0
          - 8 check cytology
            - positive cytology — 9 — malignancy
            - negative cytology
              - check amylase
                - amylase >200 U/dl
                  - pancreatitis
                  - pancreatic pseudocyst
                - amylase <200 U/dl
                  - check TB culture
                    - culture positive — 10 — tuberculosis
                    - culture negative
                      - check ANA
                        - ANA positive — lupus pleuritis
                        - ANA negative — 11
                          - drug reaction
                          - trauma
                          - uremia
                          - pericardial disease

Cecil Chapter	**69**
Harrison Chapter	**216**

Hypercarbia

1 Hypercarbia, or the increase of CO_2 in the blood, is measured by an increase in the partial pressure of CO_2 (P_{CO_2}). Hypercarbia occurs when the lungs are unable to excrete the normal 13,000 to 15,000 mmol of CO_2 produced by the body daily. Because there is rarely an increase in bodily CO_2 production, hypercarbia almost always represents decreased alveolar ventilation (hypoventilation). Hypoventilation is produced by a decrease in the minute ventilation (the amount of air exchanged by the lungs in 1 minute) or a ventilation-perfusion mismatch.

2 The equation

$$CO_2 + H_2O \rightarrow H_2CO_3 \rightarrow H^+ + HCO_3^-$$

defines how an increase in the CO_2 will increase H^+ concentration, leading to respiratory acidosis. The H^+ is then buffered by nonbicarbonate buffers such as plasma proteins and hemoglobin, causing an increase in HCO_3^- as P_{CO_2} rises (see No. 4).

3 Because none of the body's buffering systems can overcompensate for a respiratory acidosis, a pH greater than 7.40 represents a primary metabolic alkalosis with the hypercarbia as a compensatory mechanism.

4 When the P_{CO_2} rises acutely, the H^+ liberated is rapidly buffered by intercellular buffers (see No. 2). The small but significant rise in HCO_3^- partially buffers the expected fall in pH. This buffering occurs within the first 10 to 15 minutes. Usually serum HCO_3^- rises 1 mEq/L for each 10 mm Hg rise in P_{CO_2}. Over the course of several days, renal buffering mechanisms come into play and the HCO_3^- rises further. The increased HCO_3^- is the result of increased renal H^+ excretion in the form of NH_4 with consequent HCO_3^- generation. Under chronic conditions, the HCO_3^- may rise by 3.5 mEq/L for each 10 mm Hg rise in P_{CO_2}. Therefore, the HCO_3^- concentration is a useful tool in differentiating between acute and chronic respiratory acidosis.

5 Respiratory neuromuscular weakness may result from dysfunction of the motor nerves, the neuromuscular junction, or the muscle cells themselves. Lesions in the central nervous system manifest themselves according to the site of the lesion. Lesions in the motor cortex or pyramidal system produce weakness of the voluntary muscles of respiration. Lesions in the medullary reticular formation disrupt the involuntary control of respiration. Spinal cord lesions at the C1-C2 level may produce dysfunction of both voluntary and autonomic pathways. Lesions at the C3-C5 cord level produce dysfunction of the phrenic nerve and diaphragmatic paralysis, leaving only the accessory muscles of respiration functional. Lesions in the lower cervical and thoracic cord may impair expiratory and intercostal muscle function. Polio and amyotrophic lateral sclerosis (ALS) damage the anterior horn cell of the cord, whereas primary myopathies affect muscle strength directly. Many of these lesions may cause nearly total respiratory paralysis requiring ventilator support, and all are associated with the acid-base abnormalities of chronic hypoventilation. Malnutrition may contribute significantly to neuromuscular weakness.

6 Chronic obstructive pulmonary disease (COPD) is the most common cause of chronic hypercarbia. The hypoventilation results from a combination of ventilation perfusion mismatch and an increase in dead space. Hypoxemia is frequently present and is due to the same mechanism.

7 The severity of the hypoventilation seen with kyphoscoliosis is related to the degree of deformity of the spine and rib cage. The deformity causes changes in the relation and length of the diaphragm and the intercostal muscles. Ventilatory volumes fall in proportion to the degree of deformity, leading to the development of chronic hypoventilation.

8 Pickwickian syndrome, or obesity-hypoventilation syndrome, is a constellation of abnormalities including an increase in body weight of more than 50 per cent, depressed ventilatory response to increased P_{CO_2}, obstructive sleep apnea, and weaker than normal respiratory muscles.

9 Acute respiratory acidosis is the result of a decrease in alveolar ventilation to the degree that ventilation is insufficient to excrete the CO_2 load presented to the lungs. The CO_2 load presented to the lungs may be increased by increased metabolism (catabolic states), metabolic acidosis with bicarbonate buffering, and nutrition high in carbohydrate. The decrease in ventilation occurs when the work of breathing is increased or the ventilatory drive is decreased. The work of breathing includes both resistive work, which is increased in obstructive processes, and elastic work, which is increased in restrictive processes. Ventilatory drive is controlled by the respiratory center and may be decreased by a variety of mechanisms (see Nos. 5 and 15).

10 Generalized pulmonary edema with severe hypoxia and CO_2 retention constitutes adult respiratory distress syndrome (ARDS). Many conditions are associated with this disorder, including infections, trauma, aspiration, drug overdose, inhaled toxins, intravascular coagulation, uremia, pancreatitis, and increased intracranial pressure.

11 Respiratory acidosis occurs late in the course of pulmonary edema. Although the exact mechanism is unclear, one theory states that an increase in P_{CO_2} is more a function of the increased work of breathing than CO_2 retention and usually signifies the need for ventilatory support.

12 Hypoventilation is a late manifestation of pulmonary embolism and signifies respiratory muscle fatigue. Because the P_{CO_2} is usually decreased in the period immediately following pulmonary embolism, an increase in the P_{CO_2} usually means that ventilatory support is needed.

13 Respiratory muscle strength is best measured by maximum inspiratory pressure (PI max) and maximum expiratory pressure (PE max). The normal values are age- and sex-dependent. PI max ranges from -75 to -125 cm H_2O in males and -66 to -90 cm H_2O in females. PE max ranges from 130 to 215 cm H_2O in males and 105 to 135 cm H_2O in females. Both neurologic and primary muscular abnormalities affect these measurements, as does nutritional status.

14 Guillain-Barré syndrome is the prototype of the peripheral neuropathies that may produce sufficient respiratory muscle weakness to cause hypoventilation. Isolated phrenic neuropathy as well as alcoholic neuropathy, usually associated with hypophosphatemia, may also cause respiratory failure.

15 The forced expiratory volume over 1 second (FEV_1) and the peak expiratory flow rate are useful tests in the diagnosis of airflow obstruction. Respiratory acidosis in the setting of obstructive disease is an ominous sign and usually signifies profound respiratory muscle fatigue. An FEV_1 of less than 1 L/sec and a peak flow of less than 100 L/min are associated with severe airway obstruction and increased risk of hypercarbia.

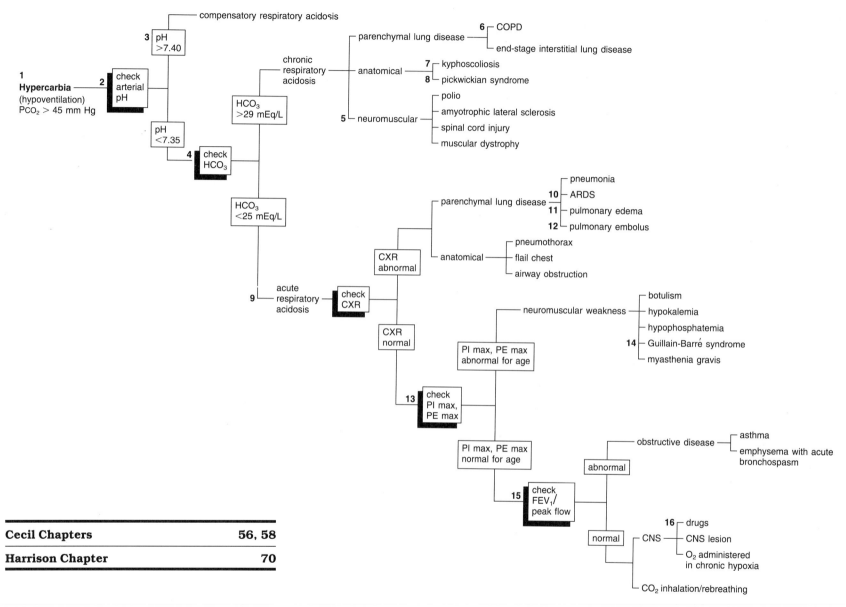

1 Hypercarbia (hypoventilation) $PCO_2 > 45$ mm Hg

2 check arterial pH

3 pH >7.40 — compensatory respiratory acidosis

4 check HCO_3

HCO_3 >29 mEq/L — chronic respiratory acidosis

parenchymal lung disease — **6** COPD / end-stage interstitial lung disease

anatomical — **7** kyphoscoliosis / **8** pickwickian syndrome

5 neuromuscular — polio / amyotrophic lateral sclerosis / spinal cord injury / muscular dystrophy

pH <7.35

HCO_3 <25 mEq/L

9 acute respiratory acidosis

check CXR

CXR abnormal

parenchymal lung disease — pneumonia / **10** ARDS / **11** pulmonary edema / **12** pulmonary embolus

anatomical — pneumothorax / flail chest / airway obstruction

CXR normal

13 check PI max, PE max

PI max, PE max abnormal for age — neuromuscular weakness — botulism / hypokalemia / hypophosphatemia / **14** Guillain-Barré syndrome / myasthenia gravis

PI max, PE max normal for age

15 check FEV_1/ peak flow

abnormal — obstructive disease — asthma / emphysema with acute bronchospasm

normal — CNS — **16** drugs / CNS lesion / O_2 administered in chronic hypoxia

CO_2 inhalation/rebreathing

Cecil Chapters	**56, 58**
Harrison Chapter	**70**

16 Drug-induced hypoventilation may be caused by depression of the respiratory center by opiates, anesthetics, tricyclic antidepressants (in large doses), tranquilizers, and barbiturates. Paralysis of the respiratory muscles may be induced by depolarizing agents such as succinylcholine.

BIBLIOGRAPHY

Braman SS (ed): Pulmonary signs and symptoms. Clin Chest Med 8(2):21–26, 1987.

O'Neil KM, Lazarus AA: Hemoptysis indications for bronchoscopy. Arch Intern Med 151:171–74, 1991.

Poe RH, Israel RH: Problems in Pulmonary Medicine for the Primary Physician. Philadelphia, Lea and Febiger, 1982.

Taylor RB: Difficult Diagnosis. Philadelphia, W. B. Saunders Company, 1985.

Vladutio AO: Pleural Effusion. New York, Futura Publishing Company, 1986.

3 ▪ Cardiovascular Disorders

Signs and symptoms:	Hypertension
Chest pain	Murmurs
Hypotension	**Labs:**
Syncope	Cardiomegaly
Edema	

Chest Pain

1 Chest pain is one of the most common medical complaints. The etiology of the pain may be obvious, but the pain may present in an atypical manner in a significant number of patients. Because the etiology of chest pain can range from trivial to life-threatening, a thorough and extensive evaluation may be necessary. Any of the structures within the chest except the lung parenchyma and the visceral pleura may be responsive to painful stimuli. The mechanism of pain from the ischemic myocardium is poorly understood but is the result of an oxygen supply-demand imbalance.

2 The diagnosis of myocardial ischemia is of great importance in patients with chest pain. A history of "typical" ischemic pain such as substernal pain, a pressure or squeezing sensation with radiation to the jaw, shoulders, or the ulnar aspect of one or both arms, requires further evaluation. In addition, pain associated with exertion, heavy meals, or emotional stress is suspicious. Rest pain, especially at night, may also represent ischemia related to coronary artery spasm. Patients with risk factors for coronary artery disease should be evaluated even if the pain is not typical for angina. These risk factors include age, family history, hyperlipidemia, hypertension, smoking, and diabetes.

3 The most reliable enzymatic indicator of myocardial infarction is creatine kinase (CK). An elevation of the myocardial specific fraction, or MB-isoenzyme, is diagnostic of myocardial damage. The CK-MB increases in the serum 1 to 3 hours after the infarction and peaks between 12 and 24 hours. The level of CK-MB may return to normal within 36 hours. Therefore, serial measurements of this enzyme should be started as soon as possible after the episode of pain. Serum glutamic-oxaloacetic transaminase (SGOT) and lactic dehydrogenase (LDH) are also elevated between 1 and 3 days after

myocardial infarction and may be measured if the first enzyme measurements are performed after the CK-MB may have peaked or returned to normal.

4 When myocardial ischemia is suspected to be a cause of the chest pain, but no supportive evidence can be obtained from the electrocardiogram (EKG) or the cardiac enzymes, exercise testing may be necessary. The standard treadmill examination is a graded exercise test in which an attempt is made to achieve 80 to 85 per cent of maximal predicted heart rate. ST segment depression of 1 to 2 mm on EKG during the treadmill examination will predict myocardial ischemia in up to 75 per cent of cases. An ST depression greater than 2 mm will predict up to 95 per cent of patients with myocardial ischemia. The sensitivity of the standard treadmill may be greatly reduced by baseline EKG abnormalities including digitalis effect, left ventricular hypertrophy (LVH), hyperventilation, left bundle branch block, mitral valve prolapse, or other conduction abnormalities. In these cases, more specific imaging using nuclear or echocardiographic techniques may be necessary. The thallium treadmill is the standard treadmill examination with the addition of injected radioactive thallium. The thallium is not taken up in poorly perfused areas of myocardium and may therefore increase the sensitivity of the standard treadmill and aid in treadmill interpretation when the baseline EKG is abnormal. Recently, the stress echocardiogram has become a useful tool in the diagnosis of ischemic cardiac disease. The test combines the standard treadmill examination with an echocardiographic image of cardiac function. This technique gives a sensitive indicator of the presence and location of the ischemia. In skilled hands, the stress echocardiogram may substitute for the thallium test, thereby eliminating the need for radionuclide administration. The Holter monitor may be useful in determining whether those patients experiencing chest pain at rest manifest any ischemic changes on EKG.

5 If, by history and the absence of risk factors, a cardiac source of chest pain is unlikely, the physical examination may help differentiate between noncardiac causes of chest pain. Positive findings on physical examination related to chest pain include dyspnea, tachypnea, wheezing, intercostal muscle retraction, use of accessory muscles of breathing, decreased or absent breath sounds, rhonchi, rales, fever, cough, hemoptysis, and cy-

anosis. It should be noted, however, that many of these same physical signs may be present with cardiac chest pain as well.

6 Lung imaging is usually begun with a nuclear ventilation-perfusion scan when pulmonary embolism is suspected. Mismatched defects in the perfusion scan are suggestive of pulmonary embolization. Many abnormalities of the lung and pleura may cause an abnormal lung scan; therefore, a positive scan indicates only a high probability of pulmonary emboli. The definitive diagnosis of pulmonary embolization must be made with a pulmonary angiogram.

7 Many patients with mitral valve prolapse complain of occasional chest pain. At times the pain associated with mitral valve prolapse may be indistinguishable from typical angina but is more often sharp and well localized. The pain is usually unrelated to exertion and may last from minutes to days. The mechanism for the pain is poorly understood, but stretching of the valve leaflets, coronary artery spasm, and increased ventricular wall tension have all been proposed as possible etiologies.

8 Herpes zoster may present as chest pain prior to the onset of typical skin lesions. The burning quality of the pain, its location, and the age of the patient are important clues to the diagnosis. Postherpetic neuralgia is common and may last well after the skin lesions have cleared.

9 Costochondritis, or Tietze's syndrome, is one of the most common causes of chest pain. The pain is due to an inflammation of the costochondral cartilage. Costochondritis may be associated with trauma or exercise and commonly occurs following viral illnesses. The most common sites for pain are over the second, third, and fourth costochondral cartilages. An important clue to the diagnosis is point tenderness elicited by palpation directly over the cartilage. A palpable enlargement of the cartilage is also common.

10 Many diseases of the gastrointestinal system may cause chest pain. Chest pain most often results from abnormalities in the esophagus, stomach, or gallbladder. Evaluation of the gastrointestinal tract may include upper gastrointestinal series, esophageal motility

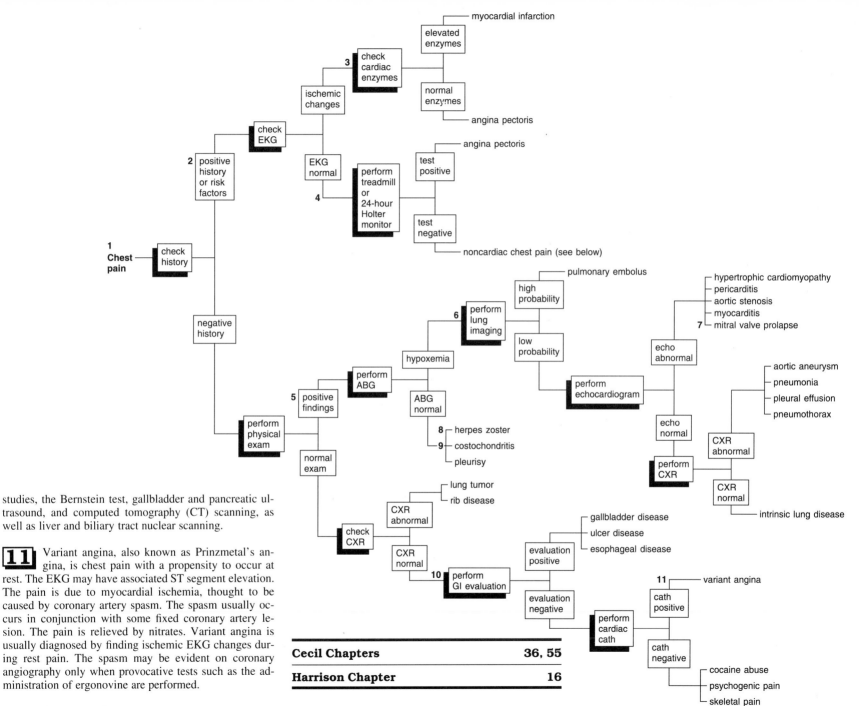

studies, the Bernstein test, gallbladder and pancreatic ultrasound, and computed tomography (CT) scanning, as well as liver and biliary tract nuclear scanning.

11 Variant angina, also known as Prinzmetal's angina, is chest pain with a propensity to occur at rest. The EKG may have associated ST segment elevation. The pain is due to myocardial ischemia, thought to be caused by coronary artery spasm. The spasm usually occurs in conjunction with some fixed coronary artery lesion. The pain is relieved by nitrates. Variant angina is usually diagnosed by finding ischemic EKG changes during rest pain. The spasm may be evident on coronary angiography only when provocative tests such as the administration of ergonovine are performed.

Cecil Chapters	36, 55
Harrison Chapter	16

Hypotension

1 Hypotension is defined as an abnormally low blood pressure accompanied by systemic symptoms. These symptoms include lightheadedness, visual changes, decreased mentation, syncope, and shock. Because blood pressure may vary so widely among various individuals, a ''low blood pressure'' in the absence of the above symptoms may be normal and should not be considered true hypotension.

2 Orthostatic hypotension is commonly defined as a drop in systolic blood pressure of 10 mm Hg or greater, accompanied by an increase in heart rate of 10 beats per minute or greater when the patient assumes a sitting or standing position. These changes must persist for more than 2 minutes. Certain drugs or cardiac conduction abnormalities may prevent the expected increase in heart rate and may make the hypotension more severe.

3 Intravascular blood volume may be evaluated by physical examination. The most reliable physical findings include skin turgor, moistness of the mucous membranes, amount of axillary perspiration, and the height of the jugular venous blood column. When these signs are not readily apparent, or when a more accurate assessment of intravascular blood volume is necessary, central venous or pulmonary artery wedge pressure may be measured.

4 Orthostatic hypotension may be caused by severe forms of peripheral neuropathy. The diseases most commonly associated with these neuropathies include diabetes mellitus, renal failure, amyloidosis, Wernicke's disease, syphilis, and porphyria.

5 Hypotension accompanied by decreased tissue perfusion is the definition of shock. Inadequate tissue perfusion is manifested by organ dysfunction and a change from aerobic to anaerobic metabolism at the cellular level. The metabolic end product of anaerobic metabolism is lactic acid with a resultant increased anion gap metabolic acidosis. The most reliable indicators of organ dysfunction due to inadequate tissue perfusion include decreased mental status, absence of peristaltic activity in the intestines, decreased pulmonary gas exchange, and cool pale skin. Any of these signs, with the exception of the lactic acidosis, may, however, be associated with other disease processes.

6 Symptomatic nonorthostatic hypotension in the absence of decreased tissue perfusion is usually due to transient vasomotor instability. The episode of hypotension is short-lived and usually related to either stimulation of the vagal nerve or increased vagal tone.

7 Decreased intravascular blood volume may be actual or relative. Actual hypovolemia is caused by the loss of red blood cells or plasma water from the vascular space. Relative hypovolemia is due to vasodilatation with subsequent inability of the circulating blood volume to maintain the blood pressure. Vasodilatation is the cause of the hypotension that occurs with sepsis, neuropathic hypotension, anaphylactic reactions, and some drugs. The clinical signs associated with actual and relative hypovolemia are similar. The determination of whether actual blood volume has been lost may require measurement of systemic vascular resistance and cardiac filling pressures by a balloon flotation catheter.

8 Neuropathic forms of hypotension are caused by interruption of the descending pathways in the spinal cord associated with spinal cord trauma, including transection and edema, syringomyelia, and spinal tumors. Epidural and spinal anesthesia may also cause profound neuropathic hypotension. Certain drugs, most notably the barbiturates, may also cause a neuropathic form of hypotension. Cerebral hemorrhage, especially in the pontine area, may interrupt the descending sympathic pathways, causing profound hypotension.

9 Valvular abnormalities that may lead to hypotension and shock include critical aortic stenosis, acute aortic insufficiency, and acute mitral insufficiency. The latter is usually caused by a ruptured papillary muscle or chordae tendineae.

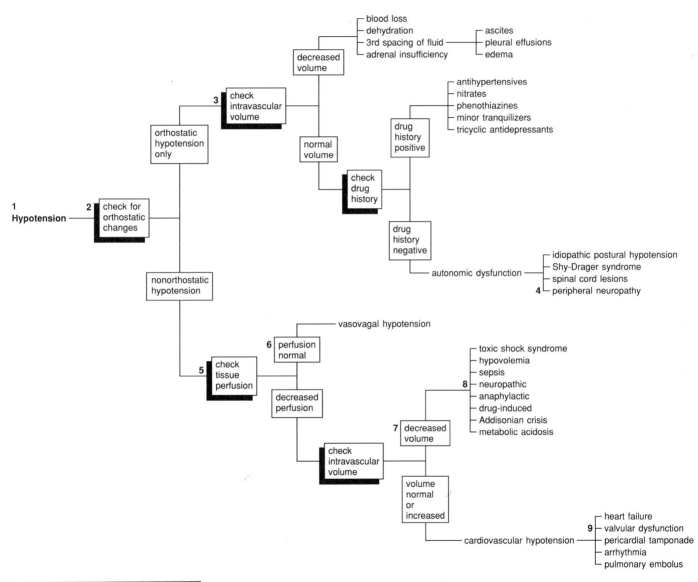

blood loss
dehydration
3rd spacing of fluid — ascites
pleural effusions
edema
adrenal insufficiency

decreased volume

3 check intravascular volume

antihypertensives
nitrates
phenothiazines
minor tranquilizers
tricyclic antidepressants

orthostatic hypotension only

drug history positive

normal volume

check drug history

1 Hypotension — 2 check for orthostatic changes

drug history negative

idiopathic postural hypotension
Shy-Drager syndrome
spinal cord lesions
4 peripheral neuropathy

autonomic dysfunction

nonorthostatic hypotension

vasovagal hypotension

6 perfusion normal

toxic shock syndrome
hypovolemia
sepsis
8 neuropathic
anaphylactic
drug-induced
Addisonian crisis
metabolic acidosis

5 check tissue perfusion

decreased perfusion

7 decreased volume

check intravascular volume

volume normal or increased

heart failure
9 valvular dysfunction
pericardial tamponade
arrhythmia
pulmonary embolus

cardiovascular hypotension

Cecil Chapters	38, 41
Harrison Chapters	39, 189

Syncope

1 Syncope is defined as a sudden loss of consciousness and vascular tone. Similar altered states of consciousness such as seizure, vertigo, coma, or narcolepsy must be excluded from this definition, as the mechanism and etiology of these disorders may be markedly different from those of true syncope. Syncope is a common disorder, with up to 30 per cent of the population reporting at least one episode in their life. Syncope must be evaluated especially in the elderly patient, because the syncopal episode may predict future life-threatening events. In patients suffering a first episode of syncope, approximately 55 per cent of episodes will have a vasovagal or psychobiologic etiology, 10 per cent of episodes will have a cardiovascular cause, 10 per cent will be a first seizure, 5 per cent of patients will have other neurologic disorders, 5 per cent of episodes will be drug-induced, and 15 per cent will remain undiagnosed.

2 Syncope is associated with numerous drugs. The mechanism may be the postural hypotension occurring with many of the antihypertensive agents, diuretics, and nitrates. Orthostatic hypotension with occasional syncope is also associated with the phenothiazines as well as some of the minor tranquilizers and the tricyclic antidepressants. Anaphylactic reactions, drug overdoses, and drug-induced arrhythmias are also causes of syncope.

3 Shy-Drager syndrome (idiopathic orthostatic hypotension) is a rare disorder occurring usually in middle age. The syndrome causes progressive autonomic dysfunction. In addition to the orthostatic hypotension, which may result in syncope, extrapyramidal symptoms, sexual impotency, urinary hesitancy, and anhidrosis may be prominent features. The illness leads to severe disability and death, usually within 5 to 15 years.

4 Subclavian steal syndrome is an unusual disorder causing syncope as well as other symptoms of vertebrobasilar insufficiency. Blood is shunted from the vertebrobasilar artery via the subclavian artery to one of the arms. The hallmark of the disorder is the finding of differences in the blood pressure and pulse between the patient's arms. Syncope may follow upper arm exercise.

5 Syncope is an uncommon presentation of a transient ischemic attack (TIA). A TIA should be suspected when syncope is associated with other neurologic symptoms, especially in the vertebrobasilar artery distribution. A TIA should also be suspected when no etiology for syncope can be found in a patient at risk for cerebrovascular disease.

6 Many forms of cardiac monitoring are available for the evaluation of the patient with syncope. The standard 12-lead EKG should be performed to rule out obvious rhythm disturbances such as heart block, other forms of bradycardia, and frequent ventricular ectopy. The brief 12-lead EKG, however, is often unrevealing, and a 24- or 48-hour continuous EKG recording may be necessary. A diagnostic study currently in use is the signal-averaged EKG. With this method, the surface EKG is computer enhanced to detect low-amplitude, high-frequency components that may predict the possibility of inducible ventricular tachycardia, especially in patients with underlying cardiac disease. If an episode of syncope occurs during continuous EKG monitoring without associated rhythm disturbances, a cardiac etiology for the syncope can be ruled out.

7 Carotid sinus massage may be useful in demonstrating carotid sinus hyperactivity as a source of syncope when other diagnostic studies have not been helpful. A positive result is obtained if an asystolic pause of greater than 3 seconds occurs or a decrease in systolic blood pressure of more than 50 mm without a change in pulse is noted. A history of syncope associated with turning of the head or tight collars may give further clues to the diagnosis. Carotid sinus massage should be performed with great caution in elderly patients, as permanent neurologic deficits have followed this maneuver.

8 Vasovagal syncope is by far the most common cause of loss of consciousness. It may occur at any age but is more common in young patients. The syncope usually occurs in response to emotional stress or injury. The syncope is usually preceded by symptoms of weakness, lightheadedness, sweating, nausea, and dimming of vision. The mechanism for the syncope is probably dilation of large vascular beds, such as the mesentery, renal, and cerebral vessels, without a compensatory increase in heart rate and cardiac output.

9 Situational syncope refers to syncope occurring during normal bodily functions such as micturition, defecation, cough, and swallowing. Micturition syncope occurs in middle-age men, usually at night and many times following consumption of large amounts of alcohol. Rarely, micturition syncope has been associated with a pheochromocytoma of the bladder wall. Cough syncope follows a paroxysm of coughing. Cough syncope most commonly occurs in obese middle-age men, many of whom also have a history of heavy alcohol use. Acute pulmonary processes like asthma, chronic obstructive pulmonary disease, and bronchiectasis have also been associated with cough syncope.

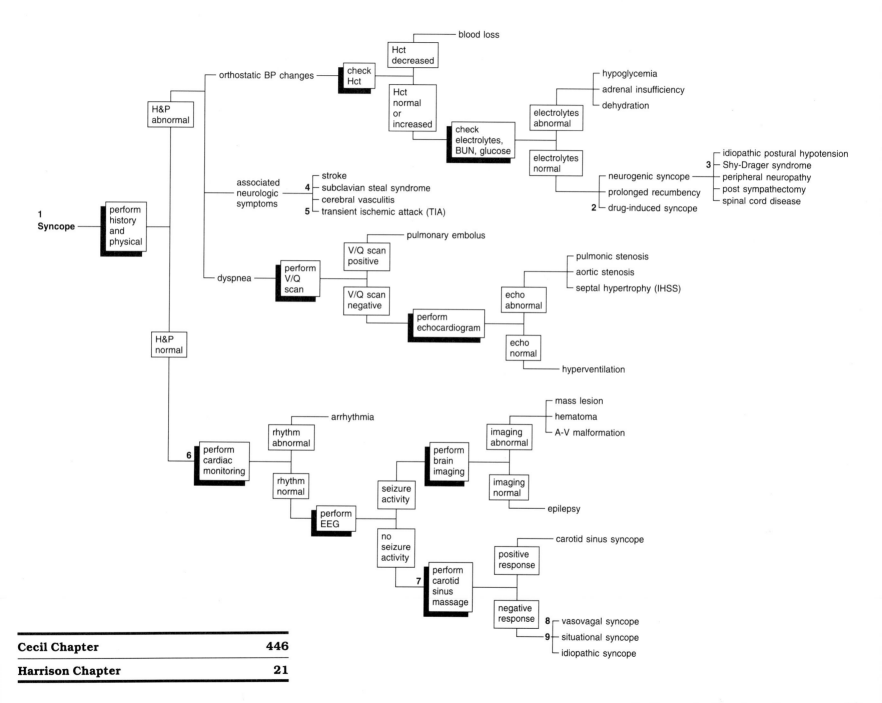

1
Syncope

perform history and physical

H&P abnormal

— orthostatic BP changes — check Hct
- Hct decreased — blood loss
- Hct normal or increased — check electrolytes, BUN, glucose
  - electrolytes abnormal
    - hypoglycemia
    - adrenal insufficiency
    - dehydration
  - electrolytes normal
    - neurogenic syncope **3**
      - idiopathic postural hypotension
      - Shy-Drager syndrome
      - peripheral neuropathy
      - post sympathectomy
      - spinal cord disease
    - prolonged recumbency
    - drug-induced syncope **2**

— associated neurologic symptoms **4**
- stroke
- subclavian steal syndrome
- cerebral vasculitis
- transient ischemic attack (TIA) **5**

— dyspnea — perform V/Q scan
- V/Q scan positive — pulmonary embolus
- V/Q scan negative — perform echocardiogram
  - echo abnormal
    - pulmonic stenosis
    - aortic stenosis
    - septal hypertrophy (IHSS)
  - echo normal — hyperventilation

H&P normal

6 perform cardiac monitoring
- rhythm abnormal — arrhythmia
- rhythm normal — perform EEG
  - seizure activity — perform brain imaging
    - imaging abnormal
      - mass lesion
      - hematoma
      - A-V malformation
    - imaging normal — epilepsy
  - no seizure activity — **7** perform carotid sinus massage
    - positive response — carotid sinus syncope
    - negative response
      - **8** vasovagal syncope
      - **9** situational syncope
      - idiopathic syncope

Cecil Chapter	446
Harrison Chapter	21

Edema

1 Edema is the excess accumulation of fluid in the tissues. The etiology of the fluid accumulation may be the result of increased filtration of fluid out of the vascular space or decreased removal of interstitial fluid by the lymphatic system. The movement of fluid out of the intravascular space is governed by the relationship of hydrostatic pressure, oncotic pressure, and capillary permeability. An increase in hydrostatic pressure or capillary permeability or a decrease in oncotic pressure will increase the movement of fluid out of the intravascular space.

2 Intracardiac filling pressure can be estimated or measured by a variety of methods. Right-sided pressures can be estimated by evaluating the height of the jugular venous blood column. True right atrial pressure, or central venous pressure, may be measured directly by placing a catheter into the right atrium through a peripheral, subclavian, or jugular vein. Left-sided intracardiac pressures can be estimated using a balloon-tip flotation catheter to measure the pulmonary capillary wedge pressure.

3 A two-dimensional echocardiogram can help differentiate between ventricular failure due to poor myocardial contractility and restriction of diastolic filling by pericardial disease. The two-dimensional echocardiogram will clearly demonstrate ventricular function and the presence of pericardial thickening or fluid. When pericardial restriction of ventricular filling becomes severe, cardiac tamponade occurs. The presence of a pulsus paradoxus of greater than 10 mm Hg on physical examination or the equalization of the right atrial, pulmonary artery diastolic, and pulmonary artery wedge pressures is diagnostic of pericardial tamponade.

4 Many drugs have been associated with the formation of edema. Various mechanisms may be involved, but the edema most often results from the retention of salt and water or changes in capillary permeability. The drugs most commonly associated with edema include hormones such as the corticosteroids, estrogen, progesterone, and testosterone; anti-inflammatory agents such as phenylbutazone, naproxen, indomethacin, and ibuprofen; antihypertensive agents such as minoxidil, clonidine, hydralazine, the rauwolfias, and some beta- and calcium channel blockers. Other drugs, including the monoamine oxidase (MAO) inhibitors and amantadine, have also been associated with edema formation.

5 Idiopathic edema occurs most commonly in women. Edema develops during the day and resolves at night from the diuresis associated with recumbency. Water excretion tests are occasionally abnormal and can aid in the diagnosis. Compulsive salt-eaters may also present with idiopathic edema.

6 Edema associated with nutritional deficiency alone is uncommon in Western cultures. When food availability is normal, anorexia nervosa is the most common cause of malnutrition and nutritionally associated edema. When edema is secondary to decreased protein synthesis from malnutrition, other signs, including cheilosis, red tongue, and severe weight loss, are usually present.

7 The venogram is the definitive test to determine the presence of venous obstruction. The test itself, however, has considerable morbidity. Adverse reactions to the venogram include infection, allergic reactions to the iodinated contrast, dye-induced renal failure, and as high as a 10 per cent incidence of new venous thrombosis associated with the procedure itself.

8 Lymphedema is usually firm and nonpitting on examination. It is usually progressive and painless, with no evidence of venous stasis. The edema may be due to inflammation from infection, surgery, trauma, or radiation. Lymphedema from malignant involvement of lymph nodes occurs most commonly with gastrointestinal or genitourinary tumors as well as lymphomas. Magnetic resonance imaging alone or combined with ^{99m}Tc colloidal sulfur lymphoscintigraphy is useful in detecting the site of the lymphatic obstruction.

9 Noninvasive vascular testing provides a specific, if somewhat less sensitive, method of detecting venous obstruction. Noninvasive testing such as impedance plethysmography and Doppler ultrasonography may be used in place of venography in order to avoid the associated morbidity (see No. 7). Impedance plethysmography measures blood volume changes in the calf produced by venous occlusion. These changes are detected by changes in electrical resistance measured by skin electrodes. Impedance plethysmography is a sensitive predictor of proximal vein thrombosis with an accuracy approaching 98 per cent. The test is much less sensitive for detecting calf vein thrombosis, as many of the distal vein thrombi are nonocclusive. Doppler ultrasonography, which measures changes in the velocity of blood flow through the veins, is also a sensitive test for the detection of proximal vein thrombosis but is more difficult to interpret than impedance plethysmography. ^{125}I-fibrinogen scanning detects thrombi that are making fibrin. This test may be useful in the detection of calf vein thrombi during their early development.

10 Edema associated with musculoskeletal disorders is frequently painful and acute in onset. Common etiologies of musculoskeletal edema include acute arthritis, tenosynovitis, Baker's cyst, calf muscle tears, and reflex sympathetic dystrophy (exaggerated edema formation following trauma).

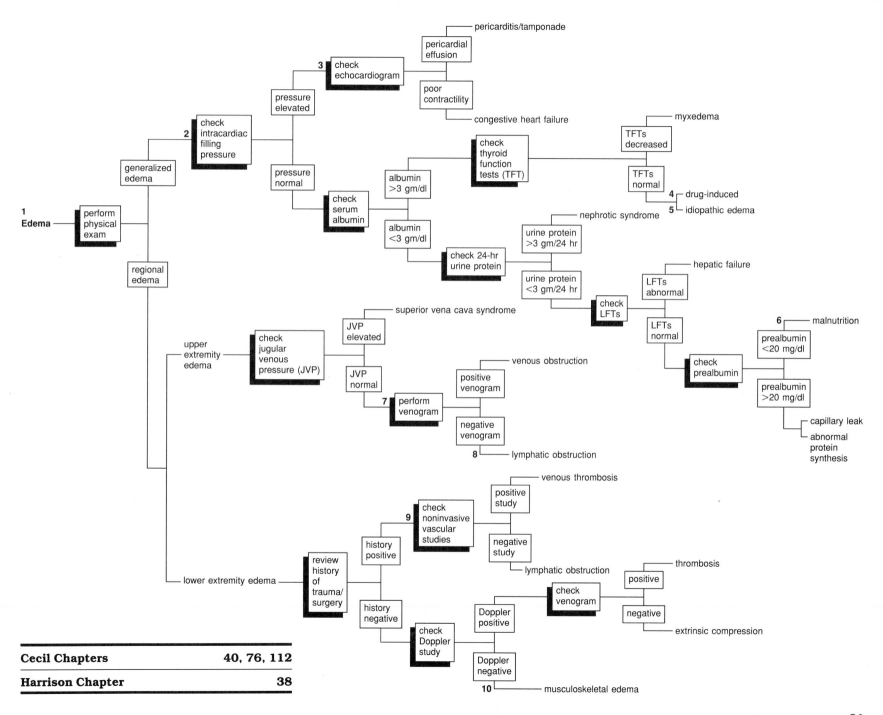

1
Edema — perform physical exam

generalized edema

- check **2** intracardiac filling pressure
  - pressure elevated
    - check **3** echocardiogram
      - pericardial effusion — pericarditis/tamponade
      - poor contractility — congestive heart failure
  - pressure normal
    - check serum albumin
      - albumin >3 gm/dl
        - check thyroid function tests (TFT)
          - TFTs decreased — myxedema
          - TFTs normal
            - **4** — drug-induced
            - **5** — idiopathic edema
      - albumin <3 gm/dl
        - check 24-hr urine protein
          - urine protein >3 gm/24 hr — nephrotic syndrome
          - urine protein <3 gm/24 hr
            - check LFTs
              - LFTs abnormal — hepatic failure
              - LFTs normal
                - check prealbumin
                  - prealbumin <20 mg/dl
                    - **6** — malnutrition
                  - prealbumin >20 mg/dl
                    - capillary leak
                    - abnormal protein synthesis

regional edema

- upper extremity edema
  - check jugular venous pressure (JVP)
    - JVP elevated — superior vena cava syndrome
    - JVP normal
      - **7** perform venogram
        - positive venogram — venous obstruction
        - negative venogram
          - **8** — lymphatic obstruction
- lower extremity edema
  - review history of trauma/surgery
    - history positive
      - check **9** noninvasive vascular studies
        - positive study — venous thrombosis
        - negative study — lymphatic obstruction
    - history negative
      - check Doppler study
        - Doppler positive
          - check venogram
            - positive — thrombosis
            - negative — extrinsic compression
        - Doppler negative
          - **10** — musculoskeletal edema

Cecil Chapters   **40, 76, 112**

Harrison Chapter   **38**

Hypertension

1 Although some controversy exists, it is generally agreed that a diastolic blood pressure of greater than 90 mm Hg on two or more measurements constitutes a diagnosis of hypertension. A systolic pressure of 140 mm Hg or more constitutes systolic hypertension. Systolic hypertension can be an isolated phenomenon or can occur in association with diastolic hypertension. The systolic blood pressure is much more sensitive to transient elevation related to stress or other external stimuli than is the diastolic blood pressure. Isolated systolic hypertension is most commonly associated with advanced age, but other factors such as the decrease in peripheral resistance seen with Paget's disease, arteriovenous shunts, and nutritional deficiencies like beriberi can result in systolic hypertension. Conditions that increase cardiac output such as anemia and thyrotoxicosis are also associated with elevated systolic blood pressure.

2 Aldosterone excretion is best determined by the measurement of 24-hour urinary aldosterone excretion after correction of hypokalemia and following 3 days of salt loading (200 mEq/day). Using this technique, an aldosterone excretion of greater than 14 μg in 24 hours has a greater than 90 per cent sensitivity and specificity for primary aldosteronism. CT and magnetic resonance imaging (MRI) of the adrenals should be performed when the workup for primary aldosteronism is positive. If these tests fail to localize the tumor, adrenal vein sampling may be helpful.

3 Primary aldosteronism accounts for only 1 per cent of the causes of hypertension. Other syndromes of mineralocorticoid excess such as congenital adrenal hyperplasia and defects in steroid synthesis are even more rare. Once the diagnosis of primary aldosteronism is made or suspected, CT or MRI of the adrenals is the most useful diagnostic study to isolate the lesion. Adrenal adenomas (60 to 85 per cent), bilateral adrenal hyperplasia (15 to 40 per cent), or, rarely, adrenal carcinoma may be responsible for the increased aldosterone synthesis. The importance of making this diagnosis lies in the fact that the hypertension is surgically curable.

4 Although secondary causes of hypertension account for only 5 per cent of the estimated 60 million hypertensive persons in the United States, the incidence is much higher when the onset of hypertension occurs before the age of 30. In these young patients, evaluation for secondary causes of hypertension is justified because not only is the incidence of secondary hypertension higher, but the morbidity and cost of life-long medical treatment may be avoided if a curable form of hypertension is found.

5 In the past, the measurement of 24-hour urinary excretion of 3-methoxy-4-hydroxymandelic acid, metanephrine, and normetanephrine were the most commonly used tests for determining excess catecholamine secretion. Currently, however, serum catecholamine determination has been found to be a more sensitive indicator. Sampling for serum catecholamine levels must be performed at least 30 minutes after venipuncture with the patient at rest in order to avoid measuring the transient elevation in serum catecholamines resulting from pain and stress. Serum catecholamine levels are extremely high in patients with pheochromocytoma, with the mean approximately 8000 ng/L.

6 Pheochromocytomas are rare tumors of neural crest tissue. Approximately 85 per cent are benign. These tumors account for 0.5 to 1 per cent of all cases of hypertension. Ninety per cent of the tumors are located in the adrenal medulla; the other 10 per cent may occur anywhere along the distribution of the neural crest (autonomic tissue). Approximately 10 per cent of pheochromocytomas are bilateral. Once a pheochromocytoma is suspected, CT scanning is the most useful diagnostic study. Tumors less than 1 cm in size may be detected using ^{131}I-metiodobenzylguanide (^{131}I-MIBG) nuclear imaging. There is a strong association between pheochromocytomas and certain genetic diseases, including multiple endocrine adenomatoses and neurocutaneous disorders like von Recklinghausen's disease.

7 The administration of central adrenergic blocking agents like clonidine may be useful when the serum catecholamine level is minimally elevated in a hypertensive patient. If the elevation in catecholamines is secondary to a pheochromocytoma, the level will not be suppressed by the drug. The test is performed by administering 0.2 to 0.3 mg of clonidine orally. If the serum catecholamine is not within the normal range after 2 to 3 hours, a pheochromocytoma should be suspected.

8 The administration of an angiotensin-converting enzyme inhibitor like captopril will cause an exaggerated rise in plasma renin activity (PRA) in patients with renal artery stenosis. The test is performed with the patient off all antihypertensive medications and on a normal sodium intake. After the patient is seated for 30 minutes, a baseline PRA is obtained. Fifty milligrams of captopril is given orally under careful BP monitoring. A PRA sample is obtained at 1 hour. A positive test is determined by a stimulated PRA of 12 ng/ml/hr and an absolute increase of 10 ng/ml/hr, or a 150 per cent increase in PRA (the PRA increase must be greater than 400 per cent if the baseline PRA is less than 3 ng/ml/hr). This test has been shown to have a sensitivity of 70 to 90 per cent in screening for renal artery stenosis and carries less morbidity than the rapid-sequence IVP. Angiotensin-converting enzyme inhibition combined with a ^{99m}Tc-diethylenetriamine pentaacetic acid (DTPA) or a ^{131}I-orthohippurate (hippuran) renal scan with or without concomitant furosemide administration has also been found to have a 95 to 98 per cent specificity and sensitivity for detecting renal artery stenosis. With these tests, a delay in the uptake of isotope by the affected kidney not only predicts the presence of renal artery stenosis, but may help to predict the patient's response to therapy.

9 Renal artery stenosis occurs in the young patient as a result of fibromuscular disease or in the elderly patient as a result of atherosclerotic disease. Among those patients with fibromuscular disease, there is a strong female predominance. Atherosclerotic disease accounts for the remaining two thirds of the cases of renal artery stenosis. Patients with rapid onset of resistant hypertension, especially in their early twenties or late fifties, are highly suspect for renal artery stenosis.

10 Because the sensitivity of the captopril challenge may be as low as 70 per cent, a renal angiogram may be necessary to completely exclude renal artery stenosis when plasma renin levels are markedly elevated. The angiogram should be performed if there is a strong clinical suspicion of renal artery stenosis or if physical findings such as a renal artery bruit are present. MRI of the renal arteries may soon approach the accuracy of the traditional arteriogram. MRI tomography is now available at many large medical centers and will soon be more widely available. It should be noted that elevated renin levels are seen in many hypertensive patients with normal renal arteries.

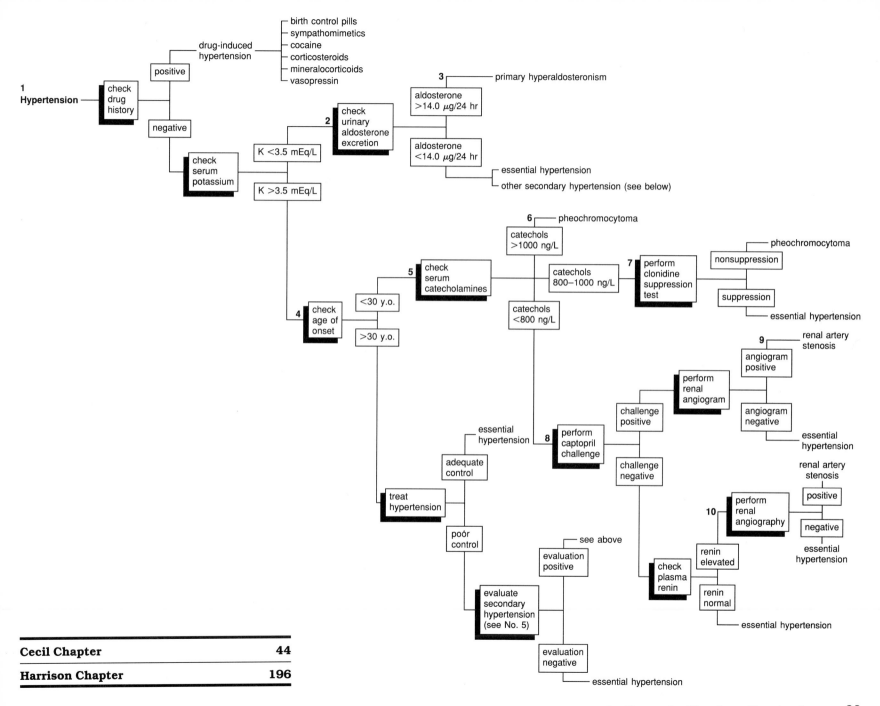

1
Hypertension

check drug history

positive → drug-induced hypertension
- birth control pills
- sympathomimetics
- cocaine
- corticosteroids
- mineralocorticoids
- vasopressin

negative → check serum potassium

K <3.5 mEq/L → **2** check urinary aldosterone excretion

3 aldosterone >14.0 μg/24 hr → primary hyperaldosteronism

aldosterone <14.0 μg/24 hr → essential hypertension / other secondary hypertension (see below)

K >3.5 mEq/L → **4** check age of onset

<30 y.o. → **5** check serum catecholamines

6 catechols >1000 ng/L → pheochromocytoma

catechols 800–1000 ng/L → **7** perform clonidine suppression test

nonsuppression → pheochromocytoma

suppression → essential hypertension

catechols <800 ng/L

>30 y.o. → treat hypertension

adequate control → essential hypertension

poor control → evaluate secondary hypertension (see No. 5)

evaluation positive → see above

evaluation negative → essential hypertension

8 perform captopril challenge

challenge positive → perform renal angiogram

9 angiogram positive → renal artery stenosis

angiogram negative → essential hypertension

challenge negative → check plasma renin

renin elevated → **10** perform renal angiography

positive → renal artery stenosis

negative → essential hypertension

renin normal → essential hypertension

Cecil Chapter	**44**
Harrison Chapter	**196**

Murmurs

1 Cardiac murmurs are caused by the abnormal flow, velocity, direction, or turbulence of blood across an intracardiac opening. Murmurs can be characterized by their location, radiation, intensity, and quality. These features are extremely useful in the diagnosis of the underlying abnormality. Murmurs may be described as high- or low-pitched. Their configuration may be crescendo, crescendo-decrescendo, even, or variable. The murmur may be heard in systole or diastole or continuously. The portion of the cardiac cycle, i.e., early, mid, late, or throughout (holo), in which the murmur is present has importance in the differential diagnosis of the cardiac abnormality. The intensity of the murmur is typically described on a scale of 1 to 6. A grade 1 murmur is barely audible with a stethoscope. A grade 2 murmur is faint but easily heard. A grade 3 murmur is prominent but not loud. Grade 4 through 6 murmurs are accompanied by a thrill.

2 The phonocardiogram is a useful adjunct to auscultation of the heart when the location of the murmur is unclear or when more than one murmur is present. The phonocardiogram provides a graphic display of the murmur, including its relationship to the normal heart sounds. Simultaneous recording of the phonocardiogram and carotid or jugular pulse waves may also provide useful information. Some laboratories may have the capacity to do simultaneous phono- and echocardiographic recordings, thereby saving an extra step in diagnosis. Pulsed-wave Doppler and color-flow Doppler ultrasonography add a further dimension to standard echocardiography. Both of these techniques can sample Doppler shifts in moving objects. This is especially useful in measuring peak velocity through stenotic lesions.

3 Acute mitral regurgitation may present as an early systolic murmur instead of the more characteristic holosystolic murmur. This phenomenon occurs because the regurgitant blood flow is into a normal-sized and less distensible left atrium. As the pressure in the atrium rises rapidly, the blood flow is stopped during the early phase of systole. Over time, as the left atrium distends, the regurgitant blood flow may last throughout systole. Papillary muscle rupture or dysfunction is the most common cause of acute mitral regurgitation.

4 When ventricular septal defects (VSDs) are large, the left-to-right shunting will cause pressure overload in the right ventricle and the pulmonary vasculature. As pressure in the right heart and pulmonary resistance increase, there is a decrease in the duration of the left-to-right blood flow through the VSD, decreasing the length of time the murmur is audible.

5 Many murmurs heard typically during midsystole are not associated with any anatomic abnormality. These murmurs may be related to increased blood flow across one or more valves, as occurs with anemia, fever, exercise, thyrotoxicosis, and occasionally in normal persons. Benign murmurs may also be due to other forms of turbulence of the blood flow through the great vessels such as the pulmonary trunk and aorta. Still's murmur is a benign murmur thought to originate from periodic vibrations of the aortic or pulmonary valve leaflets.

6 In the absence of valvular abnormalities, holosystolic murmurs are the result of intracardiac shunts between high- and low-pressure chambers or vessels. As the hemodynamic consequences of the shunt cause pressure gradients to change over time, the murmurs may change in intensity or duration (see No. 4). In murmurs without valvular abnormality, cardiac catheterization may be necessary to diagnose the etiology of the murmur.

7 Mid-diastolic murmurs may be the result of increased blood flow or velocity across normal atrioventricular (AV) valves. The murmurs may be the result of blood flow across the mitral valve in the presence of ventricular septal defects or a patent ductus arteriosus. Abnormal flow across the tricuspid valve is seen with ostium secundum atrial septal defects.

8 The mid-diastolic murmur heard in the presence of a complete heart block is due to antegrade flow across an AV valve that is in the process of closing. The blood flow occurs when atrial contraction coincides with the phase of rapid diastolic filling in the recipient ventricle.

9 Arteriovenous fistulae may occur in several areas of the heart. The most common connections are between coronary artery and vein, as a left coronary artery arising from the pulmonary trunk, and as communication between a sinus of Valsalva aneurysm and the right heart. The configuration, intensity, and location of the murmurs will vary depending on the site of the fistula.

10 Noncardiac continuous murmurs usually result from disturbances to blood flow in constricted systemic or pulmonary arteries. These murmurs most commonly occur in patients with severe peripheral vascular disease. Occasionally, continuous murmurs can be heard with normal vasculature. An example is the mammary souffle heard over the lactating breasts in late pregnancy or the early postpartum period.

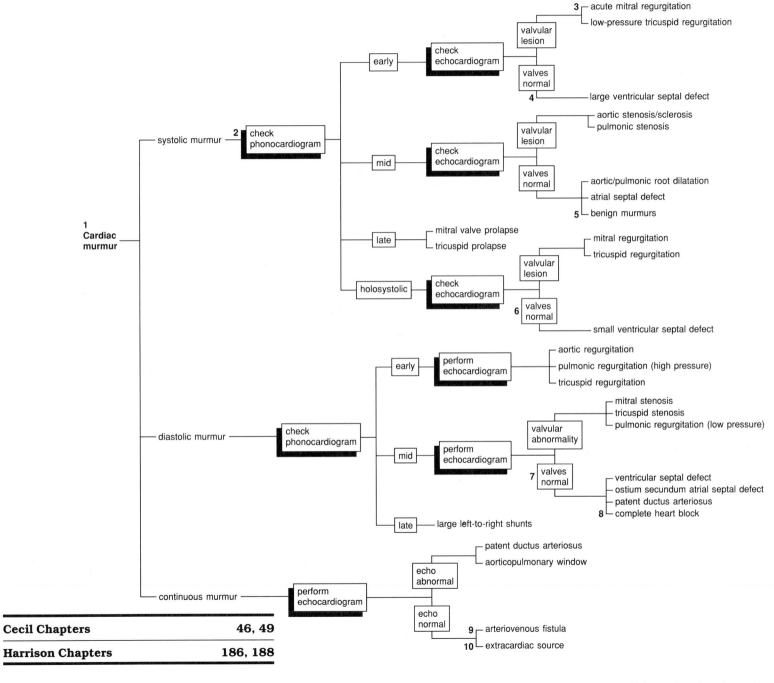

**1
Cardiac
murmur**

systolic murmur — **2 check phonocardiogram**

early — **check echocardiogram**
- valvular lesion
  - **3** ⌐ acute mitral regurgitation
  - └ low-pressure tricuspid regurgitation
- valves normal
  - **4** └ large ventricular septal defect

mid — **check echocardiogram**
- valvular lesion
  - ⌐ aortic stenosis/sclerosis
  - └ pulmonic stenosis
- valves normal
  - ⌐ aortic/pulmonic root dilatation
  - ├ atrial septal defect
  - **5** └ benign murmurs

late
- ⌐ mitral valve prolapse
- └ tricuspid prolapse

holosystolic — **check echocardiogram**
- valvular lesion
  - ⌐ mitral regurgitation
  - └ tricuspid regurgitation
- **6** valves normal
  - └ small ventricular septal defect

diastolic murmur — **check phonocardiogram**

early — **perform echocardiogram**
- ⌐ aortic regurgitation
- ├ pulmonic regurgitation (high pressure)
- └ tricuspid regurgitation

mid — **perform echocardiogram**
- valvular abnormality
  - ⌐ mitral stenosis
  - ├ tricuspid stenosis
  - └ pulmonic regurgitation (low pressure)
- **7** valves normal
  - ⌐ ventricular septal defect
  - ├ ostium secundum atrial septal defect
  - ├ patent ductus arteriosus
  - **8** └ complete heart block

late — large left-to-right shunts

continuous murmur — **perform echocardiogram**

echo abnormal
- ⌐ patent ductus arteriosus
- └ aorticopulmonary window

echo normal
- **9** ⌐ arteriovenous fistula
- **10** └ extracardiac source

Cecil Chapters	**46, 49**
Harrison Chapters	**186, 188**

Cardiomegaly

1 Cardiomegaly is defined as any abnormal increase in the size of the heart. The increase in size may be due to local or global increases in chamber size, hypertrophy or infiltrative disease of the myocardial muscle, pericardial effusion, or an aneurysm of the myocardium. Cardiomegaly may be suspected on physical examination or, more commonly, on chest radiograph. These techniques may, however, underestimate or overestimate actual heart size, because hypertrophy of less than 1 cm or single-chamber enlargement is difficult to detect by these methods alone. Techniques such as echocardiography (see No. 2) have been developed to accurately measure cardiac size. Cardiomegaly is usually the result of a chronic process; therefore, a complete evaluation is necessary in order to determine the disease process causing the cardiomegaly, as well as the physiologic consequences that may result from the cardiomegaly itself.

2 Echocardiography can provide invaluable information regarding both the anatomy and function of the heart. Chamber size, myocardial thickness, valvular motion and calcification, valve leaflet thickness, and pericardial disease can all be determined accurately. Two-dimensional and Doppler echocardiography can also give accurate assessments of overall cardiac function and regional abnormalities.

3 Asymmetric hypertrophic cardiomyopathy (idiopathic hypertrophic subaortic stenosis [IHSS]) occurs in both familial and sporadic forms. IHSS is defined as a septal–to–posterior wall thickness ratio of greater than 1.3 on echocardiogram. Although many patients are asymptomatic, the most common clinical manifestations include angina, dyspnea, syncope, and palpitations. Most patients demonstrate significant obstruction to aortic outflow, which further intensifies the left ventricular hypertrophy. A few patients will have no evidence of outflow obstruction. Drugs that increase the force of left ventricular contraction or decrease systemic resistance worsen the hemodynamic effects of the outflow obstruction and increase or precipitate symptoms.

4 High-output states cause cardiomegaly by increasing cardiac work and increasing intracardiac blood volume. Clinical conditions associated with high cardiac outputs include severe anemia, polycythemia vera, renal insufficiency, arteriovenous fistulas and anastomoses, erythroderma, Paget's disease, hyperthyroidism, and chronic hypoxemia. Both left and right heart enlargement may occur, and heart failure is common.

5 Infiltrative diseases of the myocardium include amyloidosis, sarcoidosis, hemochromatosis, and Löffler's myocarditis. The hypertrophy of the myocardium is secondary to the deposition of material within the myocardial fibers themselves. Infiltration of the myocardium with melanoma, lymphoma, leukemia, and metastatic carcinoma of the lung or breast has also been described.

6 Congestive cardiomyopathy with cardiomegaly due to primary myocardial disease accounts for approximately 1 per cent of the cardiac disease in the United States but may represent up to 15 per cent of the cardiac disease worldwide. Although the symptoms of a primary myocardial disorder are similar to those of other forms of heart disease, the diagnosis should be suspected when cardiomegaly is discovered in a patient who is young and normotensive and has no evidence of ischemic disease.

7 The mechanism of cardiac dilatation secondary to chronic ethanol ingestion is unknown but appears to be metabolic in origin. The severity of the disease is related to both the quantity and the duration of the ethanol consumption. Arrhythmias, congestive heart failure, and thromboembolic events are the hallmarks of this disorder. The 3-year mortality exceeds 40 per cent.

8 Cardiomegaly secondary to a congestive cardiomyopathy may occur following a viral myocarditis. Group B coxsackieviruses and the poliomyelitis virus are the most frequently associated agents. Other viral illnesses that have also been implicated in cardiomyopathies include measles, mumps, influenza, varicella, and infectious mononucleosis. Myocardial injury probably results from direct cellular invasion by the virus or from immunologic processes that are not yet well defined.

9 Doxorubicin (Adriamycin) myocarditis is the prototype of a drug-induced myocarditis leading to cardiomegaly. The cardiomyopathic effect may occur at any dose but occurs most commonly if the cumulative dose exceeds 400 mg/m² of body surface area. Other drugs that have been associated with cardiomyopathies include emetine, tricyclic antidepressants, the sulfonamides, and the phenothiazines.

10 The familial cardiomyopathies are rare causes of cardiomegaly. Cardiac enlargement is due to congestive cardiomyopathy. Included among this group of diseases are endocardial fibroelastosis, Fabry's disease, Pompe's disease, and Hurler syndrome.

11 Laboratory examination in the evaluation of cardiomegaly should include a complete blood count (CBC), sedimentation rate, electrolytes, glucose, Ca, Mg, PO_4, antinuclear antibodies (ANAs), blood cultures for bacteria and fungi, and thyroid function studies.

12 Several of the collagen vascular diseases are associated with congestive cardiomyopathy and resultant cardiomegaly. Progressive systemic sclerosis (scleroderma) may cause myocardial fibrosis. Systemic lupus erythematosus (SLE) may affect any area of the heart, including the myocardium. Rheumatoid arthritis usually involves the pericardium but may occasionally involve the myocardium itself.

BIBLIOGRAPHY

Alpert JS, Rippe JM (eds): Manual of Cardiovascular Diagnosis and Therapy. Boston, Little, Brown and Company, 1985.
Horwitz LD, Groves BM (eds): Signs and Symptoms in Cardiology. Philadelphia, J. B. Lippincott Company, 1985.
Kapoor WN: Diagnostic evaluation of syncope. Am J Med 90:91–103, 1991.
Taylor RB: Difficult Diagnosis. Philadelphia, W. B. Saunders Company, 1985.
Wyngaarden JB, Smith LH Jr (eds): Cecil Textbook of Medicine. 18th ed. Philadelphia, W. B. Saunders Company, 1988.

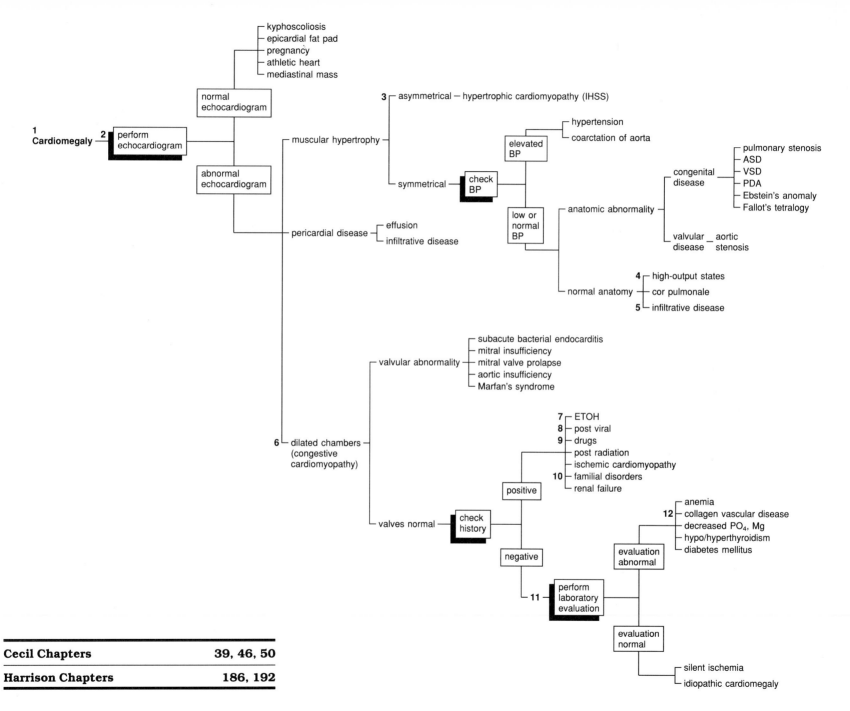

4 ▪ Gastrointestinal Disorders

Signs and symptoms:
Constipation
Diarrhea
Gastrointestinal bleeding
Dysphagia
Abdominal pain
Jaundice/hyperbilirubinemia

Hepatomegaly
Ascites
Labs:
Transaminitis
Elevated alkaline phosphatase

Constipation

1 Because bowel habits vary widely among individuals, there is no universal definition of constipation. Constipation must be discussed in the setting of change from the baseline habits of an individual. Bowel-conscious patients may report constipation because they are fixated on the amount and regularity of bowel movements they perceive as "normal," when in fact no abnormality exists. In general, fewer than three bowel movements a week is very unusual. The term constipation can be used by patients to refer to a variety of abnormalities, and the meaning should be investigated individually with each patient. Constipation is defined as decreased frequency of stools, but patients may use the term when referring to incomplete defecation, the need to strain to defecate, painful defecation, or hard stools. If constipation is of recent onset, a thorough diagnostic investigation should be undertaken. If constipation is chronic by history, a trial of bulk agents is usually indicated prior to the initiation of evaluation.

2 Although the gastrointestinal (GI) manifestations associated with diabetes mellitus are most commonly vomiting and diarrhea, autonomic neuropathy can result in altered bowel habits with constipation. The cause is not known, but the disorder is seen more commonly in association with long-standing diabetes. Autonomic denervation of the proximal gut is the likely etiology.

3 Although a very rare cause of constipation, diuretics can result in constipation by causing dehydration or hypokalemia.

4 Calcium- and aluminum-containing antacids are a frequent cause of constipation. Magnesium-containing antacids are associated with diarrhea.

5 Approximately 25 per cent of large bowel cancer occurs in the rectum so that digital rectal examination is essential in the investigation of constipation.

6 Sigmoidoscopy is the most sensitive and specific test for detecting rectal and sigmoid lesions. Direct visualization of rectal and sigmoid mucosa allows for simultaneous biopsy of any abnormality. Barium enema is unreliable as a primary diagnostic test because of poor resolution of the rectum. Barium enema should follow examination with the sigmoidoscope in order to detect lesions higher in the bowel that may not be seen with the sigmoidoscope.

7 Sigmoidoscopic examination may reveal a superficial brown pigmentation of the rectal mucosa that occurs in patients who abuse laxatives. Called melanosis coli, the pigmentation is most commonly due to the use of anthraquinone laxatives such as cascara and senna. The condition is not pathologically significant except to prevent extensive, unnecessary workup by identifying the patient who denies laxative use.

8 Cathartic colon is the consequence of prolonged use of laxatives and is a common cause of constipation. Long-term laxative abuse can destroy intramural nerve plexuses in the large bowel, resulting in constipation. This disorder is most frequently associated with the use of stimulant laxatives that act by increasing colonic propulsive motor activity and stimulating intestinal fluid secretion. Examples of stimulant laxatives include senna, castor oil, phenolphthalein, and the biguanides.

9 Megacolon can be congenital or acquired and is a frequent cause of constipation. Hirschsprung's disease is due to a congenital absence of intramural neural plexuses. The diagnosis of Hirschsprung's disease is made on full-thickness biopsy of the rectum in which ganglion cells of Meissner's and Auerbach's plexuses are absent. Acquired megacolon is much more common than congenital megacolon. The acquired form is secondary to obstruction of any etiology but usually is due to laxative abuse.

10 Metabolic abnormalities are rarely causes of constipation but must be excluded before constipation can be considered to be idiopathic.

11 The milk-alkali syndrome is due to ingestion of large amounts of antacids that contain calcium (>5 gm/day). Hypercalcemia results and, if long-standing, can lead to renal failure. The syndrome was more common in the past when milk and calcium-containing antacids were used in the treatment of peptic ulcer disease.

12 Irritable bowel syndrome is a functional cause of constipation that has no demonstrable organic etiology. The syndrome is common and presents as episodes of abdominal discomfort and alternating diarrhea and constipation. Other organic causes of constipation, diarrhea, and abdominal pain should always be sought prior to making a diagnosis of irritable bowel syndrome.

13 Poor bowel habits refers to suppression of defecation by patients who are "too busy" to defecate or who do not defecate when the urge presents at an inconvenient time.

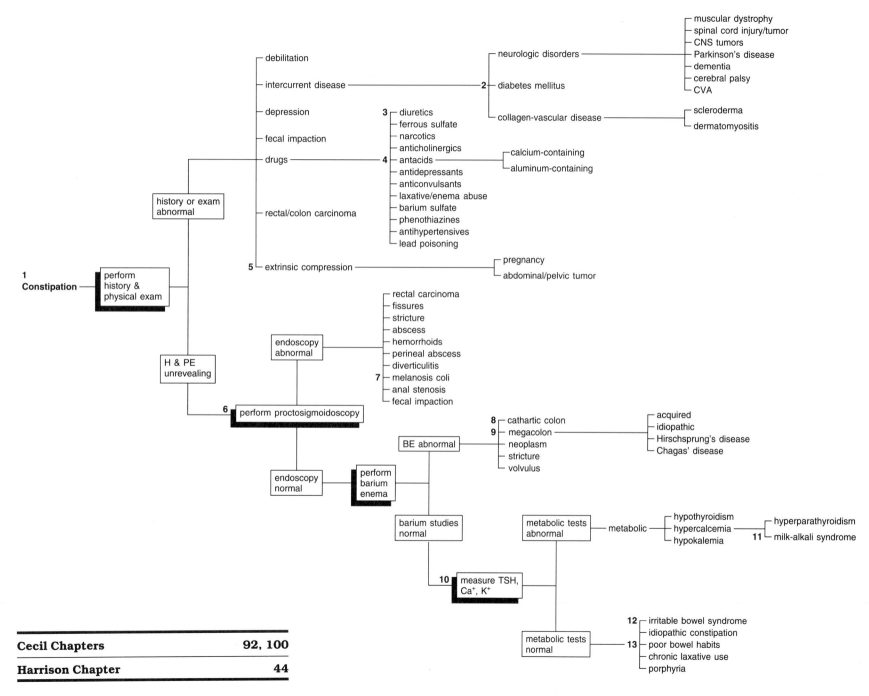

1 Constipation — perform history & physical exam

history or exam abnormal
- debilitation
- intercurrent disease — **2**
  - neurologic disorders
    - muscular dystrophy
    - spinal cord injury/tumor
    - CNS tumors
    - Parkinson's disease
    - dementia
    - cerebral palsy
    - CVA
  - diabetes mellitus
  - collagen-vascular disease
    - scleroderma
    - dermatomyositis
- depression
- fecal impaction
- drugs — **4**
  - **3** diuretics
  - ferrous sulfate
  - narcotics
  - anticholinergics
  - antacids
    - calcium-containing
    - aluminum-containing
  - antidepressants
  - anticonvulsants
  - laxative/enema abuse
  - barium sulfate
  - phenothiazines
  - antihypertensives
  - lead poisoning
- rectal/colon carcinoma
- **5** extrinsic compression
  - pregnancy
  - abdominal/pelvic tumor

H & PE unrevealing — **6** perform proctosigmoidoscopy

endoscopy abnormal
- rectal carcinoma
- fissures
- stricture
- abscess
- hemorrhoids
- perineal abscess
- diverticulitis
- **7** melanosis coli
- anal stenosis
- fecal impaction

endoscopy normal — perform barium enema

BE abnormal
- **8** cathartic colon
- **9** megacolon
  - acquired
  - idiopathic
  - Hirschsprung's disease
  - Chagas' disease
- neoplasm
- stricture
- volvulus

barium studies normal — **10** measure TSH, Ca+, K+

metabolic tests abnormal — metabolic
- hypothyroidism
- hypercalcemia
  - hyperparathyroidism
  - **11** milk-alkali syndrome
- hypokalemia

metabolic tests normal
- **12** irritable bowel syndrome
- idiopathic constipation
- **13** poor bowel habits
- chronic laxative use
- porphyria

Cecil Chapters	**92, 100**
Harrison Chapter	**44**

Diarrhea

ACUTE DIARRHEA

1 In general, one objective definition of diarrhea is based on volume. The patient is considered to have diarrhea if the stool bulk exceeds 150 ml/day. The acuteness of onset of the diarrhea and the "toxicity" of the patient (fever, chills, leukocytosis) determine whether the diarrhea should be treated symptomatically or a diagnostic evaluation initiated. Patients with diarrhea who are "nontoxic" can be treated symptomatically. Diagnostic evaluation of the "nontoxic" patient should begin if the diarrhea persists after 3 to 4 weeks of symptomatic treatment. A mild, self-limited acute diarrhea would suggest a viral etiology, and no evaluation should be undertaken. Acute bloody diarrhea with associated fever demands immediate evaluation.

2 Acute diarrhea is defined as diarrhea of less than 2 weeks' duration. The most common cause of acute diarrhea is viral gastroenteritis. Diarrhea that is chronic and persistent is less likely to be of infectious etiology.

3 A sigmoidoscopic examination should be performed in the evaluation of every patient with diarrhea. Rectal or colonic masses, such as carcinoma or impacted stool, may cause diarrhea when liquid stool passes around the obstruction. Often the liquid stool appears as fecal incontinence. Fecal impaction should be considered in elderly or debilitated patients who have diarrhea.

4 Drugs are a common cause of diarrhea. Laxatives are the most common cause of drug-induced diarrhea, and antibiotics are the second most common cause. Antibiotics most commonly cause a mild diarrhea that stops once the antibiotic is discontinued. A more serious form of antibiotic-associated diarrhea is pseudomembranous colitis. This disorder is due to the proliferation of *Clostridium difficile*. The bacteria produce a pathogenic toxin that damages the colonic mucosa and forms a pseudomembrane. The pseudomembrane is composed of fibrin, leukocytes, and epithelial debris. Diarrhea usually begins between the fifth and tenth day of antibiotic treatment but may occur when the antibiotics are instituted or as long as 3 weeks after the antibiotics have been discontinued. Broad-spectrum antibiotics have been most commonly associated with pseudomembranous colitis, especially lincomycin, clindamycin, and ampicillin. Pseudomembranous colitis can occur even when the antibiotics have been used parenterally. If pseudomembranous colitis is suspected, a fresh stool specimen should be evaluated for the presence of *C. difficile* toxin.

5 Antacids containing magnesium, carbenoxolone, and other liquorice derivatives can cause diarrhea.

6 Stool culture and examination for ova and parasites are important, especially with a history of recent travel to an endemic area. Examination for ova and parasites should be repeated on three separate occasions to be considered negative, although sensitivity of the stool examination is poor despite multiple examinations.

7 Stool examination for ova and parasites may reveal the organism in cases of parasite infestation except for *Giardia lamblia*. *Giardia lamblia* is the most common parasitic cause of traveler's diarrhea. Infection with *Giardia* is most commonly due to ingestion of contaminated water. If *Giardia* infection is suspected, examination of duodenal aspirates is usually necessary for diagnosis. Often duodenal aspirates are negative so that a therapeutic trial of metronidazole may be diagnostic if symptoms resolve.

8 Traveler's diarrhea is defined as diarrhea that occurs within 2 weeks of traveling to countries whose water supply is likely to be contaminated. The diarrhea is self-limited (lasting less than 10 days) and is most commonly due to an enterotoxin-producing *Escherichia coli*. Other common bacterial causes of traveler's diarrhea are *Salmonella* sp., *Shigella* sp., *Yersinia enterocolitica*, and *Campylobacter* sp. Most cases of bacterial diarrhea are caused by ingestion of contaminated food or water. A stool culture will screen for the common enteric pathogens and can be useful to diagnose the presence of *Salmonella*, *Shigella*, *Yersinia*, and *Campylobacter*.

9 The diagnosis of food poisoning is based on the historic aspects of the onset of the diarrhea. *Staphylococcus aureus* and *Clostridium perfringens* cause diarrhea owing to ingestion of preformed toxins in contaminated food. The symptoms of vomiting followed by diarrhea, occurring within 2 to 6 hours of eating the contaminated food, are suggestive of a toxin-induced diarrhea. If other persons eating the same food are also afflicted, the diagnosis of food poisoning is highly likely.

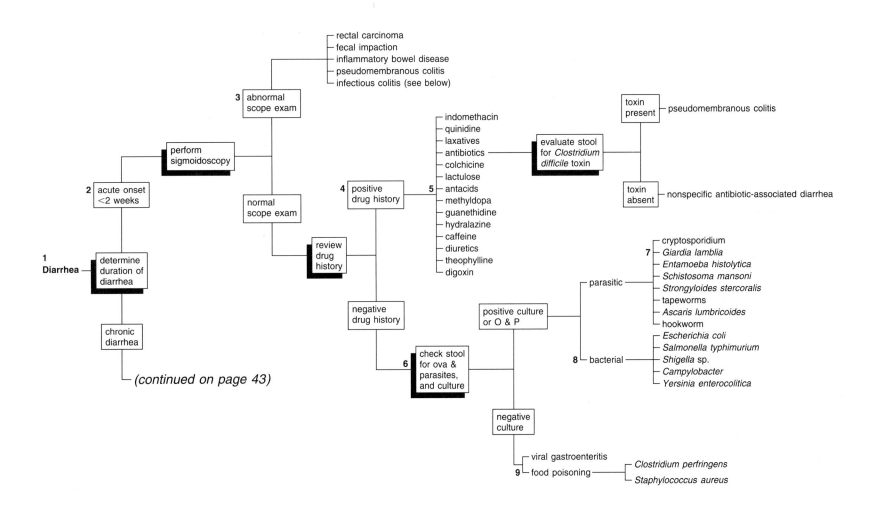

rectal carcinoma
fecal impaction
inflammatory bowel disease
pseudomembranous colitis
infectious colitis (see below)

3 abnormal scope exam

indomethacin
quinidine
laxatives
antibiotics
colchicine
lactulose
5 antacids
methyldopa
guanethidine
hydralazine
caffeine
diuretics
theophylline
digoxin

toxin present — pseudomembranous colitis

evaluate stool for *Clostridium difficile* toxin

toxin absent — nonspecific antibiotic-associated diarrhea

perform sigmoidoscopy

4 positive drug history

2 acute onset <2 weeks

normal scope exam

review drug history

cryptosporidium
7 *Giardia lamblia*
Entamoeba histolytica
Schistosoma mansoni
Strongyloides stercoralis
tapeworms
Ascaris lumbricoides
hookworm

parasitic

1
Diarrhea — determine duration of diarrhea

negative drug history

positive culture or O & P

bacterial

Escherichia coli
Salmonella typhimurium
8 *Shigella* sp.
Campylobacter
Yersinia enterocolitica

chronic diarrhea

6 check stool for ova & parasites, and culture

(continued on page 43)

negative culture

viral gastroenteritis
9 food poisoning — *Clostridium perfringens*
Staphylococcus aureus

Cecil Chapter	101
Harrison Chapter	44

Diarrhea *(Continued)*

CHRONIC DIARRHEA

10 Chronic diarrhea can be defined as diarrhea lasting for more than a month. More than 90 per cent of chronic diarrhea is due to three disorders: chronic inflammatory bowel disease, colon carcinoma, and irritable bowel syndrome. Diarrhea is less likely to be infectious when it is chronic.

11 Surreptitious ingestion of laxatives (only the phenolphthalein type) can be detected by adding sodium hydroxide to a fresh stool sample. Presence of phenolphthalein will turn the stool pink and implicates use of phenolphthalein-containing stimulant laxatives. Laxative abuse is a rare cause of chronic diarrhea, but the test can be done quickly and easily when laxative abuse is suspected. A positive test prevents unnecessary extensive evaluation.

12 Methylene blue or Wright's stains can be used to detect the presence of white cells in the stool. Blood can be detected by gross examination of the stool or by testing for occult blood. The presence of blood or pus indicates that colitis (intestinal inflammation) is present. Colitis can be due to infection with mucosal invasion and inflammation or to chronic inflammatory conditions.

13 Although infection is usually not a source of chronic diarrhea, some pathogens can cause chronic diarrhea. Therefore, stool should be cultured and examined for the presence of parasites when blood or pus is present.

14 If the stool culture and repeated (at least three) evaluations for parasitic infections are negative, proctosigmoidoscopy should be undertaken without prior bowel preparation. Direct visualization of the mucosa will identify inflammatory conditions. Mucosal biopsy can be performed simultaneously with endoscopic examination in order to confirm inflammatory disorders and will detect diseases that might not be grossly evident. Biopsy may detect evidence of inflammation that was not detected by endoscopic visualization. In addition, biopsy will aid the diagnosis in a normal-appearing mucosa, such as amyloidosis or Whipple's disease.

15 If the diagnosis of chronic diarrhea is not evident after proctosigmoidoscopy and biopsy, barium radiographic examination should be performed. Barium studies may identify the diagnosis of diarrhea-causing disease that does not involve the mucosa accessible to the sigmoidoscope. At times, a barium study is performed, even when endoscopic examination has revealed evidence of mucosal disease, in order to determine the extent of involvement. Colonoscopy is necessary when the diagnosis of inflammation or carcinoma is likely but has not been confirmed with sigmoidoscopic or radiographic examination.

16 Diarrhea of unknown origin is the term used to refer to diarrhea for which full evaluation fails to reveal a diagnosis. Patients with this condition require close follow-up and careful re-evaluation, which should include documentation of stool volumes and quantitative fecal fat determinations.

17 The malabsorption syndrome refers to a group of signs and symptoms that result when intestinal absorption of various dietary components is altered. The absorption abnormality can involve protein, fat, vitamins or minerals, or carbohydrates. Symptoms include the presence of stools that are light yellow or gray, soft, and greasy. In addition, there may be evidence of weight loss and anorexia. Celiac disease is the most common cause of malabsorption, but there are many disorders that result in malabsorption, including pancreatic insufficiency, gastrectomy, infection, and drugs. The clinical manifestations depend upon the specific absorptive defect.

18 Diarrhea of unknown origin (see No. 16) is most commonly due to irritable bowel syndrome, bile salt malabsorption, and surreptitious laxative abuse when no colonic inflammation (no blood/pus) can be documented.

19 Irritable bowel syndrome can usually be suspected on the basis of history and negative barium studies. Colonoscopy is not usually necessary. The patient has a history of intermittent diarrhea alternating with constipation, abdominal pain, and no systemic symptoms. There is no evidence of intestinal abnormality with stool examinations or proctosigmoidoscopy.

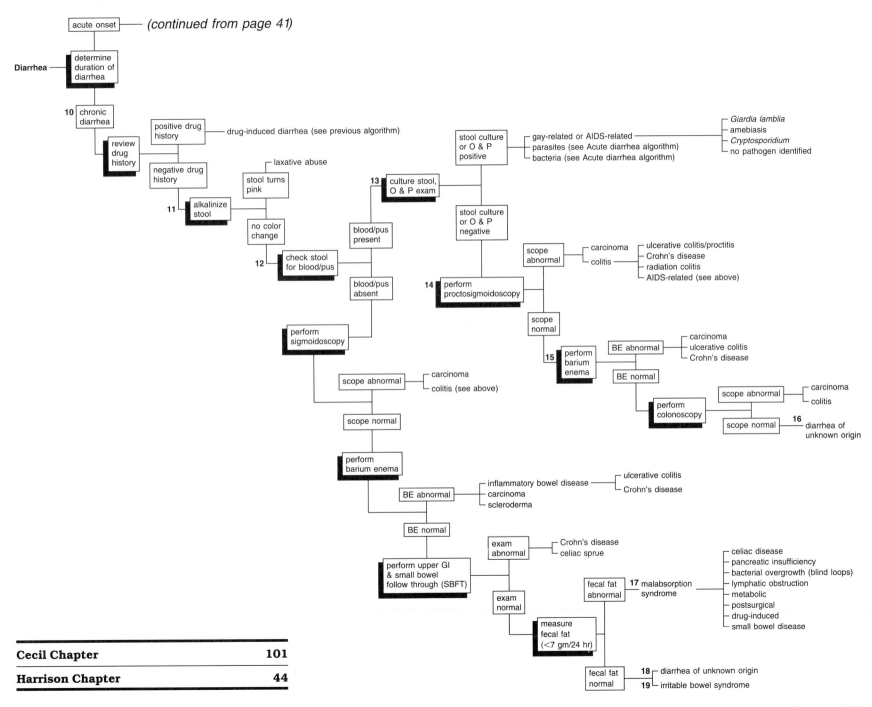

acute onset　　(continued from page 41)

Diarrhea —— determine duration of diarrhea

10 chronic diarrhea

review drug history

positive drug history —— drug-induced diarrhea (see previous algorithm)

negative drug history

stool turns pink —— laxative abuse

11 alkalinize stool

no color change

12 check stool for blood/pus

blood/pus present

blood/pus absent

13 culture stool, O & P exam

stool culture or O & P positive —— gay-related or AIDS-related —— *Giardia lamblia* / amebiasis / *Cryptosporidium* / no pathogen identified

parasites (see Acute diarrhea algorithm)

bacteria (see Acute diarrhea algorithm)

stool culture or O & P negative

14 perform proctosigmoidoscopy

scope abnormal —— carcinoma / colitis —— ulcerative colitis/proctitis / Crohn's disease / radiation colitis / AIDS-related (see above)

scope normal

15 perform barium enema

BE abnormal —— carcinoma / ulcerative colitis / Crohn's disease

BE normal

perform colonoscopy

scope abnormal —— carcinoma / colitis

scope normal —— **16** diarrhea of unknown origin

perform sigmoidoscopy

scope abnormal —— carcinoma / colitis (see above)

scope normal

perform barium enema

BE abnormal —— inflammatory bowel disease —— ulcerative colitis / Crohn's disease

carcinoma

scleroderma

BE normal

perform upper GI & small bowel follow through (SBFT)

exam abnormal —— Crohn's disease / celiac sprue

exam normal

measure fecal fat (<7 gm/24 hr)

fecal fat abnormal —— **17** malabsorption syndrome —— celiac disease / pancreatic insufficiency / bacterial overgrowth (blind loops) / lymphatic obstruction / metabolic / postsurgical / drug-induced / small bowel disease

fecal fat normal —— **18** diarrhea of unknown origin / **19** irritable bowel syndrome

Gastrointestinal Bleeding

1 Prior to attempts to localize and diagnose the source of GI bleeding, the patient must first be stabilized so that adequate blood pressure is maintained. At times blood loss is so massive and rapid that it becomes necessary to attempt to localize the bleeding source operatively without the benefit of preoperative evaluation. The evaluation presented here presumes that the patient has been stabilized.

2 The most important factor in localizing the source of GI bleeding lies in the nature of the blood loss. Hematemesis is obviously due to upper GI bleeding. Stool quality will provide the clue to further diagnostic workup. In general, the quality of the stool depends upon the volume and rapidity of bleeding and location of bleeding, as well as the length of time the blood remains in the GI tract. Blood with a long transit time through the GI tract will become black (melena) because of the breakdown of the blood by acid. Blood also acts as a cathartic, however, so that the presence of large amounts of blood will result in a decreased transit time through the GI tract, and the stool may be maroon (hematochezia) rather than black. Hematemesis and melena usually result from upper GI bleeding. Hematochezia can be due to either upper or lower GI bleeding. Bright red rectal blood (BRBPR) is usually due to lower GI bleeding. Anatomically, the ligament of Treitz is considered to be the dividing point for upper and lower GI bleeding. Black stool must be tested to document the presence of blood, because a variety of other substances may cause the stool to turn black. Ingested bismuth, charcoal, spinach, and, most commonly, iron will result in black stools in the absence of blood. Other history, such as the use of aspirin or nonsteroidal anti-inflammatory agents, gives clues to peptic ulcer disease. The presence of stigmata of liver disease such as spider angiomata, palmar erythema, and ascites indicates the likelihood of variceal bleeding.

3 Upper GI endoscopy is the most sensitive and specific test for diagnosing the source of upper GI bleeding. Endoscopy detects a definitive or a potential bleeding site only 80 per cent of the time. Detection is increased when the bleeding is more severe. In the presence of rapid bleeding such that visualization by endoscopy is impossible, angiography may help to localize the bleeding source.

4 The most common sources of upper GI bleeding are peptic ulcer, esophageal varices, and acute mucosal lesions such as acute esophagitis, gastritis, or Mallory-Weiss tears. Gastroesophageal (GE) reflux is not an endoscopic diagnosis, but the diagnosis can be suspected by the mucosal changes seen in the lower esophagus upon endoscopy.

5 Melena usually arises from upper GI bleeding. An upper endoscopy is the first test that should be performed in evaluating the source of melena. Hematochezia (maroon stool) can result from either upper or lower GI bleeding. In order for hematochezia to occur, the upper GI bleed must be of a volume of at least 1000 ml. Bleeding lesions lower in the GI tract may present as hematochezia at lower volumes of blood loss.

6 Colonoscopic examination may be difficult in the presence of active bleeding. If the patient is not actively bleeding and is stable for 48 hours, barium enema can be performed alternatively, but colonoscopy is a more sensitive and specific test. Barium enema examination is not useful in the face of active bleeding, because the barium will interfere with angiography and will also preclude subsequent endoscopic visualization of the colon.

7 Angiodysplasia, or vascular malformations, have been found to be a more common cause of lower GI bleeding than was previously suspected. In the past, bleeding from the right side of the colon was attributed to diverticula, if diverticula were demonstrated on barium enema. With the advancement of endoscopic techniques, it is now known that vascular malformations are more commonly the site of active bleeding. This observation underscores the need to confirm that a lesion is actually the site of hemorrhage by observing active bleeding with endoscopy or arteriography.

8 Primary amyloidosis results in amyloid deposition in the connective tissue and in the walls of blood vessels. GI bleeding is common and can be severe.

9 Small bowel enteroclysis is a study in which barium and air are placed in the small bowel and viewed radiographically. The procedure is similar to the air-contrast barium enema. This technique enables graphic visualization of mucosal lesions in the small bowel. This technique does not enable visualization of angioma or angiodysplasia, which can be detected only by endoscopic examination.

10 If bleeding continues but the lesion has not been directly visualized or localized by endoscopic examination, an angiogram may become necessary. An angiogram will not identify the type of lesion but will help to localize the site of the bleeding lesion. If available, a radioisotope-tagged erythrocyte study can be used prior to the more invasive angiogram.

11 Gastric mucosa, present in Meckel's diverticula 15 to 30 per cent of the time, can be detected with a technetium isotopic scan. However, only half of all bleeding Meckel's diverticula are found to contain gastric mucosa. Acid-secreting gastric mucosa–lined Meckel's diverticula may also cause adjacent ileal mucosal ulceration and bleeding. In a young patient with GI bleeding, a Meckel's scan should probably be performed prior to angiography, because 50 per cent of cases of lower GI bleeding are due to Meckel's diverticula in children, and many cases have been reported in young adults. Meckel's diverticulum is present in approximately 2 per cent of the population.

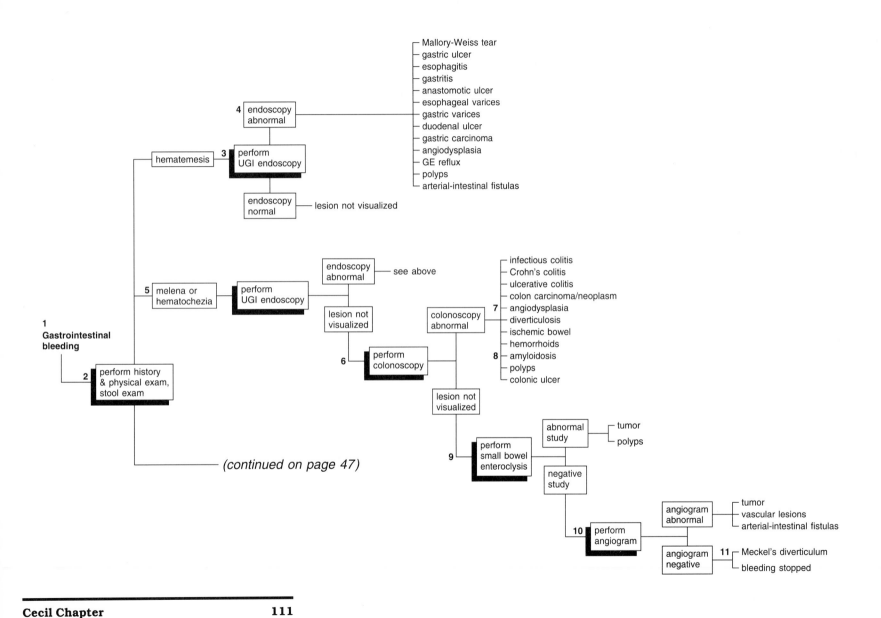

1
Gastrointestinal bleeding

2 perform history & physical exam, stool exam

hematemesis

3 perform UGI endoscopy

4 endoscopy abnormal
- Mallory-Weiss tear
- gastric ulcer
- esophagitis
- gastritis
- anastomotic ulcer
- esophageal varices
- gastric varices
- duodenal ulcer
- gastric carcinoma
- angiodysplasia
- GE reflux
- polyps
- arterial-intestinal fistulas

endoscopy normal — lesion not visualized

5 melena or hematochezia

perform UGI endoscopy

endoscopy abnormal — see above

lesion not visualized

6 perform colonoscopy

colonoscopy abnormal
7 —
- infectious colitis
- Crohn's colitis
- ulcerative colitis
- colon carcinoma/neoplasm
- angiodysplasia
- diverticulosis
- ischemic bowel
- hemorrhoids
8 — amyloidosis
- polyps
- colonic ulcer

lesion not visualized

9 perform small bowel enteroclysis

abnormal study
- tumor
- polyps

negative study

10 perform angiogram

angiogram abnormal
- tumor
- vascular lesions
- arterial-intestinal fistulas

angiogram negative
11 — Meckel's diverticulum
- bleeding stopped

(continued on page 47)

Cecil Chapter	111
Harrison Chapter	46

Gastrointestinal Bleeding
(Continued)

12 Rectal blood is usually due to lower GI bleeding, most commonly from internal hemorrhoids. A proctosigmoidoscopy is most sensitive and specific in detecting the bleeding lesion. If the lesion cannot be identified by sigmoidoscopy, a more proximal source must be investigated via colonoscopy.

13 Routine physical examination includes fecal occult blood tests to screen for occult GI blood loss. Because the cost of investigating false-positive results is considerable, the sensitivity of the screening test should be known. (Specificity should also be known to prevent patient morbidity caused by false-negative results.) A combination of screening tests, i.e., both a guaiac test and an immunologic assay, can be used to detect occult gastrointestinal bleeding with greater sensitivity and specificity prior to full GI evaluation. Additionally, some of the common sources of false-positive test results should be considered. Oral iron supplementation, which can turn stool black, is a cause of false-positive occult blood tests. Vitamin C in large doses may result in false-negative occult blood results, because it interferes with the chemical reaction in the test. In the presence of a positive stool test for occult blood, a hematocrit should also be measured. Occult blood can be measured from any source, including swallowed blood subsequent to a nosebleed. Evaluation of both the upper and lower GI tract is necessary when occult blood is discovered.

14 If diagnostic evaluation is unrevealing, stool must again be examined for the presence of occult blood within 6 months and a full endoscopic examination repeated if occult blood is present. If re-evaluation remains negative after three subsequent examinations (every 6 months over an 18-month period), it is unlikely that the lesion is significant.

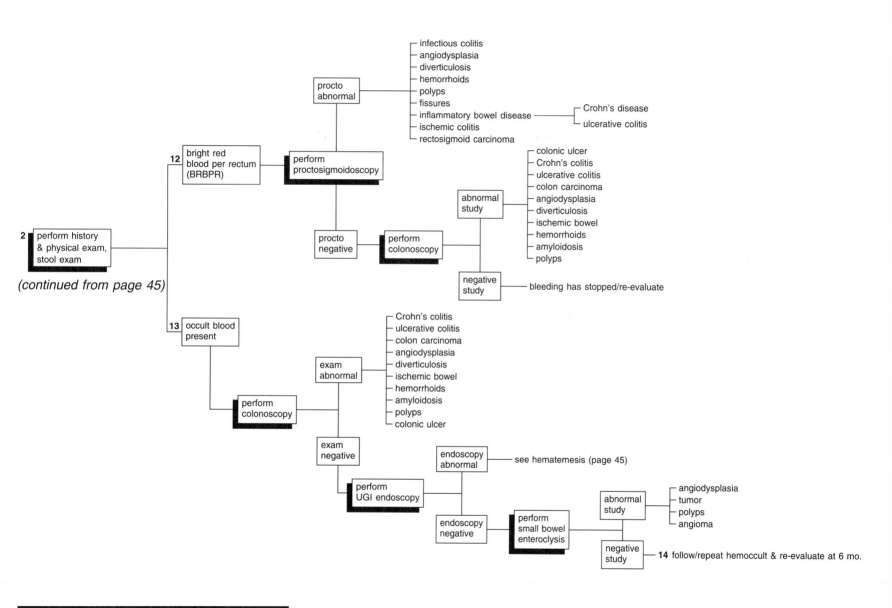

(continued from page 45)

2 perform history & physical exam, stool exam

12 bright red blood per rectum (BRBPR)

perform proctosigmoidoscopy

procto abnormal
- infectious colitis
- angiodysplasia
- diverticulosis
- hemorrhoids
- polyps
- fissures
- inflammatory bowel disease
  - Crohn's disease
  - ulcerative colitis
- ischemic colitis
- rectosigmoid carcinoma

procto negative

perform colonoscopy

abnormal study
- colonic ulcer
- Crohn's colitis
- ulcerative colitis
- colon carcinoma
- angiodysplasia
- diverticulosis
- ischemic bowel
- hemorrhoids
- amyloidosis
- polyps

negative study
- bleeding has stopped/re-evaluate

13 occult blood present

perform colonoscopy

exam abnormal
- Crohn's colitis
- ulcerative colitis
- colon carcinoma
- angiodysplasia
- diverticulosis
- ischemic bowel
- hemorrhoids
- amyloidosis
- polyps
- colonic ulcer

exam negative

perform UGI endoscopy

endoscopy abnormal
- see hematemesis (page 45)

endoscopy negative

perform small bowel enteroclysis

abnormal study
- angiodysplasia
- tumor
- polyps
- angioma

negative study
- **14** follow/repeat hemoccult & re-evaluate at 6 mo.

Dysphagia

1 Dysphagia is defined as difficulty with swallowing and refers specifically to the difficulty of passing solids or liquids from the mouth to the stomach. History and physical examination are the initial steps in the diagnosis of dysphagia. Swallowing difficulty that progresses from solids to liquids over time indicates the presence of a progressive lesion such as carcinoma. If swallowing difficulty remains fixed with a certain-sized quantity of food, a stationary obstruction such as stricture is suspected. If dysphagia occurs with both solids and liquids, a motility disorder is the likely source of the dysphagia. The patient may be able to localize the site of obstructive lesions by indicating where he or she experiences the sensation of the food being stuck. Dysphagia associated with hiccups suggests distal esophageal lesions.

2 Pain associated with swallowing is referred to as odynophagia and may or may not accompany dysphagia. Painful oral lesions can account for odynophagia and can be seen with a variety of oral infections and malignancy. With odynophagia alone, swallowing may be difficult secondary to pain, but the material can be passed easily from the oropharynx to the stomach once swallowing has occurred. The most common causes of odynophagia are herpes simplex and *Candida* stomatitis or esophagitis. Abscesses and oral carcinomas are very rare causes of odynophagia.

3 Endoscopic evaluation with biopsy is the most specific test in establishing the presence of anatomic lesions and documenting complications due to motility disorders. Endoscopy is the best test for the evaluation of dysphagia, but barium swallow is still often used as the initial test. The barium swallow is a radiographic evaluation of the pharynx and esophagus as the patient swallows a bolus of contrast medium. Cineradiography is usually performed simultaneously. Because dysphagia can be present with solids and absent with liquids, a normal study with liquid barium cannot be taken as conclusive evidence of absence of disease. Often, symptoms of solid dysphagia can be reproduced with the use of a barium capsule or marshmallow.

4 The Plummer-Vinson syndrome (also known as Paterson-Kelly syndrome and siderophagic dysphagia) is an extremely rare condition in which dysphagia is associated with hypochromic anemia. The condition is seen in women. Dysphagia is due to an esophageal web and is thought to be a premalignant condition ultimately resulting in pharyngeal carcinoma.

5 External compression of the esophagus is a possible but extremely rare cause of dysphagia. Of interest is the anomalous right subclavian artery. The right subclavian artery usually arises from the brachiocephalic artery and passes anterior to the trachea. In approximately 1 per cent of the population, the right subclavian artery arises as the last branch of the aortic arch and passes from left to right behind the esophagus and trachea. The compression of the esophagus between the anomalous artery and the semirigid trachea can result in dysphagia.

6 Esophageal stricture is likely with a history of reflux esophagitis. Rare skin disorders such as cicatricial pemphigoid and epidermolysis bullosa involve the esophagus as well, resulting in stricture.

7 Zenker's diverticulum is an outpouching of the esophagus above the upper esophageal sphincter. Patients may complain of regurgitation of food into the mouth, halitosis, and a mass in the neck. Although extremely rare, the pouch may enlarge to such a degree that compression on the adjacent esophagus is the primary cause of dysphagia.

8 Scleroderma causes a decreased esophageal peristalsis, but this dysmotility is rarely the source of dysphagia associated with scleroderma. Dysphagia in scleroderma is usually the result of the formation of inflammatory strictures from gastroesophageal reflux.

9 Motor abnormalities will be suspected by the appearance of the esophagus upon endoscopic examination, or by cineradiography or fluoroscopy. Manometric measurements are more useful in characterizing the exact nature of the motility disorder. Manometry measures intraesophageal pressures at several points simultaneously. A long catheter with pressure-sensitive transducers at various intervals is introduced into the esophageal lumen and used to measure and record the intraluminal pressure. Dysmotility can be detected by measuring muscular activity in terms of amplitude, velocity, and duration of waves. Although disorders such as scleroderma and gastroesophageal reflux will be detected by esophagoscopy, manometry is often performed subsequently in order to characterize and confirm the nature of esophageal dysmotility.

10 Diffuse esophageal spasm is the synchronous contraction of the esophagus rather than orderly peristalsis. Manometry is confirmatory.

11 Achalasia is a disorder in which the lower esophageal sphincter fails to relax, which results in the dilation of the upper esophagus. Manometry will confirm suspected achalasia by demonstrating failure of the lower esophageal sphincter to relax and reduced or absent peristalsis in the distal half of the esophagus.

12 Globus hystericus is the sensation of a lump in the throat. The disorder conveys a sense of dysphagia, but swallowing is normal. The sensation is due to the tightening of the upper esophageal sphincter. The "lump" disappears transiently when the patient swallows. The condition is benign.

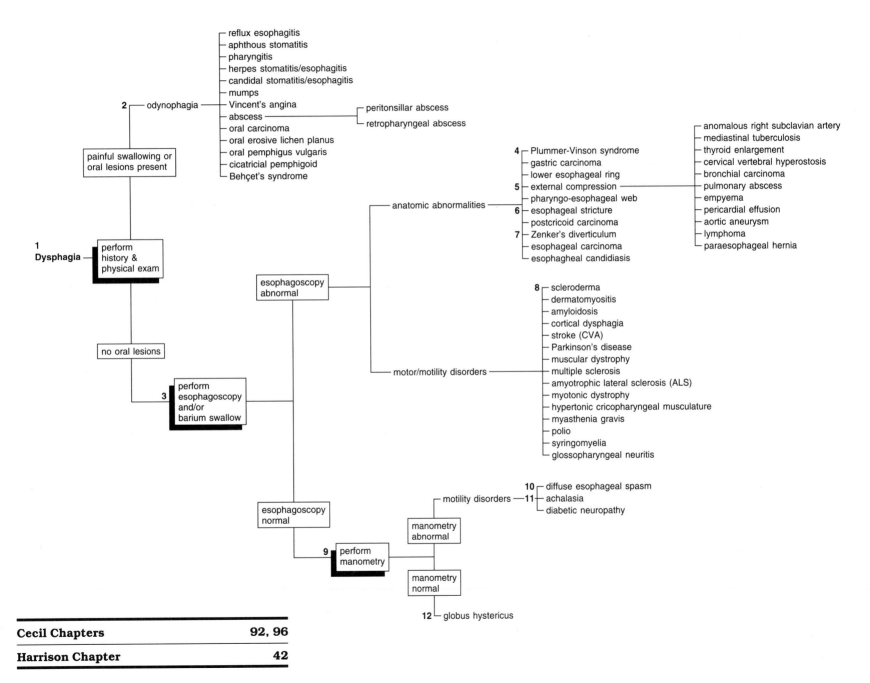

1 **Dysphagia**

2 — odynophagia
- reflux esophagitis
- aphthous stomatitis
- pharyngitis
- herpes stomatitis/esophagitis
- candidal stomatitis/esophagitis
- mumps
- Vincent's angina
- abscess
  - peritonsillar abscess
  - retropharyngeal abscess
- oral carcinoma
- oral erosive lichen planus
- oral pemphigus vulgaris
- cicatricial pemphigoid
- Behçet's syndrome

painful swallowing or oral lesions present

perform history & physical exam

no oral lesions

3 perform esophagoscopy and/or barium swallow

esophagoscopy abnormal

anatomic abnormalities
- **4** Plummer-Vinson syndrome
- gastric carcinoma
- lower esophageal ring
- **5** external compression
  - anomalous right subclavian artery
  - mediastinal tuberculosis
  - thyroid enlargement
  - cervical vertebral hyperostosis
  - bronchial carcinoma
  - pulmonary abscess
  - empyema
  - pericardial effusion
  - aortic aneurysm
  - lymphoma
  - paraesophageal hernia
- pharyngo-esophageal web
- **6** esophageal stricture
- postcricoid carcinoma
- **7** Zenker's diverticulum
- esophageal carcinoma
- esophagheal candidiasis

motor/motility disorders
- **8** scleroderma
- dermatomyositis
- amyloidosis
- cortical dysphagia
- stroke (CVA)
- Parkinson's disease
- muscular dystrophy
- multiple sclerosis
- amyotrophic lateral sclerosis (ALS)
- myotonic dystrophy
- hypertonic cricopharyngeal musculature
- myasthenia gravis
- polio
- syringomyelia
- glossopharyngeal neuritis

esophagoscopy normal

9 perform manometry

manometry abnormal

motility disorders
- **10** diffuse esophageal spasm
- **11** achalasia
- diabetic neuropathy

manometry normal

12 globus hystericus

Cecil Chapters	92, 96
Harrison Chapter	42

Abdominal Pain

1 Abdominal pain may result from intra-abdominal inflammation or abdominal wall disorders or may be pain referred from areas outside of the abdomen. Common sources of pain referred to the abdomen include retroperitoneal processes, such as renal colic, and intra-thoracic processes, such as myocardial infarction and pneumonia. Conversely, abdominal processes can refer pain to extra-abdominal sites. The pain of acute cholecystitis can be referred to the tip of the scapula. Pain associated with acute pancreatitis can be referred to the mid-back.

2 Thorough history and physical examination are the most important "tests" in diagnosing abdominal pain. The sources and severity of abdominal pain are so diverse that no one diagnostic test is available that will allow specific and rapid identification of the cause. Perhaps the most useful historical fact in the diagnosis of abdominal pain lies in the location of the pain. Despite localization of pain to one area of the abdomen, a large amount of overlap exists, so that the diagnosis usually consists of several entities of high likelihood. In addition, the nature, quality, and radiation of the pain are important aspects of the history that will aid in the differential diagnosis. Pain associated with peritoneal inflammation is aching, steady, and made worse with movement, so that the patient tends to lie very still. Pain is usually localized directly over the inflamed area. The presence of rebound tenderness confirms peritoneal inflammation. Intermittent, colicky pain causes the patient to be restless. Colic is associated with obstruction of hollow viscera. Although colic is typically intermittent, it can be constant and of low-grade intensity. Colicky pain is crampy and poorly localized. Pelvic and rectal examination should be included in every patient with abdominal pain, because pelvic disorders can cause abdominal pain, and rectal examination will add additional information to determine the diagnosis.

3 Upper abdominal pain is usually associated with intrathoracic processes or visceral pain from organs derived from the embryonic foregut. Lesions most commonly associated with upper abdominal pain include biliary colic, hepatitis, peptic ulcer disease, pancreatitis, and splenomegaly. Extra-abdominal, specifically thoracic, sources of pain should always be considered and sought in the presence of any upper abdominal pain. Chest x ray and electrocardiogram may rule out common sources of referred thoracic pain by detecting myocardial infarction, pericarditis, pleural effusion, pulmonary infarction, and pneumonia. It is important to keep in mind that any localized pain may be neurogenic in origin, e.g., herpes zoster, when there is a paucity of other physical findings such as fever and leukocytosis to indicate an intra-abdominal process.

4 Generalized abdominal pain is most difficult to diagnose because of the lack of specificity for underlying structures. Oftentimes, abdominal pain is diffuse initially and localizes to a specific area as the disease progresses. This phenomenon is particularly common with acute appendicitis in which the patient presents with diffuse abdominal pain, tenderness, fever, nausea, and vomiting. With time, appendiceal pain localizes to the right lower quadrant. This progression of pain localization underscores the importance of frequent, repeated examinations during the course of investigation in patients presenting with generalized abdominal pain.

5 Periumbilical pain is usually from the small intestine but can also result from lesions in the cecum, right colon, and appendix. Pain from abdominal aortic aneurysm is typically in the central abdomen.

6 Lower abdominal pain may arise from processes involving the abdominal structures or pelvic structures, including the female reproductive organs and the urinary bladder. Even prostatic inflammation can present with lower abdominal pain.

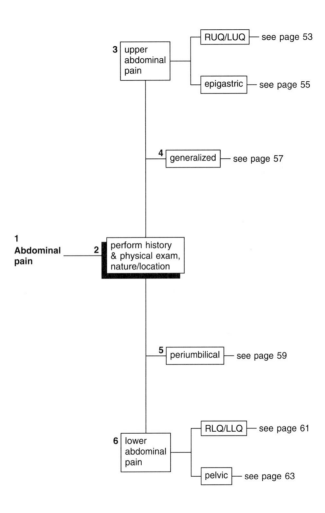

Abdominal Pain (Continued)

RIGHT UPPER QUADRANT/LEFT UPPER QUADRANT ABDOMINAL PAIN

1 Pain due to intrathoracic lesions is commonly referred to the upper abdomen. Initial examination should include routine chest film and electrocardiogram to exclude thoracic sources of abdominal pain.

2 Plain abdominal radiography is a simple, inexpensive screening test that may provide much information about the source of upper abdominal pain. Although only 20 per cent of gallstones are radiopaque, their detection on plain film is a clue to diagnosis. Renal stones may also be detected on abdominal film. Hepatomegaly may be missed on physical examination because of guarding but may be seen on abdominal film. Free air due to a perforated viscus or dilated bowel loops can also be seen on abdominal film. A plain abdominal film may reveal an enlarged spleen that could not be palpated on physical examination.

3 A common cause of acute splenic enlargement and left upper quadrant (LUQ) pain is infectious mononucleosis. Other causes of splenic enlargement associated with pain include vascular congestion, acute infections, and infiltrative diseases.

4 Elevation of serum amylase is not specific for pancreatic disease, because amylase is present in other tissues as well. An elevated serum amylase can be present with acute pancreatitis, acute cholecystitis, perforated peptic ulcer, and small bowel obstruction, especially with bowel infarction. Operable causes of abdominal pain cannot therefore be ruled out on the basis of an elevated amylase level. Serum lipase is also elevated in acute pancreatitis and may remain elevated for as long as 2 weeks after the serum amylase returns to normal. Lipase is also elevated with perforated peptic ulcer and pancreatic duct obstruction. Elevated serum transaminases are a clue to hepatic disease.

5 History and physical examination are not diagnostic for pancreatitis, but the diagnosis is less likely in the presence of right upper quadrant (RUQ) pain. Pancreatitis more commonly presents with epigastric pain with a left-sided component. In approximately 30 per cent of patients with acute pancreatitis, the serum amylase may be within normal limits early in the disease. Therefore, even with a normal amylase, pancreatitis should be considered in the appropriate clinical setting.

6 The importance of pelvic examination in all patients with abdominal pain is emphasized by gonococcal perihepatitis (Fitz-Hugh-Curtis syndrome) as a source of right upper quadrant pain. The diagnosis is suspected when adnexal tenderness is palpated on pelvic examination and is confirmed by a cervical smear revealing gonococci.

7 Hepatic inflammation and cholecystitis are the most common causes of right upper quadrant pain. If acute cholecystitis is not detected on ultrasound examination and not suspected in light of a normal amylase level, a radionuclide scan ^{99m}Tc-HIDA) can be performed. This scan is very sensitive in detecting acute cholecystitis.

8 Upper gastrointestinal disorders, although most commonly presenting as epigastric pain, can be referred to the right or left upper quadrant. An upper GI endoscopy should ultimately be performed in the evaluation of right and left upper quadrant pain if all previous tests are not diagnostic. An additional endoscopic procedure, endoscopic retrograde cholangiopancreatography (ERCP), can be performed when indicated. ERCP is not a first-line test because of cost and potential complications, but it is invaluable in further evaluation of the biliary tree and the pancreas after preliminary diagnostic testing has been performed. ERCP is especially useful when ultrasound is normal but liver function tests are abnormal or amylase levels are elevated.

9 Splenic infarction may be the source of left upper quadrant pain in patients with sickle cell disease. Right upper quadrant pain in these patients is typically due to gallstones as a result of chronic hemolysis.

10 Neurogenic causes should always be considered in the differential diagnosis of well-localized abdominal pain. Herpes zoster commonly presents with severe localized pain in the absence of skin lesions. Only as the disease progresses and typical skin lesions appear is the diagnosis suspected.

11 Although most commonly presenting as right lower quadrant pain, acute appendicitis should also be considered as a source of right upper quadrant pain. Right upper quadrant pain with appendicitis is due to a retrocecal location of the appendix. In the analysis of over 10,000 cadavers, the appendix was found in a retrocecal location in 64 per cent of the cases. The frequency of a retrocecal location of the appendix underscores the importance of rectal examination in all patients with abdominal pain.

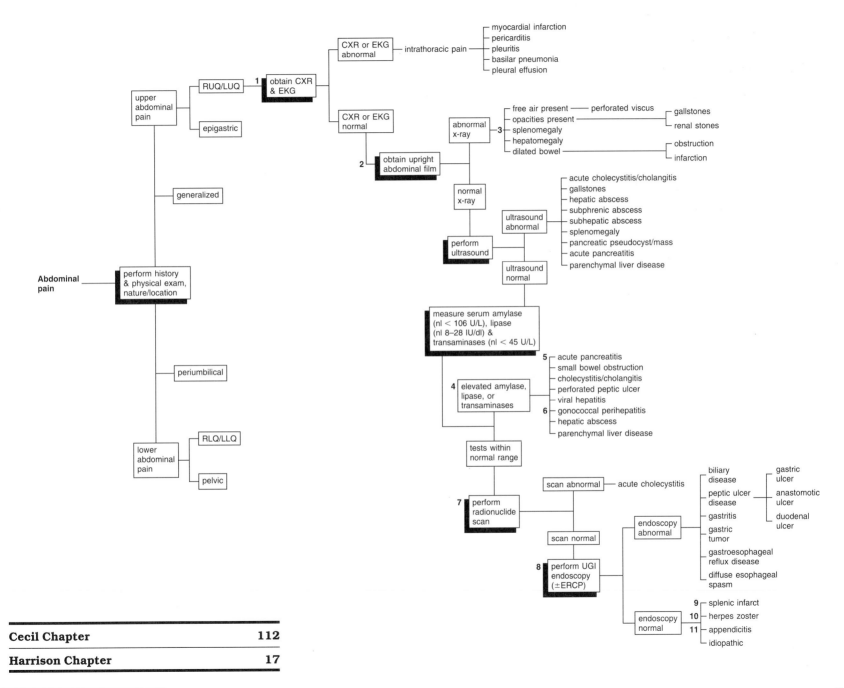

upper abdominal pain

RUQ/LUQ

1 obtain CXR & EKG

CXR or EKG abnormal — intrathoracic pain —
- myocardial infarction
- pericarditis
- pleuritis
- basilar pneumonia
- pleural effusion

epigastric

CXR or EKG normal

2 obtain upright abdominal film

abnormal x-ray
- 3 — free air present — perforated viscus
- opacities present —
  - gallstones
  - renal stones
- splenomegaly
- hepatomegaly
- dilated bowel —
  - obstruction
  - infarction

normal x-ray

perform ultrasound

ultrasound abnormal
- acute cholecystitis/cholangitis
- gallstones
- hepatic abscess
- subphrenic abscess
- subhepatic abscess
- splenomegaly
- pancreatic pseudocyst/mass
- acute pancreatitis
- parenchymal liver disease

ultrasound normal

measure serum amylase (nl < 106 U/L), lipase (nl 8–28 IU/dl) & transaminases (nl < 45 U/L)

4 elevated amylase, lipase, or transaminases
- 5 — acute pancreatitis
- small bowel obstruction
- cholecystitis/cholangitis
- perforated peptic ulcer
- viral hepatitis
- 6 — gonococcal perihepatitis
- hepatic abscess
- parenchymal liver disease

tests within normal range

7 perform radionuclide scan

scan abnormal — acute cholecystitis

scan normal

8 perform UGI endoscopy (±ERCP)

endoscopy abnormal
- biliary disease
- peptic ulcer disease —
  - gastric ulcer
  - anastomotic ulcer
  - duodenal ulcer
- gastritis
- gastric tumor
- gastroesophageal reflux disease
- diffuse esophageal spasm

endoscopy normal
- 9 — splenic infarct
- 10 — herpes zoster
- 11 — appendicitis
- idiopathic

Abdominal pain

perform history & physical exam, nature/location

generalized

periumbilical

lower abdominal pain
- RLQ/LLQ
- pelvic

Abdominal Pain (Continued)

EPIGASTRIC ABDOMINAL PAIN

1 Pain from intrathoracic processes can be referred to the upper abdomen, most commonly the mid-epigastrium. The evaluation of upper abdominal pain should always include a chest radiograph and an electrocardiogram.

2 Although an upper GI series including a barium swallow with cineradiography is a good screening test in the evaluation of epigastric pain, upper GI endoscopy is more specific. Upper endoscopy can identify mucosal evidence of gastroesophageal reflux esophagitis as well as gastritis, which will not be identified by barium studies. Conversely, diffuse esophageal spasm will not be identified with upper endoscopy, whereas cineradiography may capture and identify diffuse spasm (see No. 5).

3 Acute cholecystitis typically begins with right upper quadrant pain but may present initially as left upper quadrant or epigastric pain. As the disease progresses, the pain usually shifts to localize in the right upper quadrant. Ultrasound is the simplest and most reliable method to identify gallstones as a cause of cholecystitis, because abdominal radiographs will reveal opacities in only about 20 per cent of patients with gallstones. Radionuclide scanning is the most reliable method to confirm acute cholecystitis if the diagnosis is suspected.

4 Acute pancreatitis is a common cause of mid-epigastric pain. A left upper quadrant component to the pain is a useful clue to the diagnosis of pancreatitis.

Measurement of amylase may not always be useful in the diagnosis, because elevated amylase levels are nonspecific and may be found in association with other inflammatory conditions associated with epigastric pain. Elevated serum amylase levels may occur in association with peptic ulcer disease, acute cholecystitis, and intestinal obstruction. Conversely, amylase levels may be normal, especially in the early stages of pancreatic inflammation. In addition to abdominal processes, ruptured ectopic pregnancy and ruptured ovarian cysts can result in elevated amylase, but the pain with these conditions is more likely to be located in the lower abdomen.

5 Diffuse esophageal spasm will not be identified with upper GI endoscopy but may be suspected on barium swallow with fluoroscopy or cineradiography (see No. 2). Esophageal manometry is the best test to confirm the diagnosis of diffuse esophageal spasm.

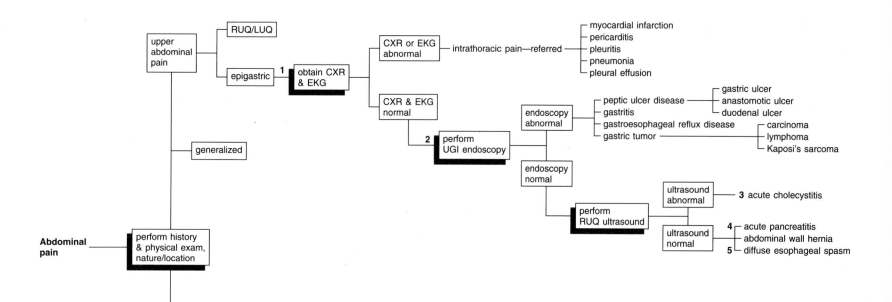

upper abdominal pain

RUQ/LUQ

epigastric **1** obtain CXR & EKG

CXR or EKG abnormal — intrathoracic pain — referred
- myocardial infarction
- pericarditis
- pleuritis
- pneumonia
- pleural effusion

CXR & EKG normal **2** perform UGI endoscopy

endoscopy abnormal
- peptic ulcer disease
  - gastric ulcer
  - anastomotic ulcer
  - duodenal ulcer
- gastritis
- gastroesophageal reflux disease
- gastric tumor
  - carcinoma
  - lymphoma
  - Kaposi's sarcoma

endoscopy normal **3** perform RUQ ultrasound

ultrasound abnormal **3** acute cholecystitis

ultrasound normal
4 acute pancreatitis
abdominal wall hernia
5 diffuse esophageal spasm

Abdominal pain perform history & physical exam, nature/location

generalized

periumbilical

lower abdominal pain

RLQ/LLQ

pelvic

Cecil Chapter	112
Harrison Chapter	17

Abdominal Pain *(Continued)*

GENERALIZED ABDOMINAL PAIN

1 Generalized abdominal pain is the most difficult to diagnose because it is so nonspecific. Determining the nature of the pain is helpful in the diagnosis by identifying the presence or absence of peritoneal inflammation (peritonitis). In general, peritoneal inflammation will localize to an area directly over the inflamed lesion, but with generalized abdominal pain, the differential diagnosis is broad.

2 Dilated loops of bowel can be seen on plain abdominal films and are a clue to the diagnosis of bowel obstruction.

3 Only 20 per cent of gallstones are radiopaque and visible on abdominal films. Renal stones can be visible on abdominal films but rarely are a cause of generalized abdominal pain.

4 Bowel ischemia and infarction can result from venous or arterial occlusion (thrombosis or embolism) and can cause generalized abdominal pain. Because vascular disease is more common in the elderly, bowel infarcts are more common in elderly patients. Despite the severity of the condition, symptoms may be mild initially, especially in elderly patients. Severe, poorly localized abdominal pain is generally the hallmark of intestinal ischemia, with pain often out of proportion to the objective findings. Initially, there may be no abdominal abnormalities upon examination. Abdominal tenderness and peritonitis may be late findings.

5 Porphyria (especially acute intermittent porphyria) and lead colic frequently cause abdominal pain due to severe hyperperistalsis. The pain may be localized to the midline or may be generalized. Lead poisoning may be associated with signs of peripheral neuropathy and a blue ''lead-line'' on the gums.

6 Metabolic disturbances such as diabetic ketoacidosis (DKA) and uremia may result in diffuse, generalized abdominal pain. It is important to remember that DKA is often the result of infection, so acute appendicitis must not be overlooked in a patient with DKA and generalized abdominal pain. If the metabolic disturbance is corrected in DKA but the pain persists, further investigation should be undertaken to determine the source of the abdominal pain.

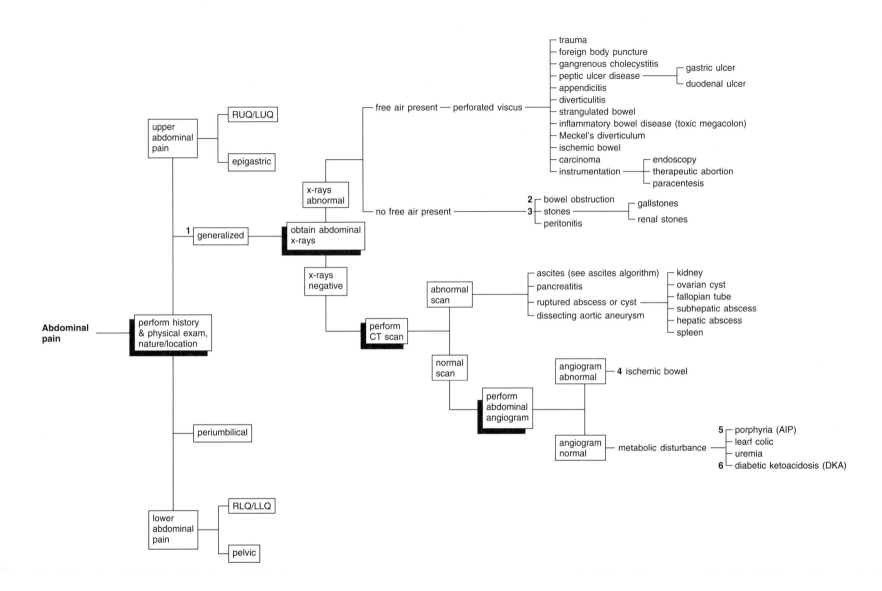

- **Abdominal pain** — perform history & physical exam, nature/location

  - upper abdominal pain
    - RUQ/LUQ
    - epigastric
  - **1** generalized — obtain abdominal x-rays
    - x-rays abnormal
      - free air present — perforated viscus
        - trauma
        - foreign body puncture
        - gangrenous cholecystitis
        - peptic ulcer disease
          - gastric ulcer
          - duodenal ulcer
        - appendicitis
        - diverticulitis
        - strangulated bowel
        - inflammatory bowel disease (toxic megacolon)
        - Meckel's diverticulum
        - ischemic bowel
        - carcinoma
        - instrumentation
          - endoscopy
          - therapeutic abortion
          - paracentesis
      - no free air present
        - **2** bowel obstruction
        - **3** stones
          - gallstones
          - renal stones
        - peritonitis
    - x-rays negative — perform CT scan
      - abnormal scan
        - ascites (see ascites algorithm)
        - pancreatitis
        - ruptured abscess or cyst
          - kidney
          - ovarian cyst
          - fallopian tube
          - subhepatic abscess
          - hepatic abscess
          - spleen
        - dissecting aortic aneurysm
      - normal scan — perform abdominal angiogram
        - angiogram abnormal — **4** ischemic bowel
        - angiogram normal — metabolic disturbance
          - **5** porphyria (AIP)
          - lead colic
          - uremia
          - **6** diabetic ketoacidosis (DKA)
  - periumbilical
  - lower abdominal pain
    - RLQ/LLQ
    - pelvic

Cecil Chapter	112
Harrison Chapter	17

Abdominal Pain (Continued)

PERIUMBILICAL ABDOMINAL PAIN

1 Plain radiographs and ultrasound examination of the abdomen are the simplest and most effective screening tests in investigating the source of periumbilical abdominal pain.

2 Evidence of dilated bowel loops and the presence of "fingerprinting" of the bowel mucosa on radiographs are indicative of obstruction and edema of the bowel. Obstruction can be secondary to a variety of lesions, including volvulus, adhesions, intrinsic or extrinsic tumor, or intussusception. Pain referred to the periumbilical area can arise from the jejunum, ileum, cecum, or right colon.

3 Vascular occlusion of the superior mesenteric artery is a catastrophic event caused by the extensive contribution of this artery to the blood supply of both the large and small bowel. Subsequent infarction of bowel may occur in the transverse colon, jejunum, cecum, and ileum, all of which will cause periumbilical pain.

4 Acute appendicitis characteristically begins as generalized or periumbilical abdominal pain and later localizes to the right lower quadrant.

5 The pain associated with metabolic diseases such as acute intermittent porphyria (AIP) and lead colic is due to the induction of hyperperistalsis. The associated pain can be diffuse or localized to the periumbilical area.

6 Meckel's diverticulum is a congenital abnormality of the gut that occurs in approximately 2 per cent of the population. The diverticulum is located 30 to 90 cm proximal to the iliocecal sphincter and therefore is not visualized with an enema contrast study. Gastric mucosa, which is present in the lumen of approximately 15 to 30 per cent of Meckel's diverticula, can be detected by a technetium isotope scan. Most symptomatic Meckel's diverticula contain gastric mucosa, and a Meckel's scan can be useful when enema contrast studies are negative.

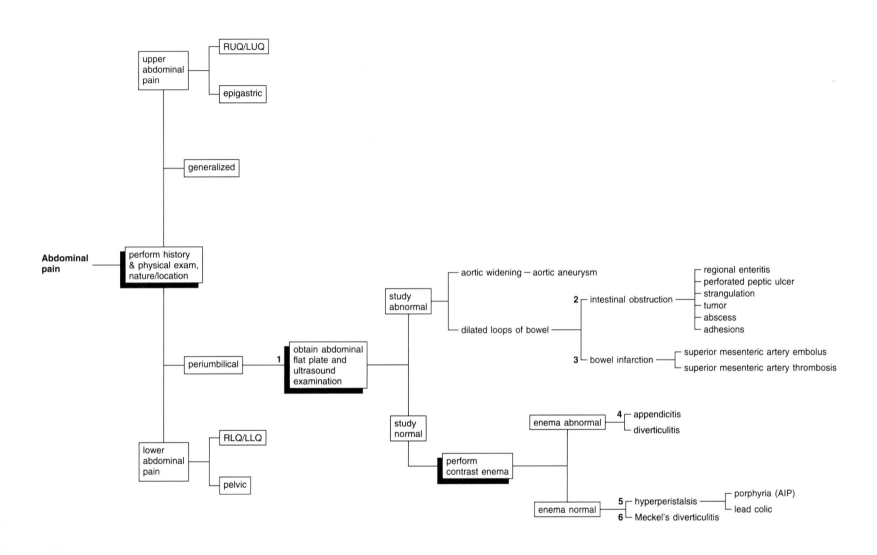

Abdominal
pain

upper
abdominal
pain

RUQ/LUQ

epigastric

generalized

perform history
& physical exam,
nature/location

periumbilical

1 obtain abdominal
flat plate and
ultrasound
examination

lower
abdominal
pain

RLQ/LLQ

pelvic

study
abnormal

aortic widening − aortic aneurysm

dilated loops of bowel

2 intestinal obstruction

regional enteritis
perforated peptic ulcer
strangulation
tumor
abscess
adhesions

3 bowel infarction

superior mesenteric artery embolus
superior mesenteric artery thrombosis

study
normal

perform
contrast enema

enema abnormal

4 appendicitis
diverticulitis

enema normal

5 hyperperistalsis
6 Meckel's diverticulitis

porphyria (AIP)
lead colic

Cecil Chapter   112

Harrison Chapter   17

Abdominal Pain (Continued)

RIGHT LOWER QUADRANT/LEFT LOWER QUADRANT ABDOMINAL PAIN

1 Pelvic and rectal examination is mandatory in the evaluation of lower quadrant pain. Inflammation of the ovaries or fallopian tubes can be suspected on pelvic examination. Ruptured ectopic pregnancy should be considered in women with right lower quadrant (RLQ) or left lower quadrant (LLQ) pain regardless of menstrual history.

2 The most common cause of right lower quadrant pain is acute appendicitis.

3 Diverticulitis is the most common cause of left lower quadrant pain. Often a mass can be palpated in the left lower quadrant in the presence of diverticulitis. Complications include abscess formation, perforation, and fistula formation. Diagnosis can be confirmed on sigmoidoscopy with minimal preparation. If diverticulitis is strongly suspected, barium enema is not used for fear of increasing intraluminal pressure and causing perforation.

4 Regional enteritis, also known as Crohn's disease, commonly involves the distal ileum. Although pain may be referred to the periumbilical region, the right lower quadrant is most often tender and painful, and, at times, a mass can even be palpated in the right lower quadrant. The diagnosis of Crohn's ileitis can be suspected on the clinical pattern of recurrent abdominal pain and right lower quadrant tenderness in which dilated loops of small bowel can be demonstrated on plain films of the abdomen, suggesting partial obstruction. The diagnosis can be confirmed with upper and lower GI barium studies.

5 Inguinal hernia with entrapment and strangulation is a rare cause of left lower quadrant pain. Complete physical examination is adequate to make the diagnosis.

6 Herpes zoster can cause severe localized abdominal pain in the absence of skin lesions. The diagnosis becomes apparent as typical skin lesions develop within days of the first occurrence of the pain.

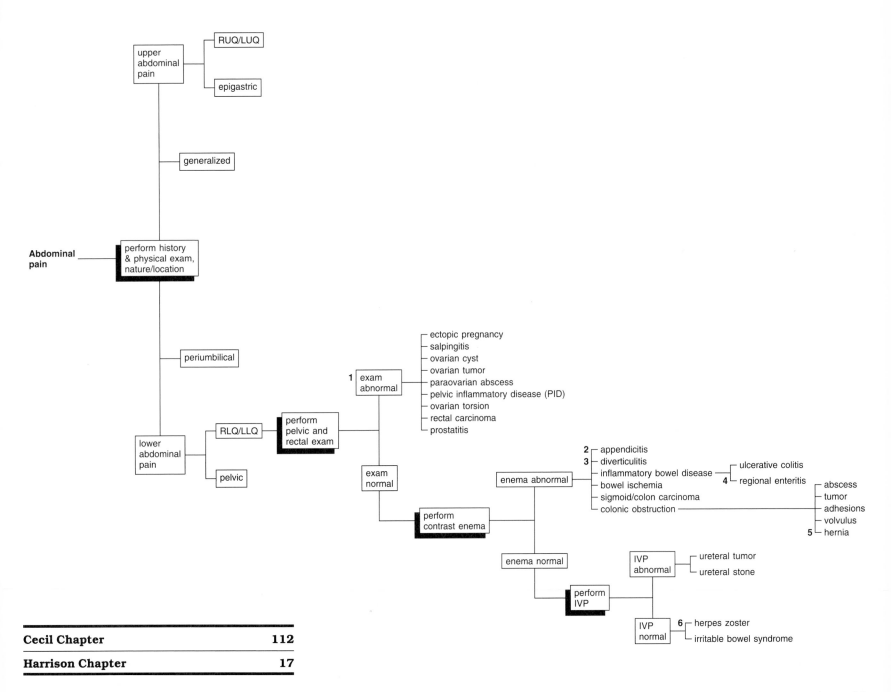

upper abdominal pain
- RUQ/LUQ
- epigastric

generalized

Abdominal pain — perform history & physical exam, nature/location

periumbilical

lower abdominal pain
- RLQ/LLQ — perform pelvic and rectal exam
- pelvic

1 exam abnormal
- ectopic pregnancy
- salpingitis
- ovarian cyst
- ovarian tumor
- paraovarian abscess
- pelvic inflammatory disease (PID)
- ovarian torsion
- rectal carcinoma
- prostatitis

exam normal — perform contrast enema

enema abnormal
- **2** appendicitis
- **3** diverticulitis
- inflammatory bowel disease
  - ulcerative colitis
  - **4** regional enteritis
- bowel ischemia
- sigmoid/colon carcinoma
- colonic obstruction
  - abscess
  - tumor
  - adhesions
  - volvulus
  - **5** hernia

enema normal — perform IVP

IVP abnormal
- ureteral tumor
- ureteral stone

IVP normal
- **6** herpes zoster
- irritable bowel syndrome

Abdominal Pain *(Continued)*

PELVIC PAIN

1 The hypogastrium, or suprapubic region, is the area in which pain localizes from lesions in the pelvis or hindgut structures. Thorough physical examination, including pelvic examination in females and rectal examination in both sexes, will provide the most information regarding the source of the pain. However, clinical examination by itself results in significant error in the evaluation of pelvic pain. If pelvic pathology remains highly likely despite a normal pelvic examination, careful consideration must be given to further diagnostic intervention such as laparoscopy. Laparoscopy can also be used to establish a definite diagnosis when the pelvic examination is abnormal but the diagnosis is not readily apparent. Distention of the urinary bladder is the most common cause of suprapubic pain and can be suspected upon percussion of the lower abdomen.

2 Prostatitis, proctitis, acute cervicitis, and rectal carcinoma can produce both pelvic and posterior midsacral pain.

3 Although innervation of the ovaries and fallopian tubes is unilateral, pain from these structures can be referred to the hypogastrium. Bilateral inflammation of the ovaries or fallopian tubes is usually experienced as midline pain. Examples include pelvic inflammatory disease and acute salpingitis. Pelvic ultrasound may be a useful adjunctive test.

4 If distention of the urinary bladder is suspected on abdominal percussion, catheterization of the bladder will be both diagnostic and curative.

5 Fiberoptic sigmoidoscopy is the most sensitive and specific test available to diagnose the various sigmoid colon lesions that give rise to pelvic pain. Diverticulitis is a focal inflammation of a colonic diverticulum that commonly occurs in the sigmoid colon. The pain of diverticulitis is more commonly localized to the left lower quadrant but can occur in the hypogastrium.

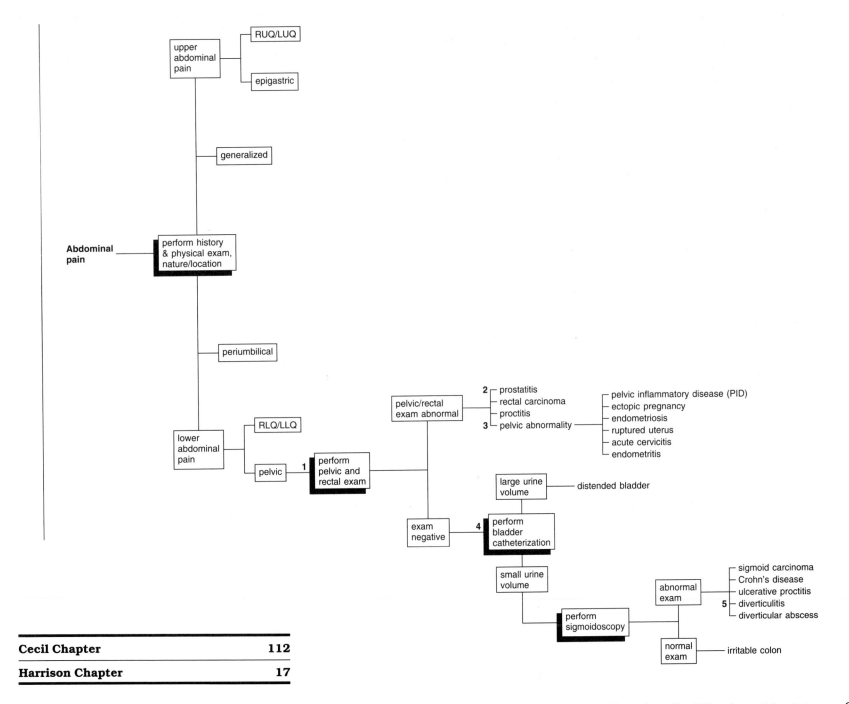

upper abdominal pain
- RUQ/LUQ
- epigastric

generalized

Abdominal pain — perform history & physical exam, nature/location

periumbilical

lower abdominal pain
- RLQ/LLQ
- pelvic — **1** perform pelvic and rectal exam

pelvic/rectal exam abnormal
- **2** prostatitis
- rectal carcinoma
- proctitis
- **3** pelvic abnormality
  - pelvic inflammatory disease (PID)
  - ectopic pregnancy
  - endometriosis
  - ruptured uterus
  - acute cervicitis
  - endometritis

exam negative — **4** perform bladder catheterization

large urine volume — distended bladder

small urine volume — perform sigmoidoscopy

abnormal exam
- sigmoid carcinoma
- Crohn's disease
- ulcerative proctitis
- **5** diverticulitis
- diverticular abscess

normal exam — irritable colon

Jaundice/Hyperbilirubinemia

1 Jaundice refers to the yellow coloration of the skin and sclerae due to deposition of bile pigments. Beta-carotene and quinacrine are two substances that can color the skin yellow and may be mistaken for jaundice. These substances, however, do not color the sclerae. Because unconjugated bilirubin stains fat heavily, jaundice due primarily to unconjugated bilirubin results in yellow staining in areas where fat accumulates. Conjugated bilirubin concentrates more easily in elastic tissues. Jaundice due primarily to conjugated bilirubin is more evident in the skin, mucous membranes, and sclerae. In general, when the total bilirubin level is greater than 2 mg/dl, jaundice will be clinically evident. However, unless the patient is observed in bright daylight, jaundice may not be detected unless the total bilirubin level is greater than 4 mg/dl.

2 The unconjugated or indirect bilirubin level rises when there is excess bilirubin production or a defect in bilirubin conjugation. Hemolytic anemia is the most common source of increased bilirubin production. In general, the liver is able to accommodate the excess bilirubin by increasing the rate of conjugation to six times its normal rate. Therefore, hemolysis alone causes only a minimal increase in the total bilirubin level, to 2 to 3 mg/dl. If the bilirubin level rises to 4 to 5 mg/dl, hemolysis is most likely accompanied by hepatocellular dysfunction. It is important to remember that the entire clinical picture must be taken into account when evaluating hyperbilirubinemia. If obstructive jaundice occurs in the presence of hemolytic disease, marked elevations of both conjugated and unconjugated bilirubin would occur. For example, gallstones can complicate chronic hemolytic diseases such as sickle cell anemia and result in a mixed hyperbilirubinemia. Direct bilirubin is water-soluble, so any excess in the serum will be excreted in the urine. Absent bilirubinuria in a jaundiced patient indicates unconjugated bilirubinemia.

3 Gilbert's disease is an autosomal dominant disorder in which the transport of free bilirubin from the blood to the site of conjugation is impaired. The intermittent episodes of jaundice (unconjugated hyperbilirubinemia) that occur in Gilbert's disease may be mistaken for viral hepatitis. The total serum bilirubin usually remains below 3 mg/dl. Increases in bilirubin may occur with concurrent illness. Gilbert's disease is not associated with any other liver abnormality.

4 Drugs such as propranolol, rifampin, and probenecid can interfere with the microsomal conjugation of bilirubin and result in an unconjugated hyperbilirubinemia.

5 Measurement of the alkaline phosphatase level (alk phos) is most useful in distinguishing whether the source of jaundice is an obstructive process (cholestatic jaundice) or acute hepatocellular damage. Marked elevation of alkaline phosphatase (greater than three times normal) suggests extrahepatic obstruction. Lesser elevations of alkaline phosphatase may accompany hepatocellular disease without biliary obstruction. Although the source of alkaline phosphatase is mainly the cells that line the biliary tree, alkaline phosphatase may also be released from bone osteoblasts, the small intestine, and the placenta. In the presence of jaundice and suspected liver disease, the source of alkaline phosphatase is fairly clear.

6 Cholestasis can be due to "intrahepatic" obstruction in which there is an interference with the flow or transport of bile in the canalicular system or to "extrahepatic" obstruction when cholestasis is caused by obstruction of the larger bile ducts and channels. Clues to extrahepatic obstruction include hepatomegaly with right upper quadrant tenderness, as well as fever and leukocytosis if secondary infection occurs. Intrahepatic cholestasis is rarely accompanied by hepatomegaly or tenderness.

7 Noninvasive tests such as ultrasonography or computed tomography (CT) can be used to determine the presence of dilation of the intra- or extrahepatic biliary system. Increased biliary pressure due to obstruction is implied if dilation is present. In addition to demonstrating biliary dilation, these tests may demonstrate the presence of a stone or a mass. If biliary dilation is demonstrated, direct ductal visualization is indicated to localize the site of obstruction. Investigation may include the use of special tests such as percutaneous transhepatic cholangiography or endoscopic retrograde cholangiopancreatography. If ultrasonography is negative, however, further invasive testing may still be indicated if extrahepatic obstruction is highly suspected, because ultrasonography is only 85 per cent sensitive. False-negative ultrasound examination may occur in the presence of gallstones, which may cause only partial or intermittent biliary obstruction so that bile ducts are not significantly dilated. Sclerosing cholangitis usually causes stricture and beading of the intrahepatic ducts as well as narrowing of the extrahepatic biliary ductal system. This disorder is another common source of false-negative ultrasound examinations.

8 Drugs are a common cause of intrahepatic cholestatic jaundice, presumably on the basis of interference with conjugated bilirubin transport.

9 Multifocal deposits of metastatic tumor or granulomas can result in intrahepatic cholestasis. CT scan or magnetic resonance imaging (MRI) is useful in diagnosing tumor and granuloma and in addition may reveal the presence of infiltrative diseases such as amyloid or lymphoma that also cause intrahepatic cholestasis. Liver biopsy is the definitive test to diagnose these disorders.

10 If a sudden fall in blood pressure is superimposed on chronic passive liver congestion, hepatic necrosis and jaundice can occur in the post-shock period.

11 Primary biliary cirrhosis is a disease of unknown etiology in which there is a progressive destruction of the small intrahepatic biliary ducts. The disorder is seen primarily in middle-aged women. Bile duct injury is thought to be due to an immunologically mediated mechanism. The presence of antimitochondrial antibody can be found in 85 to 95 per cent of patients with this disorder.

12 Although the alkaline phosphatase level is the most useful test to determine the cause of the jaundice, in reality liver transaminases are measured simultaneously. The overall pattern of these tests helps determine the diagnosis. Extremely high (>500 U/L) transaminase levels are associated with acute cellular necrosis of the liver.

13 Viral serologies are the most useful specific tests that aid in the diagnosis of hepatitis A and hepatitis B. The finding of IgM anti–hepatitis A virus (HAV) in the presence of acute disease is presumptive evidence for acute viral hepatitis A, whereas IgG anti-HAV reflects previous infection. The presence of IgM anti-HBc or HB_xAg in association with symptoms of acute hepatitis is diagnostic of acute hepatitis B. The pattern of liver function test abnormalities in viral hepatitis is distinctive. Serum transaminases rise first, with serum glutamate pyruvate transaminase (SGPT) elevated to a greater extent than the serum glutamic-oxaloacetic transaminase (SGOT). Transaminitis is followed shortly by elevated

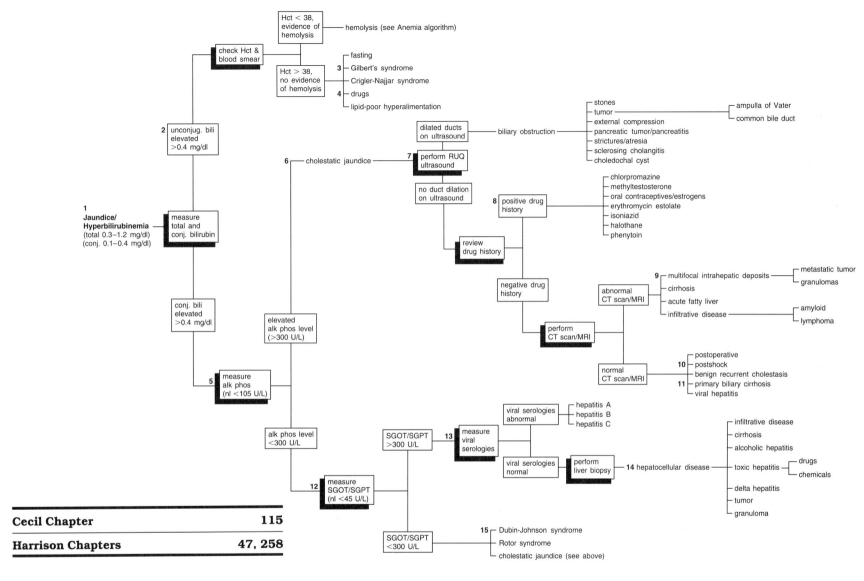

check Hct & blood smear

Hct < 38, evidence of hemolysis —— hemolysis (see Anemia algorithm)

Hct > 38, no evidence of hemolysis

—— fasting
3 Gilbert's syndrome
—— Crigler-Najjar syndrome
4 drugs
—— lipid-poor hyperalimentation

2 unconjug. bili elevated >0.4 mg/dl

1
Jaundice/
Hyperbilirubinemia
(total 0.3–1.2 mg/dl)
(conj. 0.1–0.4 mg/dl)

measure total and conj. bilirubin

conj. bili elevated >0.4 mg/dl

5 measure alk phos (nl <105 U/L)

6 cholestatic jaundice —— **7** perform RUQ ultrasound

dilated ducts on ultrasound —— biliary obstruction
—— stones
—— tumor —— ampulla of Vater
—— common bile duct
—— external compression
—— pancreatic tumor/pancreatitis
—— strictures/atresia
—— sclerosing cholangitis
—— choledochal cyst

no duct dilation on ultrasound

8 positive drug history
—— chlorpromazine
—— methyltestosterone
—— oral contraceptives/estrogens
—— erythromycin estolate
—— isoniazid
—— halothane
—— phenytoin

review drug history

negative drug history

perform CT scan/MRI

abnormal CT scan/MRI
9 multifocal intrahepatic deposits —— metastatic tumor
—— granulomas
—— cirrhosis
—— acute fatty liver
—— infiltrative disease —— amyloid
—— lymphoma

normal CT scan/MRI
10 postoperative
—— postshock
—— benign recurrent cholestasis
11 primary biliary cirrhosis
—— viral hepatitis

elevated alk phos level (>300 U/L)

alk phos level <300 U/L

12 measure SGOT/SGPT (nl <45 U/L)

SGOT/SGPT >300 U/L

13 measure viral serologies

viral serologies abnormal
—— hepatitis A
—— hepatitis B
—— hepatitis C

viral serologies normal —— perform liver biopsy —— **14** hepatocellular disease
—— infiltrative disease
—— cirrhosis
—— alcoholic hepatitis
—— toxic hepatitis —— drugs
—— chemicals
—— delta hepatitis
—— tumor
—— granuloma

SGOT/SGPT <300 U/L
15 Dubin-Johnson syndrome
—— Rotor syndrome
—— cholestatic jaundice (see above)

Cecil Chapter	115
Harrison Chapters	**47, 258**

conjugated bilirubin and clinical jaundice, as well as a moderate increase in the serum alkaline phosphatase level.

14 Intrahepatic cholestasis and jaundice may accompany severe hepatocellular disease owing to the acute damage to the hepatocyte and impairment of the mechanical or metabolic transport of conjugated bilirubin to the biliary canaliculi. Hepatocellular damage occurs most frequently with viral hepatitis but can accompany a variety of infections or ethanol intoxication. Toxins such as carbon tetrachloride and phosphorus can also result in hepatocellular disease.

15 Dubin-Johnson syndrome and Rotor's syndrome are both benign, autosomal recessively inherited diseases that can manifest with jaundice clinically. A conjugated hyperbilirubinemia exists, but other liver function tests, including serum transaminases and alkaline phosphatase, are normal. The two syndromes are rare and can be distinguished from each other on the basis of liver biopsy.

Hepatomegaly

1 The liver edge may be palpable without the presence of true hepatic enlargement. Therefore, the liver span must be estimated on physical examination by percussion. The normal liver span is 6 to 12 cm in the midclavicular line and 4 to 8 cm in the midsternal line. Apparent hepatomegaly on examination can be confirmed by plain abdominal radiography, ultrasonography, liver/spleen scan, or CT scan. Although ultrasound is probably the simplest and most cost-effective test to determine liver size, a CT scan will also provide detailed information with respect to parenchymal consistency and focal defects in addition to size.

2 Acute viral hepatitis can be suspected on the basis of the pattern of liver function abnormalities in addition to the clinical symptoms, including tender hepatomegaly. In acute viral hepatitis, the transaminases rise rapidly to levels greater than 300 U/L, followed by a lesser rise in alkaline phosphatase (to levels less than three times normal) and bilirubin levels. Viral serologies are the most useful specific tests that aid in the diagnosis of hepatitis A, B, C, and D, as well as hepatitis due to cytomegalovirus (CMV) and Epstein-Barr virus (EBV). Tests for viral hepatitis include IgM anti-HAV, HBsAg, anti-HBc, IgM anti-HBc, anti–hepatitis C virus (HCV), anti–hepatitis D virus (HDV), CMV, and EBV serologic assays. The current test system appears to detect only chronic (not acute) hepatitis C, and the length of time from infection to antibody development is unknown. The major cause of hepatitis C is transmission via blood and blood products. The incubation period ranges from 2 to 20 weeks, with an average of 8 weeks.

3 Chronic active hepatitis (CAH) can progress to cirrhosis and liver failure. Chronic hepatitis B infection (with HBsAg positivity) is associated with chronic active hepatitis in approximately 20 per cent of cases and is presumably the cause of the disease. Viral hepatitis caused by non-A non-B can also cause chronic active hepatitis (see No. 12).

4 Chronic persistent hepatitis (CPH) is a nonprogressive inflammatory liver disease. Like CAH, serologies positive for HBsAg are found in approximately 20 to 30 per cent of cases of CPH. Unlike CAH, CPH rarely progresses to liver failure. Abnormalities suggestive of CPH include transaminase levels less than 100 U/L and positive HBsAg, but liver biopsy is confirmatory. Liver biopsy is necessary to distinguish between CAH and CPH.

5 Central venous pressure can be estimated via observation of the jugular venous pressure (JVP) on physical examination. Vascular congestion can cause mild transaminitis and hepatomegaly.

6 Both acute and chronic congestive heart failure may result in elevated serum transaminases and an enlarged, tender liver. If an episode of hypotension is superimposed on chronic hepatic venous congestion, severe centrilobular necrosis may result with acute tenderness, marked elevation of serum transaminases, and hyperbilirubinemia. At times, it may be difficult to clinically distinguish centrilobular necrosis from acute viral hepatitis except by the subsequent course. The serum transaminase levels should fall rapidly following a hypotensive episode, whereas with viral hepatitis, transaminase levels decrease much more slowly.

7 Tricuspid insufficiency is most commonly due to right ventricular hypertrophy. In addition, trauma, bacterial endocarditis, and congenital heart disease may all cause isolated tricuspid regurgitation. In the setting of an acute myocardial infarction, right heart failure and tricuspid insufficiency may result in acute hepatic enlargement and tenderness.

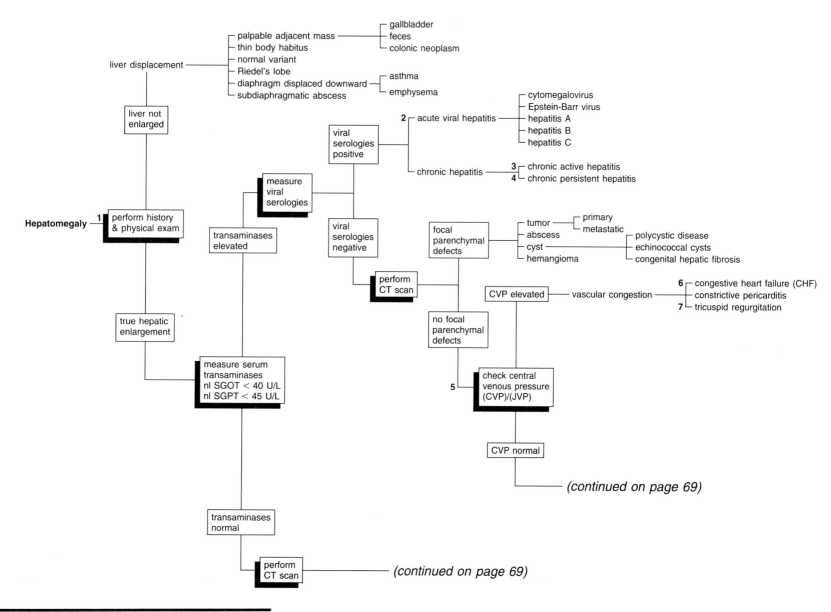

Hepatomegaly **1** perform history & physical exam

liver displacement

- palpable adjacent mass
  - gallbladder
  - feces
  - colonic neoplasm
- thin body habitus
- normal variant
- Riedel's lobe
- diaphragm displaced downward
  - asthma
  - emphysema
- subdiaphragmatic abscess

liver not enlarged

true hepatic enlargement

measure serum transaminases
nl SGOT < 40 U/L
nl SGPT < 45 U/L

transaminases elevated

transaminases normal

measure viral serologies

viral serologies positive

2 acute viral hepatitis
- cytomegalovirus
- Epstein-Barr virus
- hepatitis A
- hepatitis B
- hepatitis C

chronic hepatitis
- **3** chronic active hepatitis
- **4** chronic persistent hepatitis

viral serologies negative

perform CT scan

focal parenchymal defects
- tumor
  - primary
  - metastatic
- abscess
- cyst
  - polycystic disease
  - echinococcal cysts
  - congenital hepatic fibrosis
- hemangioma

no focal parenchymal defects

5 check central venous pressure (CVP)/(JVP)

CVP elevated — vascular congestion
- **6** congestive heart failure (CHF)
- constrictive pericarditis
- **7** tricuspid regurgitation

CVP normal

perform CT scan — *(continued on page 69)*

(continued on page 69)

Cecil Chapters	116–121
Harrison Chapter	**47**

Hepatomegaly (Continued)

8 Fat infiltration of the liver is due to the collection of triglycerides in the hepatocytes. Liver function can be well-preserved in the presence of fatty infiltration so that liver function tests are normal. Common causes of fatty liver infiltration are uncontrolled diabetes mellitus, obesity, protein-calorie malnutrition, corticosteroids, alcohol, jejunoileal bypass operations, hyperalimentation, and fatty liver of pregnancy.

9 Toxic hepatitis may be due to a variety of drugs and chemicals. The amount of hepatic injury can be drug- and dose-dependent or can be idiosyncratic. One drug may induce different types of hepatic injury in different individuals. Examples of drugs that commonly cause hepatitis include acetaminophen, erythromycin estolate, rifampin, oral contraceptives, aspirin, chlorpromazine, halothane, isoniazid, and methyldopa. If drug-induced hepatitis is suspected, the drug should be withdrawn, with further evaluation if hepatomegaly and liver function abnormalities persist despite drug withdrawal. Drugs can be a common cause for chronic hepatitis; however, diagnosis may be difficult, even with the added benefit of liver biopsy, because drug-induced liver injury is usually not associated with a specific histopathology. Nevertheless, liver biopsy may provide information that may rule out a drug as a cause of liver injury.

10 Cirrhosis refers to progressive hepatic fibrosis, which may be due to a variety of pathologic processes. Although the liver may be initially enlarged, in its end stage a cirrhotic liver becomes shrunken. Cirrhosis is a final common pathway, so that causes of cirrhosis include all the previously mentioned etiologies, i.e., hepatic injury due to drugs and toxins, viral hepatitis, biliary obstruction, metabolic and storage diseases, cardiac failure, and venous thrombosis.

11 A large number of infections other than viral hepatitis can result in hepatomegaly and liver inflammation. EBV, CMV, and yellow fever, as well as other infectious agents and parasites such as leptospirosis, salmonellosis, malaria, secondary syphilis, toxoplasmosis, Q fever, ascariasis, schistosomiasis, echinococcosis, and entamebiasis, can result in chronic hepatitis with hepatomegaly.

12 CAH is associated with chronic hepatitis B infection in only 20 to 30 per cent of cases (see No. 3). Other causes of this syndrome (negative HBsAg) include hepatitis C, other non-A non-B hepatitis, and drugs. Many cases are idiopathic. Drugs associated with CAH include isoniazid, methyldopa, sulfonamides, dantrolene, and nitrofurantoin. A variety of antibodies can be found in association with CAH, including antinuclear antibodies (ANAs) in 50 per cent of cases, anti–smooth muscle antibodies in 60 per cent of cases, and antimitochondrial antibodies in 30 per cent of cases. The significance of these antibodies is not known but is suggestive of an autoimmune basis for the disease.

13 Thrombosis or occlusion of the hepatic veins may result from hypercoagulable states, including polycythemia rubra vera, from the use of birth control pills, and from hemoglobinopathies. Also known as the Budd-Chiari syndrome, this condition manifests itself clinically with mild elevations of transaminases and bilirubin, as well as an enlarged, tender liver. Nonthrombotic occlusion of the hepatic veins may also cause a Budd-Chiari–like syndrome. This so-called veno-occlusive disease can occur in patients with alcoholic hepatitis and cirrhosis, in patients who have been treated with certain chemotherapeutic agents, in patients who have eaten plants containing pyrrolidizine alkaloids, and in patients following bone marrow transplantation.

14 Obstruction of the inferior vena cava (IVC) presents in a clinically similar fashion to hepatic vein obstruction, with ascites and hepatomegaly. Tumor is a common cause of IVC obstruction. Definitive diagnosis of hepatic vein or IVC obstruction depends on direct demonstration of the site of venous occlusion by venography.

15 Although most infiltrative and inflammatory liver diseases are associated with elevated transaminases, isolated measurements may be normal. Liver biopsy may be necessary to confirm the diagnosis.

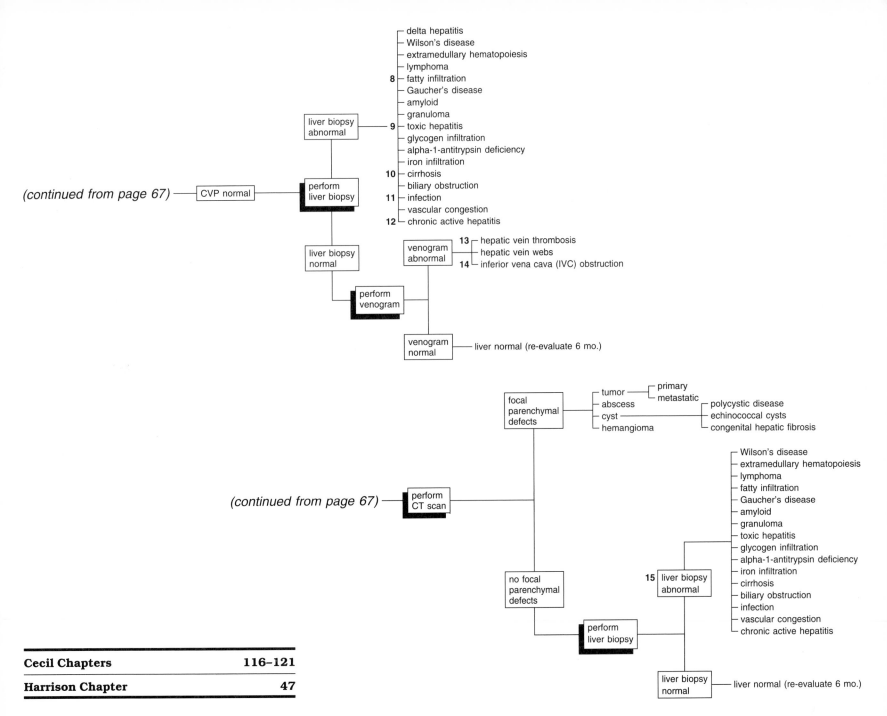

delta hepatitis
Wilson's disease
extramedullary hematopoiesis
lymphoma
8 fatty infiltration
Gaucher's disease
amyloid
granuloma
9 toxic hepatitis
glycogen infiltration
alpha-1-antitrypsin deficiency
iron infiltration
10 cirrhosis
biliary obstruction
11 infection
vascular congestion
12 chronic active hepatitis

liver biopsy abnormal

perform liver biopsy

CVP normal

(continued from page 67)

liver biopsy normal

perform venogram

venogram abnormal
13 hepatic vein thrombosis
hepatic vein webs
14 inferior vena cava (IVC) obstruction

venogram normal — liver normal (re-evaluate 6 mo.)

focal parenchymal defects
tumor — primary / metastatic
abscess
cyst — polycystic disease / echinococcal cysts / congenital hepatic fibrosis
hemangioma

perform CT scan

(continued from page 67)

no focal parenchymal defects

perform liver biopsy

15 liver biopsy abnormal
Wilson's disease
extramedullary hematopoiesis
lymphoma
fatty infiltration
Gaucher's disease
amyloid
granuloma
toxic hepatitis
glycogen infiltration
alpha-1-antitrypsin deficiency
iron infiltration
cirrhosis
biliary obstruction
infection
vascular congestion
chronic active hepatitis

liver biopsy normal — liver normal (re-evaluate 6 mo.)

Cecil Chapters	116–121
Harrison Chapter	47

Ascites

1 Abdominal distention, although commonly a result of ascites, can be due to a variety of other disorders. Obesity, large ovarian cysts, abdominal abscesses, hematomas, abdominal malignancies, and intestinal obstruction may mimic ascites. Patients with ascites may complain of an increase in clothing size, a feeling of abdominal tightness or pulling, low back pain, or the new appearance of umbilical or inguinal hernias. Examination of the abdomen in the presence of ascites may reveal bulging flanks and an everted umbilicus. It is difficult to detect less than 1.5 L of abdominal fluid upon physical examination. Tests to confirm the presence of abdominal fluid include the demonstration of a fluid wave and of dullness to percussion that shifts with change in position of the patient. With the patient positioned on the hands and knees, dullness with percussion of the central abdomen is sensitive enough to detect as little as 400 ml of abdominal fluid. This test is particularly useful in the presence of obesity because other physical tests become less sensitive. The most common causes of ascites are cirrhosis, congestive heart failure (CHF), malignancy, and tuberculosis. These conditions account for over 90 per cent of the ultimate diagnosis of ascites.

2 If ascites is strongly suspected, a diagnostic paracentesis should be performed. Although paracentesis will confirm the presence of ascites and may allow differentiation of the underlying cause, adjunctive tests are often necessary to identify or confirm the suspected diagnosis (see No. 9). At least 50 to 100 ml of fluid should be withdrawn and analyzed for the presence of protein, lactate dehydrogenase (LDH), amylase, specific gravity, cell count and differential, Gram's stain and bacterial culture, acid-fast stain and mycobacterial culture, fungal culture, and cytologic examination. Turbid fluid may be due to infection with a large number of inflammatory cells or to chylous ascites with which the triglyceride level is markedly elevated. Triglycerides should be measured if turbid fluid is withdrawn. Tests such as ultra-sound, CT, and laparoscopy are often necessary for diagnosis. In addition to pelvic and rectal examination, ultrasound or CT will aid in the diagnosis of abdominal carcinomas or ovarian masses.

3 Although overlap exists between the various diagnostic categories, the protein level of the ascitic fluid is a convenient method to distinguish between the causes of ascites. In general, the fluid is considered a transudate if the measured protein is less than 2.5 gm/dl of fluid. An exudate contains greater than 2.5 gm/dl of protein.

4 Meigs' syndrome is a transudative ascites and hydrothorax associated with ovarian tumors. Most commonly associated with ovarian cystadenomas, Meigs' syndrome was originally described in association with ovarian fibromas.

5 Tuberculous peritonitis can cause ascites. The mycobacteria can be detected on acid-fast stain and culture of ascitic fluid. Elevated white cell count (>250/ml) in the ascitic fluid is a useful clue to tuberculous infection but is also associated with other infections and malignancy.

6 Spontaneous bacterial peritonitis (SBP) occurs in approximately 10 per cent of cirrhotic patients with ascites. In two thirds of the cases, the infective organism is the gram-negative rod, *Escherichia coli.* Other common causative organisms include pneumococci, *Listeria monocytogenes, Neisseria meningitidis, Haemophilus influenzae,* and anaerobic organisms. The mechanism of infection is not known but is thought to be an "autoinfection" such as leakage of bacteria from the intestines or hematogenous bacterial seeding of ascitic fluid.

7 Several clues to the presence of intra-abdominal malignancy can be gleaned from analysis of ascitic fluid. Bloody ascitic fluid is a common indication of tumor but may also be present with tuberculous ascites, pancreatitis, abdominal trauma, endometriosis, and perforated viscus. A high LDH level is indicative of intra-abdominal malignancy. The ratio of ascitic LDH to serum LDH is more useful than an isolated LDH measurement and is suggestive of malignancy at a ratio greater than 0.6. However, 15 per cent of cirrhotic ascites may be found to have a high LDH ratio in the absence of malignancy. Other tumor markers have been measured in ascitic fluid, including the carcinoembryonic antigen (CEA). The CEA level is increased in only about half the cases of malignant ascites, but is very specific for malignancy when present.

8 Chronic pancreatic disease can result in massive ascites. The ascitic fluid contains high levels of amylase that may exceed 20,000 Somogyi units. Pancreatic ascites accounts for approximately 3 per cent of all causes of ascites and is usually associated with pancreatic disease due to alcohol or abdominal trauma.

9 Recovery of a turbid fluid on paracentesis should prompt the measurement of triglyceride levels. An elevated level of triglycerides is diagnostic for chylous ascites. Chylous ascites is due to malignancy in about 30 per cent of cases. Another 30 per cent of cases are due to various inflammatory conditions, including infection. The remaining cases are due to congenital disorders, trauma, or lymphangiectasia, or they are idiopathic.

10 An exudative ascites with a high protein level may accompany myxedema. The ascitic fluid may be gelatinous. The ascites will clear rapidly once thyroid replacement has begun.

11 Despite extensive diagnostic evaluation of ascites in some acquired immunodeficiency syndrome (AIDS) patients, the source of the ascites has not been diagnosed. Unidentified infection is suspected to be the cause of this chronic nonspecific peritonitis, and perhaps the peritonitis is due to the human immunodeficiency virus (HIV) itself.

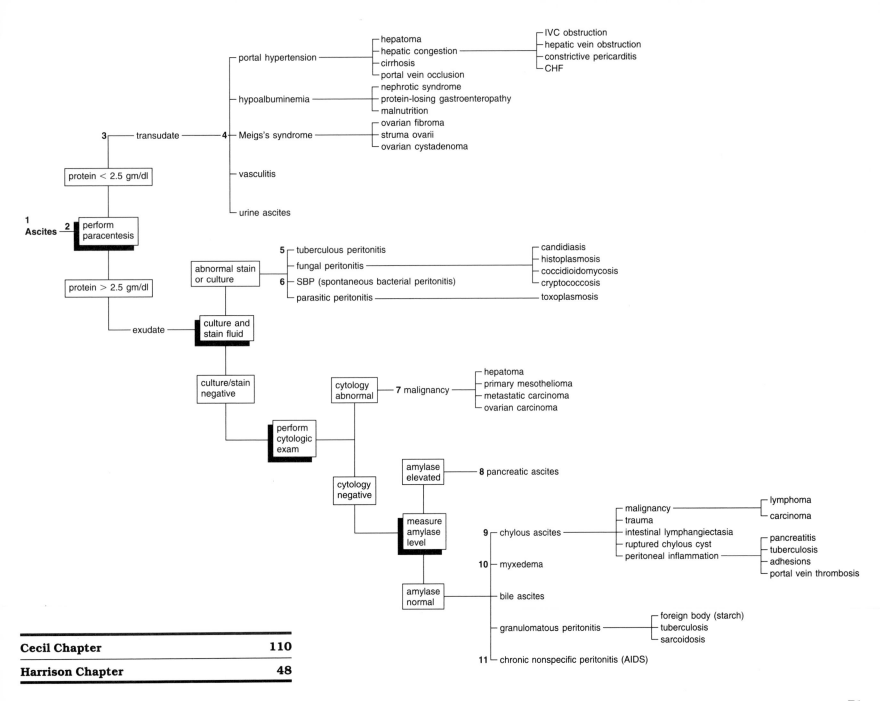

portal hypertension
— hepatoma
— hepatic congestion
  — IVC obstruction
  — hepatic vein obstruction
  — constrictive pericarditis
  — CHF
— cirrhosis
— portal vein occlusion

hypoalbuminemia
— nephrotic syndrome
— protein-losing gastroenteropathy
— malnutrition

3 — transudate — **4** — Meigs's syndrome
— ovarian fibroma
— struma ovarii
— ovarian cystadenoma

vasculitis

urine ascites

protein < 2.5 gm/dl

1
Ascites — **2** — perform paracentesis

abnormal stain or culture
5 — tuberculous peritonitis
— fungal peritonitis
  — candidiasis
  — histoplasmosis
  — coccidioidomycosis
  — cryptococcosis
6 — SBP (spontaneous bacterial peritonitis)
— parasitic peritonitis — toxoplasmosis

protein > 2.5 gm/dl

exudate — culture and stain fluid

culture/stain negative

cytology abnormal — **7** malignancy
— hepatoma
— primary mesothelioma
— metastatic carcinoma
— ovarian carcinoma

perform cytologic exam

cytology negative

amylase elevated — **8** pancreatic ascites

measure amylase level

9 — chylous ascites
— malignancy
  — lymphoma
  — carcinoma
— trauma
— intestinal lymphangiectasia
— ruptured chylous cyst
— peritoneal inflammation
  — pancreatitis
  — tuberculosis
  — adhesions
  — portal vein thrombosis

10 — myxedema

amylase normal — bile ascites

granulomatous peritonitis
— foreign body (starch)
— tuberculosis
— sarcoidosis

11 — chronic nonspecific peritonitis (AIDS)

Cecil Chapter	**110**
Harrison Chapter	**48**

Transaminitis

1 The most commonly measured transaminases are SGOT and SGPT. Although elevated levels of these enzymes are sensitive indicators of hepatocellular injury, the tests are not specific. Transaminases are present in significant quantities in other tissues, including skeletal muscle, kidney, myocardium, pancreas, and small intestine. When hepatocellular disease is suspected, however, measurement of the serum transaminase levels, along with other tests of liver function, can be helpful in diagnosing the presence of liver disease. In addition, the degree to which the transaminases are elevated is a useful clue for diagnosis. The SGPT elevation generally parallels the level of SGOT. In acute hepatitis with liver necrosis, the elevation of SGPT may be marked. When transaminase levels are elevated to greater than 300 U/L, hepatocellular disease should be suspected. Transaminase levels of 500 U/L can be seen with acute hepatic necrosis due to drugs, toxins, or ischemia. If transaminase elevations are less marked, further evaluation is required.

2 Serum creatine phosphokinase (CK or CPK) is elevated with acute atrophy or necrosis of striated muscle. CK levels remain normal in liver disease and biliary obstruction. In addition, CK enzymes can be fractionated to determine the source of their release. The CK-MB isoenzyme elevation is specific for myocardial injury. CK-MM fraction elevation is specific for striated muscle injury. Although not specific for myocardial infarction, the SGOT will be elevated with acute myocardial injury. If the myocardium is not damaged, as with angina pectoris, coronary insufficiency, and pericarditis, the serum transaminases, as well as the CK, will remain within normal levels.

3 Approximately 50 per cent of patients with extensive cerebral infarctions (cerebrovascular accidents [CVAs]) have elevated levels of CK and SGOT. The CK-MB isoenzyme is not elevated with brain injury or infarction.

4 Measurement of the alkaline phosphatase level (alk phos) is most useful in distinguishing whether the source of jaundice is an obstructive process (cholestatic jaundice) or acute hepatocellular damage. Marked elevation of alkaline phosphatase (greater than three times normal) suggests extrahepatic obstruction. Lesser elevations of alkaline phosphatase may accompany hepatocellular disease without biliary obstruction. Although the source of alkaline phosphatase is mainly the cells that line the biliary tree, alkaline phosphatase may also be released from bone osteoblasts, the small intestine, and the placenta. In the presence of transaminitis and suspected liver disease, the source of alkaline phosphatase is fairly clear.

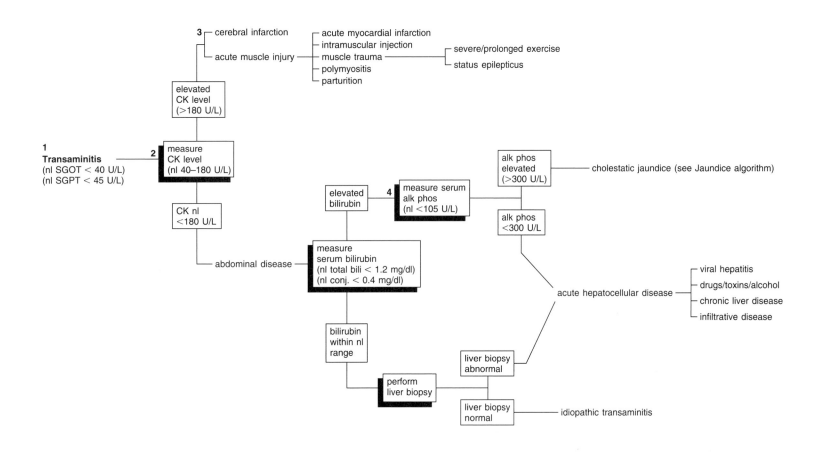

3 ⎡ cerebral infarction   ⎡ acute myocardial infarction
    │   ├ intramuscular injection
    └ acute muscle injury ───┼ muscle trauma ─────────── ⎡ severe/prolonged exercise
                             ├ polymyositis   └ status epilepticus
                             └ parturition

elevated
CK level
(>180 U/L)

1
Transaminitis   **2** ⎡ measure
(nl SGOT < 40 U/L)   │ CK level
(nl SGPT < 45 U/L)   │ (nl 40–180 U/L)

                                                                    alk phos
                                                                    elevated ──────────── cholestatic jaundice (see Jaundice algorithm)
                                                    elevated   **4** ⎡ measure serum   (>300 U/L)
                                                    bilirubin   │ alk phos
CK nl   │ (nl <105 U/L)
<180 U/L   alk phos
                                                                                         <300 U/L

                                                                                                          ⎡ viral hepatitis
                                                                                                          ├ drugs/toxins/alcohol
                            ⎡ measure   acute hepatocellular disease ────┤ chronic liver disease
abdominal disease ──────────│ serum bilirubin   └ infiltrative disease
                            │ (nl total bili < 1.2 mg/dl)
                            │ (nl conj. < 0.4 mg/dl)

                            bilirubin
                            within nl
                            range
                                                       liver biopsy
                                                       abnormal
                                    ⎡ perform
                                    │ liver biopsy
                                                       liver biopsy
                                                       normal ──────────── idiopathic transaminitis

Cecil Chapter	**116**
Harrison Chapters	**249, 252, 253**

Elevated Alkaline Phosphatase

1 Serum alkaline phosphatase is derived mainly from the cells of the biliary tract, the mucosal cells of the small intestine, the placenta, and bone osteo-blasts. The most valuable use of the alkaline phosphatase measurement lies in distinguishing an obstructive biliary process (cholestasis) from hepatocellular damage (see Jaundice algorithm, page 64). The alkaline phosphatase level is measured on routine chemistry panel and may be found as an isolated abnormality. Alkaline phosphatase from the intestine can account for as much as 60 per cent of the total serum value in some individuals but is an unlikely source for elevated serum levels in the absence of overt intestinal disease. The highest levels of serum alkaline phosphatase occur with biliary obstruction and Paget's disease. The alkaline phosphatase may be elevated to three or more times the normal level.

2 The main sources of alkaline phosphatase in the nonpregnant adult are bone and liver. Serum al-kaline phosphatase can be elevated normally with preg-nancy and growth, or with space-occupying and infiltra-tive diseases of the liver in the absence of significant bilirubin elevation. The measurement of the serum level of the enzyme 5'-nucleotidase will distinguish between a bone and liver source of the alkaline phosphatase. 5'-Nucleotidase is found mainly in the bile canaliculi of the liver and is not present in bone. Another enzyme used to determine the presence of liver disease is serum gamma-glutamyl transpeptidase. This enzyme is absent in bone and placenta and is sensitive for liver disease but is not very specific. Although the 5'-nucleotidase is not as sen-sitive, it is very specific for hepatobiliary disease. Alter-natively, heat inactivation (fractionation) of alkaline phos-phatase can be used to determine its source. The differentiation between a hepatic and bone source is based on the fact that alkaline phosphatase derived from bone is heat-labile (hence the phrase ''bone-burns'') and that liver alkaline phosphatase is heat-stable.

3 The placenta is an active source of alkaline phos-phatase, and serum levels become elevated in late pregnancy. The serum alkaline phosphatase level returns to normal by 3 weeks post partum. The Regan isozyme is an isozyme of alkaline phosphatase that is identical to the placental isozyme but is found in the presence of certain malignancies, especially lung carcinoma (see No. 6).

4 Any bone lesions that produce increased osteo-blastic activity will result in elevated serum al-kaline phosphatase levels. At times, bone lesions such as osteogenic sarcoma and metastatic carcinoma may be sus-pected on the basis of an elevated alkaline phosphatase level obtained on a routine chemistry panel.

5 An elevated alkaline phosphatase, resulting from normal bone growth, is often found on routine blood chemistry panels in children and adolescents.

6 Malignancy not involving the bone or the liver can produce an isozyme of alkaline phosphatase and result in an elevated level of serum alkaline phospha-tase. One such isozyme, the Regan isozyme, has been found to be identical to the placental isozyme and is associated most commonly with lung carcinoma. The Re-gan isozyme is found rarely in normal persons.

BIBLIOGRAPHY

Coffman DA, Chalstrey J, Smith-Laing G: Gastrointestinal Dis-orders. New York, Churchill Livingstone, 1986.

Cohen S: Clinical Gastroenterology: A Problem-Oriented Ap-proach. New York, John Wiley & Sons, 1983.

Frank BB: Clinical evaluation of jaundice. JAMA 262(21):3031–3034, 1989.

Lancaster-Smith MJ, Chapman C (eds): Gastroenterology. Little-ton, MA, PSG Publishing Company, 1985.

Lancaster-Smith MJ, Williams K: Problems in Gastroenterology. Philadelphia, F. A. Davis Company, 1982.

Schmidt E, Schmidt FW: Progress in the enzyme diagnosis of liver disease: reality or illusion? Clin Biochem 23:375–382, 1990.

Sleisenger MH, Fordtran JS (eds): Gastrointestinal Disease. Phil-adelphia, W. B. Saunders Company, 1989.

Stelling HP, Maimon HN, et al.: A comparative study of fecal occult blood tests for early detection of gastrointestinal pathol-ogy. Arch Intern Med 150:1001–1005, 1990.

Wilcox CM, Forsmark CE, et al.: High-protein ascites in patients with the acquired immunodeficiency syndrome. Gastroenter-ology 100:745–748, 1991.

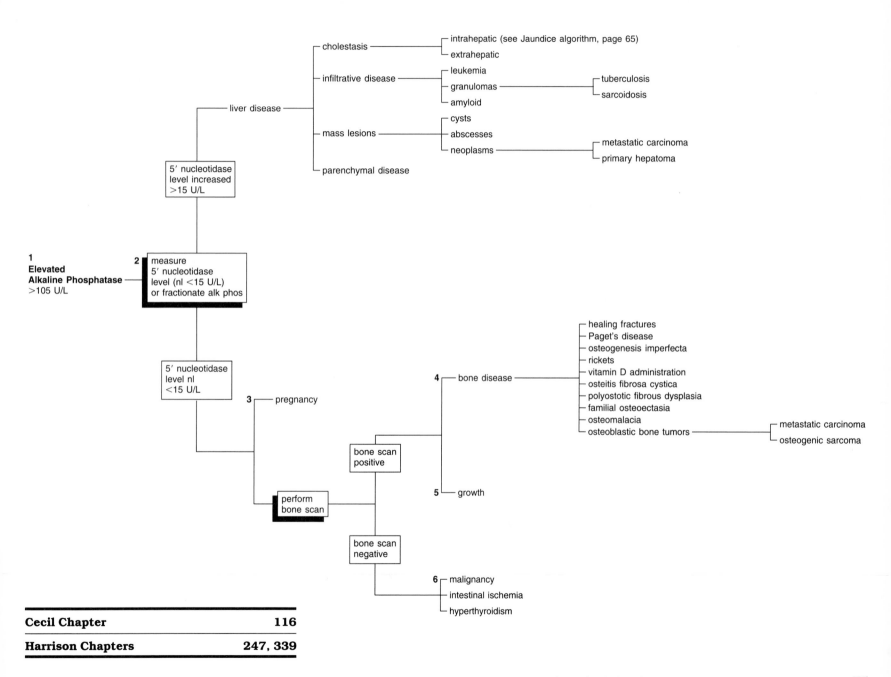

cholestasis
— intrahepatic (see Jaundice algorithm, page 65)
— extrahepatic

infiltrative disease
— leukemia
— granulomas —— tuberculosis
—— sarcoidosis
— amyloid

liver disease

mass lesions
— cysts
— abscesses
— neoplasms —— metastatic carcinoma
—— primary hepatoma

parenchymal disease

5' nucleotidase
level increased
>15 U/L

1
**Elevated
Alkaline Phosphatase**
>105 U/L

2 measure
5' nucleotidase
level (nl <15 U/L)
or fractionate alk phos

5' nucleotidase
level nl
<15 U/L

3 — pregnancy

bone scan
positive

perform
bone scan

4 bone disease
— healing fractures
— Paget's disease
— osteogenesis imperfecta
— rickets
— vitamin D administration
— osteitis fibrosa cystica
— polyostotic fibrous dysplasia
— familial osteoectasia
— osteomalacia
— osteoblastic bone tumors —— metastatic carcinoma
—— osteogenic sarcoma

5 — growth

bone scan
negative

6 — malignancy
— intestinal ischemia
— hyperthyroidism

Cecil Chapter	116
Harrison Chapters	247, 339

5 ▪ Renal Disorders

Signs and symptoms:	Labs:
Oliguria	Hematuria
	Proteinuria

Oliguria

1 Oliguria is defined as a urine output of less than 400 ml per 24 hours. Urine output below this quantity is usually evidence of a decrease in glomerular filtration rate (GFR). Normal metabolism produces between 400 and 500 mOsm of solute per day. The kidneys cannot concentrate the urine to greater than 1200 mOsm/kg, so that a urine output of less than 400 ml per 24 hours will not allow for excretion of the entire daily solute load. The simultaneous accumulation of nitrogenous wastes and an increase in the blood urea nitrogen (BUN) are commonly seen in the setting of oliguria.

2 Urine sodium (U_{Na}) is a sensitive indicator of renal perfusion. As long as tubular function is intact, the kidneys will maximally reabsorb sodium when renal perfusion is decreased. The source of the decreased perfusion is not important; the decrease may result from true intravascular volume depletion or decreased renal blood flow as seen with cardiac insufficiency or vascular obstruction. The fractional excretion of sodium (FE_{Na}) relates the excretion of sodium to the GFR and is thought to be an even more sensitive indicator of renal perfusion than U_{Na} alone. The FE_{Na} is defined by the formula

$$FE_{Na} = \frac{U_{Na}/P_{Na}}{U_{Cr}/P_{Cr}} \times 100$$

where P_{Na} is plasma sodium, U_{Cr} is urine creatinine, and P_{Cr} is plasma creatinine.

3 Prerenal oliguria is decreased urine output resulting from underperfusion of the kidney and is the most common form of oliguria. Cardiac insufficiency and overuse of diuretics are the most commonly associated causes. The kidneys are perfectly normal, and correction of the underlying condition will restore renal function to normal. Several newer classes of drugs, especially the prostaglandin synthesis inhibitors and the converting enzyme inhibitors, have been associated with oliguric renal failure. Inhibitors of prostaglandin synthesis such as propionic acid derivatives (ibuprofen, fenoprofen, naproxen) and indolacetic acid derivatives (indomethacin, tolmetin sodium) decrease renal blood flow and GFR, especially in patients with decreased effective arterial volumes or renal vascular disease.

4 A nephritic urine sediment contains the products of glomerular inflammation. These include red blood cells, white blood cells, red blood cell casts, hyalin casts, and cellular debris. Individual elements of nephritic urine, with the exception of red blood cell casts, may be seen in other renal disorders, but this combination usually signifies glomerulonephritis.

5 Oliguria is most commonly associated with the rapidly progressive forms of glomerulonephritis (RPGN). RPGN may be seen in immune disorders such as anti–glomerular basement membrane antibody disease (anti-GBM) or idiopathic crescentic glomerulonephritis. RPGN can also occur following infection with some forms of streptococci and hepatitis B virus and during the course of bacterial endocarditis. Certain systemic disorders may also cause RPGN. The most commonly associated disorders are systemic lupus erythematosus, polyarteritis, cryoglobulinemia, allergic angiitis, Henoch-Schönlein purpura, and systemic necrotizing vasculitis.

6 The renal ultrasound is a sensitive noninvasive way to image the intrarenal collecting system. Dilation of the calyces and the renal pelvis is indicative of extrarenal obstruction. The renal ultrasound may be negative in the first 24 to 36 hours after obstruction has occurred and should be repeated if a strong suspicion of obstruction exists.

7 Vasculitis resulting in oliguric renal failure may occur without associated glomerular injury. Among the vasculitides that do not usually affect the glomeruli are idiopathic systemic vasculitis, scleroderma vasculitis, malignant hypertension, and drug-related vasculitis.

8 The gallium scan is usually positive in inflammatory processes of the kidney such as interstitial nephritis. The scan should be interpreted with caution, however, because it may also be positive in other noninterstitial disorders such as infections.

9 Allergic forms of interstitial nephritis are usually drug-related. The prototype of this form of interstitial nephritis is seen with the semisynthetic penicillins such as nafcillin. Other antibiotics including the cephalosporins, sulfa drugs, tetracycline, rifampin, and ethambutol have been implicated as causes of interstitial nephritis. Nonsteroidal anti-inflammatory agents, thiazide diuretics, allopurinol, aspirin, cimetidine, methyldopa, phenytoin, and clofibrate among others have also been associated with allergic forms of interstitial nephritis.

10 Nonallergic forms of interstitial nephritis are usually due to infectious agents. Interstitial nephritis may be caused by streptococcal infections, toxoplasmosis, infectious mononucleosis, measles, syphilis, mycoplasma infections, legionnaires' disease, and Rocky Mountain spotted fever.

11 The ischemic form of acute tubular necrosis (ATN) is due to the underperfusion of the renal tubules. The most common cause of tubular ischemia is hypotension due to volume loss, poor cardiac output, or the vasodilation seen with sepsis. Prerenal forms of oliguria may progress to ischemic ATN if not adequately treated.

12 Many substances are toxic to the renal tubules. Common toxins include the aminoglycoside antibiotics, amphotericin B, heavy metals such as lead and mercury, endotoxin, myoglobin, Bence Jones protein, iodinated contrast media, fluorinated anesthetics, organic solvents, ethylene glycol, acetaminophen, and paraquat.

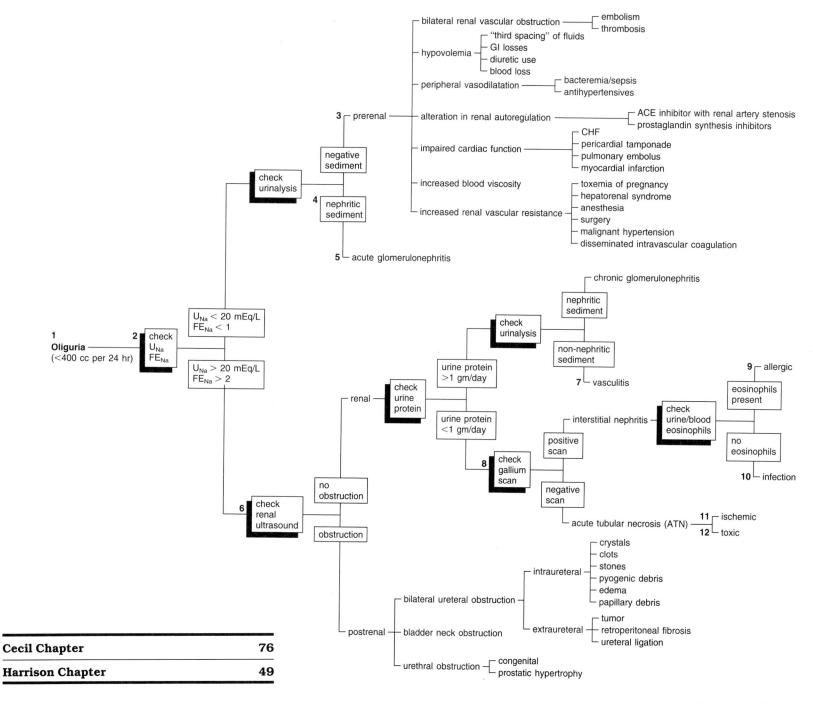

bilateral renal vascular obstruction —— embolism
                                       —— thrombosis

hypovolemia —— "third spacing" of fluids
            —— GI losses
            —— diuretic use
            —— blood loss

peripheral vasodilatation —— bacteremia/sepsis
                          —— antihypertensives

3 — prerenal — alteration in renal autoregulation —— ACE inhibitor with renal artery stenosis
                                                      —— prostaglandin synthesis inhibitors

impaired cardiac function —— CHF
                          —— pericardial tamponade
                          —— pulmonary embolus
                          —— myocardial infarction

increased blood viscosity

increased renal vascular resistance —— toxemia of pregnancy
                                    —— hepatorenal syndrome
                                    —— anesthesia
                                    —— surgery
                                    —— malignant hypertension
                                    —— disseminated intravascular coagulation

negative sediment

check urinalysis

4 nephritic sediment

5 — acute glomerulonephritis

chronic glomerulonephritis

nephritic sediment

check urinalysis

non-nephritic sediment

7 — vasculitis

9 — allergic

eosinophils present

check urine/blood eosinophils

no eosinophils

10 — infection

urine protein >1 gm/day

check urine protein

urine protein <1 gm/day

interstitial nephritis

positive scan

8 **check gallium scan**

negative scan

acute tubular necrosis (ATN) —— **11** — ischemic
                                 —— **12** — toxic

$U_{Na} < 20$ mEq/L
$FE_{Na} < 1$

1
Oliguria
(<400 cc per 24 hr)

2 **check U_{Na} FE_{Na}**

$U_{Na} > 20$ mEq/L
$FE_{Na} > 2$

renal

no obstruction

6 **check renal ultrasound**

obstruction

postrenal

bilateral ureteral obstruction —— intraureteral —— crystals
                                                 —— clots
                                                 —— stones
                                                 —— pyogenic debris
                                                 —— edema
                                                 —— papillary debris

                              —— extraureteral —— tumor
                                                —— retroperitoneal fibrosis
                                                —— ureteral ligation

bladder neck obstruction

urethral obstruction —— congenital
                     —— prostatic hypertrophy

Hematuria

1 Hematuria is the presence of abnormal numbers of red blood cells (RBCs) in the urine. Normally, up to 1,000,000 RBCs per day may appear in the urine. The presence of more than 2 or 3 RBCs per high power field on routine urinalysis, however, warrants further investigation. Cigarette smoking, strenuous exercise, and fever have been reported to cause hematuria without any underlying pathologic change. A positive test for blood on a urine dipstick in the absence of RBCs may indicate the presence of myoglobin resulting from muscle necrosis, free hemoglobin resulting from intravascular hemolysis, or lysis of RBCs in the bladder due to hypotonic urine. Hemoglobinuria has been associated with the ingestion or inhalation of certain toxins such as carbon monoxide, poisonous mushrooms, naphthalene, sulfonamides, and tin-containing compounds. The appearance of RBC casts is indicative of intrarenal pathology. Glomerulonephritis and renal vasculitis are most commonly associated with RBC casts.

2 Although spontaneous bleeding in the urinary tract can occur with the use of anticoagulant drugs and with coagulopathies, several studies have reported that more than 50 per cent of patients with this disorder have underlying urinary tract pathology. Further evaluation of the urinary tract with cystoscopy or intravenous pyelography is advisable for these patients.

3 Hematuria is more common in patients with sickle cell trait (Hb AS) than in patients with the homozygous form of the disease (Hb SS). The hematuria is painless and 80 per cent of the time comes from the left kidney only. As with other coagulopathies, there is a high incidence of associated urinary tract pathology (see No. 2).

4 Urinary protein excretion of more than 1 gm per day usually indicates glomerular damage. Some glomerular lesions or dysproteinemias such as multiple myeloma may be associated with a protein excretion of less than 1 gm per day, but these diseases are not usually associated with hematuria.

5 Renal cell carcinoma accounts for 85 per cent of all renal tumors, with the highest incidence in the sixth decade of life. Hereditary, viral, hormonal, and environmental factors have all been implicated in the etiology of this tumor. There is a two- to eight-fold increase in renal cell carcinoma in tobacco users. Certain foods containing nitrosamines, as well as coffee and high-fat diets, have also been suspected as etiologic factors.

6 Isolated renal cysts rarely cause hematuria. Ten to 15 per cent of patients with polycystic kidney disease, however, will present with gross or microscopic hematuria. Bleeding into a renal cyst in polycystic kidney disease may at times cause massive hematuria.

7 Four per cent of all urinary tumors are urothelial. The most common, transitional cell carcinoma, accounts for more than 90 per cent of the ureteral tumors. The remaining 8 to 10 per cent of tumors are squamous cell carcinomas. Adenocarcinomas are also occasionally found. These tumors occur most frequently in the sixth decade of life, with a 4:1 male predominance.

8 Tumors of the bladder have a strong male predominance. There is a greatly increased incidence of bladder carcinoma in tobacco users. The highest incidence of bladder carcinoma occurs in cigarette smokers, but pipe and cigar smoking as well as the use of chewing tobacco are all associated with an increased incidence of carcinoma of the bladder.

9 Both acute and chronic forms of glomerulonephritis are associated with hematuria. Smoky urine and red cell casts are indicative of hematuria of renal parenchymal origin. Hematuria is not specific for any form of glomerulonephritis, but membranoproliferative glomerulonephritis, focal glomerular sclerosis, and IgA nephritis (Berger's disease) are the most common glomerular diseases associated with hematuria.

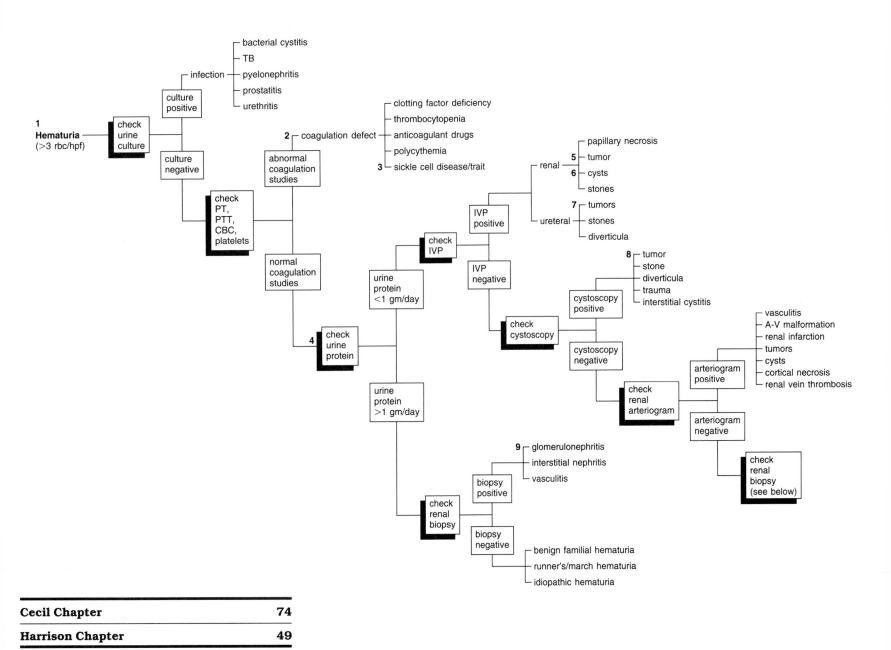

1
Hematuria
(>3 rbc/hpf)

check
urine
culture

culture
positive — infection
- bacterial cystitis
- TB
- pyelonephritis
- prostatitis
- urethritis

culture
negative

check
PT,
PTT,
CBC,
platelets

abnormal
coagulation
studies

2 ┌ coagulation defect
- clotting factor deficiency
- thrombocytopenia
- anticoagulant drugs
- polycythemia

3 └ sickle cell disease/trait

normal
coagulation
studies

check
urine
protein

4

urine
protein
<1 gm/day

check
IVP

IVP
positive

renal
5 ┌ papillary necrosis
├ tumor
6 ├ cysts
└ stones

ureteral
7 ┌ tumors
├ stones
└ diverticula

IVP
negative

check
cystoscopy

cystoscopy
positive

8 ┌ tumor
├ stone
├ diverticula
├ trauma
└ interstitial cystitis

cystoscopy
negative

check
renal
arteriogram

arteriogram
positive
- vasculitis
- A-V malformation
- renal infarction
- tumors
- cysts
- cortical necrosis
- renal vein thrombosis

arteriogram
negative

check
renal
biopsy
(see below)

urine
protein
>1 gm/day

check
renal
biopsy

biopsy
positive
9 ┌ glomerulonephritis
├ interstitial nephritis
└ vasculitis

biopsy
negative
- benign familial hematuria
- runner's/march hematuria
- idiopathic hematuria

Proteinuria

1 Most healthy persons excrete between 45 and 150 mg of urinary protein daily. Values as high as 300 mg/day have been found after exercise. About 30 per cent of the protein in the urine of normal persons is albumin, with the remainder a variety of filtered and secreted globulins. Dye-impregnated strips are the most common method of detecting proteinuria. The intensity of the color change is proportional to the concentration of protein in the urine, with trace = 10 mg/dl, 1+ = 30 mg/dl, 2+ = 100 mg/dl, 3+ = 300 mg/dl, and 4+ = >1000 mg/dl. The dipsticks may underestimate the proteinuria if large amounts of globulins or light chains are present, because the sticks are much more sensitive to albumin than to other proteins.

2 The 24-hour urine collection is the simplest method of quantifying urinary protein excretion. Simultaneous 24-hour creatinine excretion should also be measured to assess the completeness of the collection. Proteinuria can be divided into three etiologic types. Overflow proteinuria results from an increase in the concentration of a plasma protein, usually because of overproduction. Tubular proteinuria is the result of the impairment of tubular reabsorption of the smaller molecular weight proteins normally filtered at the glomerulus. Glomerular proteinuria is the result of increased permeability of the glomerular capillary wall to protein. Tubular and overflow proteinuria rarely exceed 2 gm/24 hr.

3 Monoclonal light chains, either kappa or lambda, are commonly seen in the urine in multiple myeloma. The proteinuria may be a result of overflow from the increased production of both myeloma paraprotein and light chains, or due to direct glomerular or tubular damage from the paraprotein itself. Amyloidosis occurs in approximately 10 per cent of patients with multiple myeloma and may also cause proteinuria, usually in excess of 3 gm/24 hr. The urine dipstick may be falsely negative in this disorder because the light chains or paraproteins do not react with the chemical impregnated on the stick.

4 Beta-2 microglobulin with a molecular weight of 12,000 is the standard marker in the urine for tubular proteinuria. The normal urinary excretion of 100 μg/24 hr may be increased 10- to 100-fold in tubular disease.

5 Hereditary forms of tubular disease causing proteinuria include Wilson's disease, cystinosis, oxalosis, and medullary cystic disease.

6 Congenital forms of tubular disease causing proteinuria include some forms of renal tubular acidosis and all forms of Fanconi's syndrome.

7 Acquired tubular diseases causing proteinuria include heavy metal toxicity, pyelonephritis, interstitial nephritis, obstructive uropathy, radiation nephritis, and vitamin D intoxication.

8 Several infectious diseases are associated with nephrotic-range proteinuria. Poststreptococcal glomerulonephritis, bacterial endocarditis, ''shunt'' nephritis, and syphilis are associated with nephrotic-range proteinuria.

9 Drugs that have been associated with proteinuria of greater than 3 gm/day include nonsteroidal anti-inflammatory agents, penicillamine, Mesantoin, and probenecid.

10 Familial disorders associated with nephrotic-range proteinuria include Alport's syndrome, sickle cell disease, Fabry's disease, and nail-patella syndrome.

11 Neoplastic diseases may cause proteinuria by direct toxicity to the kidney, as seen in some lymphomas and leukemias as well as Wilms' tumor and pheochromocytoma. Neoplasia can also cause proteinuria by secondary glomerular damage, as in the case of the membranous nephropathy associated with carcinomas of the lung, breast, and colon.

12 At least two abnormalities have been identified that account for the increased glomerular capillary wall permeability to protein seen in glomerulonephritis. First, there is a loss of the normal negative charge on the capillary wall. The loss of a negative charge eliminates the repelling forces between the negative charge on the protein molecule and the capillary wall. Second, there is alteration in the size barrier to passage of large molecules. The alteration may be the result of gaps in the glomerular basement membrane, detachment of epithelial cells, and the deposition of materials along the basement membrane that further disrupt the integrity of the capillary wall.

13 The glomerular injury seen in multisystem disorders may be the result of direct trauma to the renal vascular system, the deposition of antibodies directly in the glomerulus, or the deposition of circulating antigen-antibody complexes within the glomerulus. The mechanism of the proteinuria is the same as that described above (see No. 12).

BIBLIOGRAPHY

Brenner BM, Rector FC: The Kidney. Philadelphia, W. B. Saunders Company, 1986.
Glassock RJ: Current Therapy in Nephrology and Hypertension 1984–1985. St. Louis, C. V. Mosby Company, 1984.
Kurtzman NA, Batlle DC: Acid-base disorders. Med Clin North Am 67:4, 1983.
Narins RG, Jones ER, et al.: Diagnostic strategies in disorders of fluid, electrolyte, and acid-base homeostasis. Am J Med 72:496–520, 1982.
Schrier RW: Renal and Electrolyte Disorders. Boston, Little, Brown and Company, 1986.
Stein JH: Nephrology: The Science and Practice of Clinical Medicine. Vol 7. New York, Grune and Stratton, 1980.
Taylor RB: Difficult Diagnosis. Philadelphia, W. B. Saunders Company, 1985.

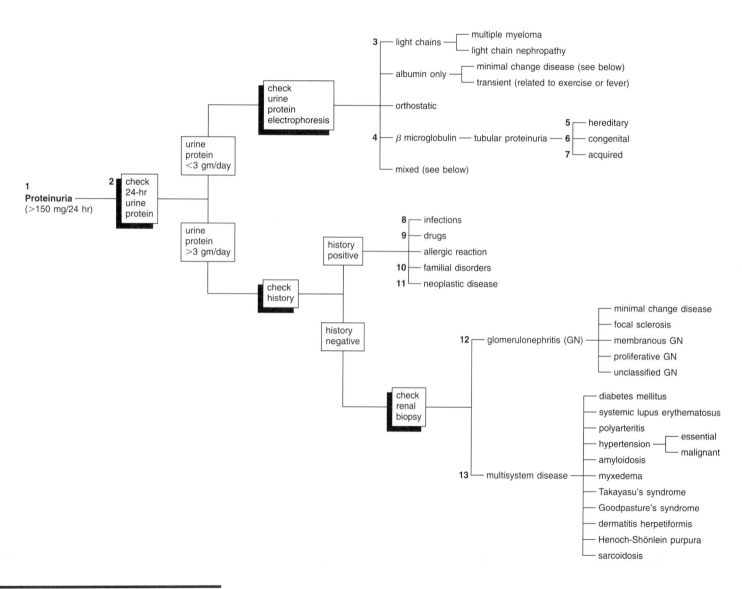

1
Proteinuria
(>150 mg/24 hr)

2 check
24-hr
urine
protein

urine
protein
<3 gm/day

**check
urine
protein
electrophoresis**

3 — light chains —— multiple myeloma
—— light chain nephropathy

albumin only —— minimal change disease (see below)
—— transient (related to exercise or fever)

orthostatic

4 — β microglobulin — tubular proteinuria — **5** — hereditary
6 — congenital
7 — acquired

mixed (see below)

urine
protein
>3 gm/day

check
history

history
positive

8 — infections
9 — drugs
— allergic reaction
10 — familial disorders
11 — neoplastic disease

history
negative

check
renal
biopsy

12 — glomerulonephritis (GN)
— minimal change disease
— focal sclerosis
— membranous GN
— proliferative GN
— unclassified GN

13 — multisystem disease
— diabetes mellitus
— systemic lupus erythematosus
— polyarteritis
— hypertension —— essential
—— malignant
— amyloidosis
— myxedema
— Takayasu's syndrome
— Goodpasture's syndrome
— dermatitis herpetiformis
— Henoch-Shönlein purpura
— sarcoidosis

Cecil Chapter	**74**
Harrison Chapter	**49**

6 ▪ Acid-Base and Electrolyte Disorders

Labs:

Hyponatremia

Hypernatremia

Hypokalemia

Hyperkalemia

Hypocalcemia

Hypercalcemia

Hypophosphatemia

Hyperphosphatemia

Hypomagnesemia

Hypermagnesemia

Acidosis

Alkalosis

Hyponatremia

1 Hyperglycemia, by osmotically shifting water into the intravascular space, will decrease the serum sodium (Na) 1.6 mEq/L for each 100-mEq/dl increase in serum glucose greater than 100 mEq/dl. If the Na is decreased out of proportion to the expected decrease owing to hyperglycemia alone, another osmolar substance may be present or true hyponatremia may coexist.

2 A low serum osmolality implies a relative or absolute water excess and overhydration of the extracellular fluid compartment. The total body Na (TB_{Na}), however, may be normal, increased, or low. Hyponatremia is the most common electrolyte abnormality in hospitalized patients.

3 Useful clinical clues to determine the patient's volume status include orthostatic blood pressure and pulse changes, the moistness of the mucous membranes, the presence or absence of axillary perspiration, skin turgor, jugular venous distention, and the presence or absence of an hepatojugular reflux.

4 Disorders in which the kidneys perceive a decreased ''effective arterial volume'' cause avid Na reabsorption by the kidneys. Effective arterial volume is synonymous with renal perfusion. The decreased ''effective volume'' may be due to decreased cardiac output in the case of congestive heart failure, or to the loss of plasma volume into a third space, such as the massive ascites that may be seen with hepatic cirrhosis. Increased antidiuretic hormone (ADH) is released in this setting and leads to the hyponatremia.

5 Sodium excretion at the level of the individual nephron is increased when total kidney glomerular filtration rate (GFR) is decreased. The ability of each nephron to increase the percentage of filtered Na, along with tubular inability to reabsorb much of the filtered Na, accounts for the increased urinary Na concentration seen in renal failure. Increased ADH is released in this setting, contributing to the hyponatremia.

6 Psychogenic polydipsia is usually seen in females with a history of psychiatric or eating disorders. When water intake is greater than 1 L per hour, the kidney's ability to excrete free water is exceeded and hyponatremia results. The urine is maximally dilute and urine osmolality is low.

7 Common iatrogenic causes of hyponatremia include the administration of hypotonic intravenous solutions, excessive water intake by persons on sodium-restricted diets, tap water enemas, and the use of large amounts of distilled water for irrigation during prostatic or bladder surgery.

8 The syndrome of inappropriate [secretion of] ADH (SIADH) is the result of either a defect in the osmoregulation of ADH or the secretion of ectopic ADH or ADH-like substances. There are many causes of SIADH, but pulmonary infections, oat cell carcinoma of the lung, and some central nervous system (CNS) lesions are the most common. SIADH should be considered in the euvolemic, hyponatremic patient when other causes of impaired water excretion have been eliminated.

9 Various drugs impair water excretion by releasing ADH or potentiating the action of ADH in the distal tubule. Drugs most commonly associated with hyponatremia include chlorpropamide and other sulfonylureas, nonsteroidal anti-inflammatory drugs, opiates, cyclophosphamide, haloperidol, tricyclic antidepressants, clofibrate, nicotine, both inhaled or delivered transdermally, and high doses of acetaminophen.

10 Several mechanisms have been implicated in the hyponatremia associated with hypothyroidism. Increased ADH levels, as well as enhanced reabsorption of sodium and water in the proximal tubule, occur with hypothyroidism. Avid sodium retention is not seen unless the patient is also volume-depleted. Urinary sodium concentration is, therefore, usually greater than 20 mEq/L.

11 Glucocorticoids have an important function in the normal control of ADH release. Patients with isolated glucocorticoid deficiency may have a profound impairment in water excretion. The hyponatremia and increased ADH levels are corrected with the administration of physiologic amounts of cortisol.

12 Hyponatremia in the setting of extrarenal volume loss is the result of the stimulation of ADH release. Water excretion is impaired even in the presence of avid sodium reabsorption by the kidney.

13 When the kidney is the source of abnormal fluid and electrolyte losses, sodium reabsorption may be impaired even in the presence of volume depletion and hyponatremia.

14 The combination of decreased Na reabsorption due to the lack of mineralocorticoid and the impaired water excretion resulting from decreased glucocorticoid levels (see No. 11) accounts for the hyponatremia seen with adrenal insufficiency.

15 Diuretic use is the most common cause of hyponatremia in the volume-depleted patient. Sodium is lost by impaired renal tubular reabsorption, whereas water excretion is impaired by both ADH secretion and the decrease of fluid delivery to the diluting portions of the nephron. Hyponatremia is most common with the thiazide diuretics.

16 Salt-losing nephritis is most commonly seen in advanced forms of renal disease with the GFR less than 10 ml/min. Medullary cystic disease, polycystic disease, obstructive nephropathy, analgesic nephropathy, and chronic pyelonephritis are the most commonly associated conditions. Salt wasting occurs because of tubular dysfunction, whereas water excretion is impaired by the same mechanism seen in other forms of renal failure (see No. 5).

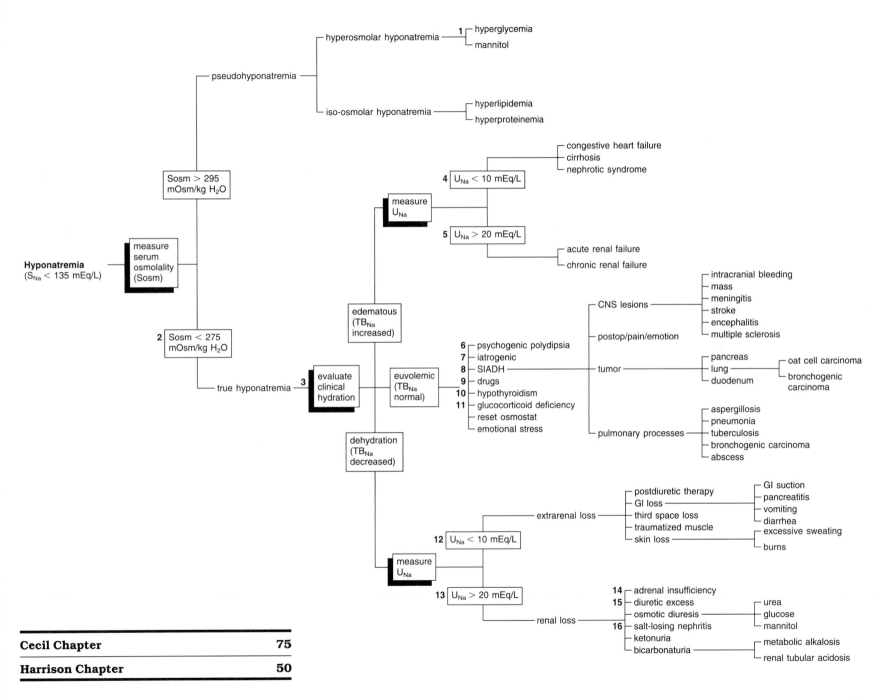

Hyponatremia
(S_{Na} < 135 mEq/L)

measure serum osmolality (Sosm)

pseudohyponatremia

Sosm > 295 mOsm/kg H_2O

hyperosmolar hyponatremia — **1** ⌐ hyperglycemia
└ mannitol

iso-osmolar hyponatremia — ⌐ hyperlipidemia
└ hyperproteinemia

2 Sosm < 275 mOsm/kg H_2O

true hyponatremia — **3** evaluate clinical hydration

edematous (TB_{Na} increased)

measure U_{Na}

4 U_{Na} < 10 mEq/L ⌐ congestive heart failure
├ cirrhosis
└ nephrotic syndrome

5 U_{Na} > 20 mEq/L ⌐ acute renal failure
└ chronic renal failure

euvolemic (TB_{Na} normal)

6 ⌐ psychogenic polydipsia
7 ├ iatrogenic
8 ├ SIADH
9 ├ drugs
10 ├ hypothyroidism
11 ├ glucocorticoid deficiency
├ reset osmostat
└ emotional stress

CNS lesions ⌐ intracranial bleeding
├ mass
├ meningitis
├ stroke
├ encephalitis
└ multiple sclerosis

postop/pain/emotion

tumor ⌐ pancreas
├ lung ⌐ oat cell carcinoma
└ duodenum └ bronchogenic carcinoma

pulmonary processes ⌐ aspergillosis
├ pneumonia
├ tuberculosis
├ bronchogenic carcinoma
└ abscess

dehydration (TB_{Na} decreased)

measure U_{Na}

12 U_{Na} < 10 mEq/L

extrarenal loss ⌐ postdiuretic therapy
├ GI loss ⌐ GI suction
│ ├ pancreatitis
│ ├ vomiting
│ └ diarrhea
├ third space loss
├ traumatized muscle
└ skin loss ⌐ excessive sweating
└ burns

13 U_{Na} > 20 mEq/L

renal loss **14** ⌐ adrenal insufficiency
15 ├ diuretic excess
├ osmotic diuresis ⌐ urea
│ ├ glucose
│ └ mannitol
16 ├ salt-losing nephritis
├ ketonuria
└ bicarbonaturia ⌐ metabolic alkalosis
└ renal tubular acidosis

Cecil Chapter   **75**

Harrison Chapter   **50**

Hypernatremia

1 Hypernatremia always represents a state of hyperosmolality. The serum osmolality can be calculated using the following formula:

$$(1.95)(P_{Na} + P_K) + BUN/2.8 + Glucose/18 = \text{calculated osmolality}$$

where P_{Na} is plasma sodium and P_K is plasma potassium. If the measured osmolality deviates by more than 10 mOsm from the calculated osmolality, the source of the unmeasured osmolality must be sought. Examples of commonly unmeasured osmolar substances include mannitol, alcohol, and ethylene glycol.

2 In the disorders associated with a urine/plasma osmolality of greater than 0.7, the total body sodium is usually low, with the hypernatremia a result of a free water deficit.

3 The hypernatremia often associated with hypercatabolic states such as severe burns is secondary to the osmotic diuresis caused by the production of excess urea. Hypercatabolic patients, along with those patients receiving the protein hydrolysate contained in hyperalimentation solutions, may develop hypernatremia unless sodium and free water are adequately replaced.

4 In the disorders in which the urine/plasma osmolality is variable, the urine sodium concentration is usually greater than 20 mEq/L. Urine sodium in this range is usually associated with normal or increased total body sodium.

5 The slight increases in serum sodium seen in Cushing's disease and primary hyperaldosteronism, although common, are rarely of clinical significance.

6 If urine/plasma osmolality is less than 0.7, the total body sodium is normal or slightly elevated. The hypernatremia results from a deficit of free water.

7 Polydipsia, the excessive intake of water, causes expansion and dilution of the extracellular fluids. As serum osmolality falls, ADH is suppressed and hypernatremia can result. Primary polydipsia may result from an abnormality in the osmolar regulation of thirst but more commonly is associated with psychiatric disorders.

8 Central diabetes insipidus is a primary failure of ADH production in the pituitary gland. Although approximately 50 per cent of the cases are idiopathic, central diabetes insipidus has several known etiologies. Disorders associated with central diabetes insipidus include trauma, a primary tumor in the sellar area (pinealoma, craniopharyngioma, and metastatic disease, most commonly from breast and lung), infections of the central nervous system (Guillain-Barré syndrome and syphilis), granulomatous diseases (sarcoidosis, tuberculosis, and Wegener's granulomatosis), histiocytic diseases, vascular events associated with sickle cell disease, aneurysms, cerebral vascular accidents, and postpartum necrosis (Sheehan's syndrome). Rarely, central diabetes insipidus can occur during, or as a sequela of, infections of the central nervous system.

9 Osmoreceptor ablation can occur when a lesion involves the area of the hypothalamus where the osmoreceptors are located. Many lesions involving this area of the hypothalamus have been implicated, including granulomas, hydrocephalus, vascular occlusion, tumors, and degenerative disorders.

10 Congenital nephrogenic diabetes insipidus is a rare X-linked disorder in which the distal tubule is unresponsive to ADH. The mechanism of the ADH resistance is not known but may represent an abnormality of ADH-mediated cyclic adenosine monophosphate.

11 Acquired nephrogenic diabetes insipidus is most commonly associated with renal diseases such as polycystic disease, chronic pyelonephritis, and ureteral obstruction. Other causes of acquired diabetes insipidus include direct drug effects on the renal tubules and collecting system as seen with alcohol, lithium, demeclocycline, sulfonylureas, amphotericin, iodinated dyes, fluorinated anesthetics, and various antibiotics, as well as sickle cell disease, multiple myeloma, amyloidosis, sarcoidosis, and Sjögren's disease.

12 The hypernatremia associated with paroxysmal atrial tachycardia appears to be caused by a primary suppression of ADH release with a resultant water diuresis.

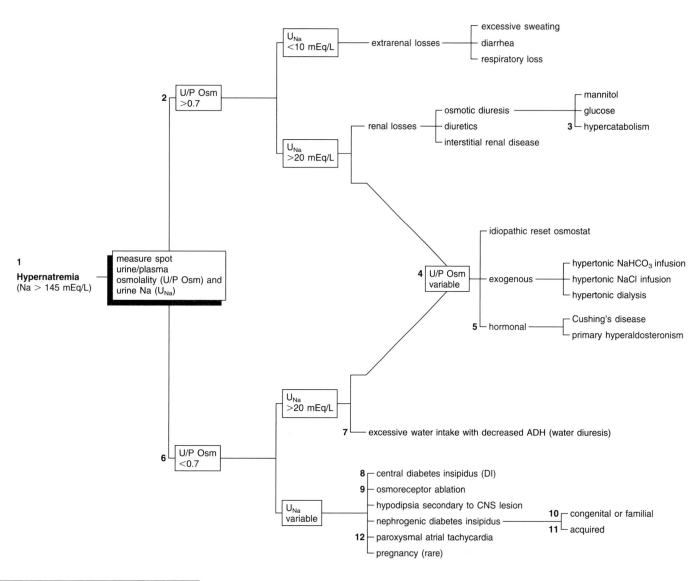

1

Hypernatremia
(Na > 145 mEq/L)

measure spot
urine/plasma
osmolality (U/P Osm) and
urine Na (U$_{Na}$)

2 U/P Osm
>0.7

U$_{Na}$
<10 mEq/L

extrarenal losses

excessive sweating

diarrhea

respiratory loss

U$_{Na}$
>20 mEq/L

renal losses

osmotic diuresis

mannitol

glucose

3 hypercatabolism

diuretics

interstitial renal disease

4 U/P Osm
variable

idiopathic reset osmostat

exogenous

hypertonic NaHCO$_3$ infusion

hypertonic NaCl infusion

hypertonic dialysis

5 hormonal

Cushing's disease

primary hyperaldosteronism

6 U/P Osm
<0.7

U$_{Na}$
>20 mEq/L

7 excessive water intake with decreased ADH (water diuresis)

U$_{Na}$
variable

8 central diabetes insipidus (DI)

9 osmoreceptor ablation

hypodipsia secondary to CNS lesion

nephrogenic diabetes insipidus

10 congenital or familial

11 acquired

12 paroxysmal atrial tachycardia

pregnancy (rare)

Cecil Chapter	**75**
Harrison Chapter	**50**

Hypokalemia

1 Elevated renin production resulting in elevated aldosterone levels will cause hypokalemia by increasing renal secretion of potassium. Malignant hypertension, renovascular hypertension, and renin-secreting tumors are the most common disorders associated with elevated renins.

2 Increased aldosterone production of any etiology can cause hypokalemia by enhancing distal tubular secretion of potassium. The hypokalemia can develop, however, only if distal fluid delivery is adequate. Disorders associated with increased aldosterone production such as congestive heart failure, cirrhosis, and nephrotic syndrome may also cause decreased renal perfusion, and the hypokalemia may not occur until diuretic therapy increases distal tubule fluid delivery.

3 Pseudohyperaldosteronism, or Liddle's syndrome, has all the clinical manifestations of aldosterone excess including hypertension, metabolic alkalosis, and hypokalemia as a result of renal potassium wasting. The etiology, however, is tubular, with hyperabsorption of sodium (Na) and volume expansion with resulting hypersecretion of potassium and H^+.

4 Hypokalemia is commonly associated with renal tubular acidosis (RTA). In proximal RTA, the potassium loss is due to increased delivery of Na and HCO_3 to the distal tubule. In distal RTA, increased potassium secretion is due at least in part to decreased H^+ secretion and the need to maintain cationic balance. Hyperaldosteronism is also seen in this disorder and may contribute to the hypokalemia.

5 Protracted vomiting is a common cause of hypokalemia. The potassium loss, however, is not from the loss of gastric fluid itself. Because gastric fluid contains only 5 to 10 mEq/L of potassium, massive losses would be necessary to deplete the body's potassium stores. Vomiting can, however, cause volume contraction that stimulates aldosterone production and the development of hypochloremic metabolic alkalosis. Both of these factors increase the renal excretion of potassium (see No. 2 and No. 12).

6 Bartter's syndrome, a disorder of uncertain etiology, consists of muscle weakness, polyuria, metabolic alkalosis, potassium wasting, and elevated renin in the absence of hypertension. The syndrome occurs most commonly in children. Although the mechanism of the disorder is uncertain, increased aldosterone and increased urinary prostaglandins appear to play a role.

7 Hypokalemia is seen commonly in association with magnesium (Mg) depletion. The mechanism is not known. Like the hypocalcemia seen with Mg depletion, the hypokalemia cannot be corrected until the Mg is repleted.

8 Diuretics, whose site of action is proximal to the sites of potassium secretion in the distal tubule, may cause profound potassium wasting. Several factors enter into the mechanism of potassium loss. These factors include increased delivery of fluid to the distal tubule, volume contraction with stimulation of aldosterone secretion, and the metabolic alkalosis seen with volume contraction (see No. 12).

9 Several drugs have been associated with hypokalemia. The most common of these are the semisynthetic penicillins such as carbenicillin, piperacillin, and ticarcillin. The hypokalemia is caused by the delivery of large quantities of Na and nonresorbable anions to the distal tubule. The aminoglycosides, most notably gentamicin, can also cause renal potassium wasting. Intracellular potassium depletion in the renal tubule is thought to play a part in the mechanism of nephrotoxicity of these drugs.

10 Hypokalemia can be seen in certain forms of both acute and chronic leukemia and is most commonly associated with lysozymuria.

11 Osmotic diuresis, most commonly associated with glycosuria, may cause profound potassium wasting and hypokalemia. The hypokalemia is secondary to increased delivery of fluid past the distal tubular potassium secretory sites, thereby increasing potassium loss. Diabetic ketoacidosis may be associated with a potassium deficit of as much as 200 to 300 mEq. The acidosis and insulin deficiency may mask this deficit, but severe life-threatening hypokalemia may develop when treatment is begun if potassium is not adequately repleted.

12 Alkalosis may cause mild hypokalemia by shifting potassium from the extracellular to the intracellular space. The effect is not nearly as profound as that seen with the hyperkalemia associated with acidosis. Respiratory alkalosis by itself causes little change in the serum potassium.

13 Hypokalemic periodic paralysis is an uncommon and usually familial disorder. Sporadic cases have also been described, and there appears to be an occasional association with thyrotoxicosis. Episodes of paralysis due to a rapid redistribution of potassium into the cells can be precipitated by various factors known to have a direct or indirect effect on potassium balance. These include carbohydrate-rich foods, insulin, glucose, beta-adrenergic agonists, adrenocorticotropic hormone (ACTH), and some mineralocorticoids. During an attack, plasma potassium may fall to 1 to 2 mEq/L. Diazoxide, propranolol, spironolactone, and acetazolamide have been shown to abort attacks.

14 Although the kidneys are efficient at conserving potassium, prolonged decreased intake of potassium will lead to total body potassium depletion and hypokalemia. Protein- and calorie-poor diets will also be lacking in potassium. True starvation and decreased intake secondary to psychological causes (anorexia nervosa) may lead to profound potassium depletion. Elderly patients with limited access to food or the inability to prepare balanced diets may become potassium depleted, hence the name "tea and toast syndrome."

15 Geophagia, a form of pica most common in the southern United States, may lead to profound hypokalemia. In this syndrome, large quantities of red clay are ingested. The red clay binds potassium in the intestine and prevents adequate absorption.

16 Perspiration contains a high concentration of potassium. Chronic loss such as is seen with routine vigorous exercise and work in hot environments can lead to excessive loss of potassium, especially if the fluid is replaced with solutions containing low or no potassium. Hypokalemia of mild-to-moderate degree has been reported in women during the perimenopausal period if flushing with heavy perspiration is extreme. Replacement fluids high in potassium, such as certain juices or sports drinks, may prevent this problem.

17 Large amounts of potassium can be lost in diarrheal stools. The stool water itself may be high in potassium. In addition, the volume contraction may increase renal potassium losses (see No. 5).

18 Villous adenomas, which constitute 2 to 12 per cent of colonic tumors, are commonly associated with hypokalemia. Potassium concentration in the se-

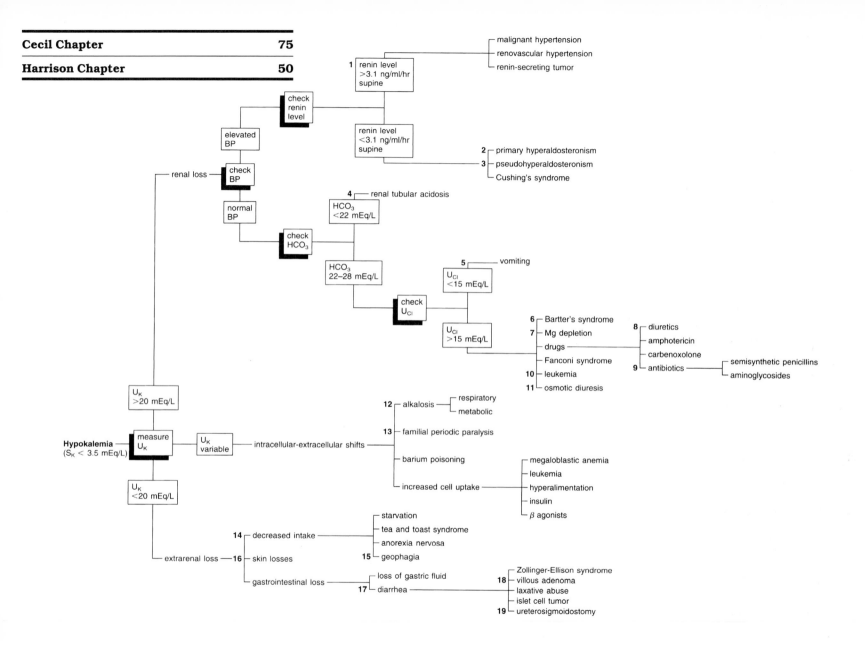

creted mucus may be as high as 80 mEq/L. Volumes of diarrhea may reach 1 to 3 liters per day. This direct loss of potassium, along with the volume contraction seen in this disorder, leads to the hypokalemia.

19 Ureterosigmoidostomy is now an uncommon urinary diversion procedure in which the ureters are implanted in an isolated portion of the sigmoid colon. Secretion of potassium and bicarbonate into the lumen of the sigmoid loop leads to both metabolic acidosis and hypokalemia. The now more common ileal loop allows for a more rapid transit time of the urine in the loop of bowel and less potassium loss.

Hyperkalemia

1 Pseudohyperkalemia is caused by the in vitro release of potassium from leukocytes, platelets, or red cells. The potassium is released when the walls of these potassium-rich cells rupture during the clotting process, which occurs after the blood has been collected. If pseudohyperkalemia is suspected, plasma potassium should be measured. Under normal circumstances, there should be no more than a 0.3-mEq/L difference between serum and plasma potassium.

2 Hyperkalemia from increased dietary potassium in the absence of renal insufficiency or hypoaldosteronism is rare. The administration of high doses of the potassium salts of various antibiotics such as potassium penicillin, or the treatment of hypokalemia with oral or intravenous potassium, has, however, been associated with life-threatening hyperkalemia.

3 The release of potassium from endogenous sources is more likely than increased dietary intake of potassium alone to cause hyperkalemia. Large quantities of potassium may be released from the hemolysis of transfused red blood cells. A large potassium load can be avoided by using blood that has been stored a short time or saline-washed prior to transfusion.

4 The relationship between acidosis and hyperkalemia is well known and until recently was believed to be relatively constant, with potassium rising 0.6 mEq/L for each fall of 0.1 pH unit. It is now known, however, that the type of acidosis, the duration of the acidosis, and the anion associated with the elevated hydrogen ion concentration are important factors influencing potassium concentration. Respiratory acidosis has a much smaller effect on serum potassium than does metabolic acidosis. Metabolic acidosis associated with mineral acids such as chloride, phosphate, and sulfate causes a greater shift of potassium out of the cells than do organic acids such as lactate or the ketoacids. This effect is caused by the impermeability of the cells to the mineral anions, forcing a greater shift of potassium out of the cells in order to maintain electrical neutrality. The profound hyperkalemia that can be seen in diabetic ketoacidosis is more a reflection of the insulin deficiency (see No. 5) and the hypoaldosteronism (see No. 15) than the actual acidosis.

5 Insulin has great importance in the maintenance of potassium homeostasis. When insulin secretion either is inhibited chemically with somatostatin or is absent in type 1 diabetes mellitus, both basal serum potassium and serum potassium after a potassium load rise. Hyperkalemia may occur in the setting of insulin deficiency alone, but a variety of other factors contribute to the hyperkalemia associated with diabetes. These factors include acidemia during episodes of ketoacidosis, hypertonicity associated with elevated blood glucose, diabetes-associated renal insufficiency, and the selective hypoaldosteronism that can be seen with diabetes mellitus.

6 The digitalis glycosides have been associated with life-threatening hyperkalemia when taken in toxic amounts. The hyperkalemia is thought to be due to inhibition by digitalis of the cellular uptake of potassium. Although hyperkalemia is a consistent finding in severe digitalis intoxication, therapeutic digitalis levels have little effect on serum potassium.

7 The muscle relaxant and paralyzing agent succinylcholine may cause mild hyperkalemia in normal patients because of increases in the ionic permeability of the muscle cells with consequent movement of potassium into the extracellular space. In many neuromuscular disorders, however, severe hyperkalemia may develop after administration of drugs like succinylcholine.

8 The treatment of metabolic alkalosis with arginine or lysine hydrochloric acid (HCl) may cause severe hyperkalemia. Patients with impaired renal function appear especially susceptible. The etiology of the hyperkalemia is thought to be due to movement of potassium from the intracellular to the extracellular space caused by the amino acids themselves rather than the actual change in pH.

9 The hyperkalemia associated with heparin administration is due to impaired aldosterone production. Heparin acts directly on the adrenal zona glomerulosa. The synthesis of aldosterone is impaired by heparin's inhibition of 18-hydroxylase activity. The hyperkalemic effect of heparin may be seen within 2 to 4 days after its initiation.

10 The hyperkalemia seen with the angiotensin-converting enzyme (ACE) inhibitors is multifactorial. Decreased aldosterone synthesis as well as a derangement of the tubular potassium secretory mechanism has been implicated. Severe hyperkalemia in the absence of impaired renal function is rare.

11 Hyperkalemia has occasionally been observed following the use of nonsteroidal anti-inflammatory drugs (NSAIDs). The inhibition of certain prostaglandins may inhibit aldosterone production as well as altering renal hemodynamics and reducing GFR. The effect is reversible within 1 to 2 weeks after discontinuing the drug.

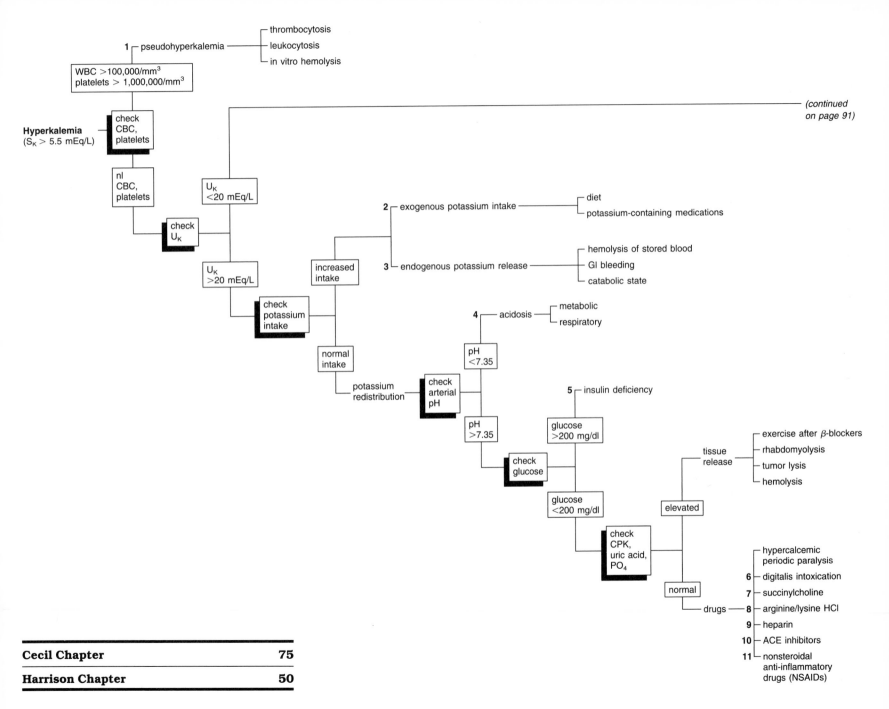

1 ┬ pseudohyperkalemia ─┬ thrombocytosis
                        ├ leukocytosis
                        └ in vitro hemolysis

WBC >100,000/mm³
platelets > 1,000,000/mm³

(continued on page 91)

Hyperkalemia
(S_K > 5.5 mEq/L)

check CBC, platelets

nl CBC, platelets

check U_K

U_K <20 mEq/L

U_K >20 mEq/L

2 ┬ exogenous potassium intake ─┬ diet
                                 └ potassium-containing medications

3 └ endogenous potassium release ─┬ hemolysis of stored blood
                                    ├ GI bleeding
                                    └ catabolic state

increased intake

check potassium intake

normal intake

4 ┬ acidosis ─┬ metabolic
             └ respiratory

pH <7.35

potassium redistribution

check arterial pH

pH >7.35

5 ┬ insulin deficiency

glucose >200 mg/dl

check glucose

glucose <200 mg/dl

tissue release ─┬ exercise after β-blockers
                ├ rhabdomyolysis
                ├ tumor lysis
                └ hemolysis

elevated

check CPK, uric acid, PO_4

normal

drugs ─┬ hypercalcemic periodic paralysis
       6 ├ digitalis intoxication
       7 ├ succinylcholine
       8 ├ arginine/lysine HCl
       9 ├ heparin
       10 ├ ACE inhibitors
       11 └ nonsteroidal anti-inflammatory drugs (NSAIDs)

Cecil Chapter	75
Harrison Chapter	50

Hyperkalemia (Continued)

12 Acute oliguric renal failure is usually associated with hyperkalemia. The hyperkalemia is due to a combination of interrelated factors. First, the GFR usually approaches zero, causing decreased potassium filtration. Second, the markedly decreased GFR decreases exchangeable sodium and fluid delivery to the distal tubule where potassium is secreted. Third, if the etiology of the acute renal failure is tubular damage, there is a reduction in the number of tubular cells available for potassium secretion. Finally, most of the patients with acute renal failure also have increased tissue catabolism, releasing more potassium into the extracellular space.

13 Hyperkalemia is unusual in chronic renal failure until the GFR approaches 10 to 15 ml/min. At this level of GFR, there is inadequate delivery of fluid to the distal tubular sites of potassium secretion. Acute potassium loads, however, can cause life-threatening hyperkalemia even with moderate renal failure. Patients with interstitial nephritis or diabetic nephropathy may develop hyperkalemia at a higher GFR because of more extensive tubular damage or associated hypoaldosteronism.

14 Hypoaldosteronism is usually associated with a renin deficiency, most commonly occurring in the elderly and in patients with diabetes mellitus. A significant proportion of patients with evidence of hypoaldosteronism, however, have no detectable reduction in renin production. These patients have a selective decrease in aldosterone production because of a generalized adrenal insufficiency, as seen in Addison's disease, or an alteration in some portion of the synthetic pathway for aldosterone, such as deficiencies in C-21-hydroxylase.

15 Renin deficiency is usually a result of damage to the juxtaglomerular cells. The damage may be due to the sclerosis accompanying aging or destruction of the cells seen in interstitial nephritis. Hydronephrosis is also a common cause of decreased renin production, and hyperkalemia may be a presenting sign of this condition. The hyperkalemia often associated with diabetes mellitus is partially due to the high frequency of decreased renin production causing hypoaldosteronism.

16 Several drugs may cause hyperkalemia by reductions in plasma renin activity and aldosterone. Several of the drugs may also change renal hemodynamics or alter prostaglandin synthesis. Cyclosporine, a widely used antirejection drug, is typical of drugs with these effects.

17 A number of drugs may decrease renal tubular secretion of potassium independent of any effect on aldosterone production or action. Triamterene and amiloride are potent inhibitors of potassium secretion. These drugs are usually combined with other diuretics to prevent excessive potassium losses. The use of these drugs in the setting of renal insufficiency or hypoaldosteronism may lead to life-threatening hyperkalemia.

18 Several primary renal diseases, as well as certain systemic diseases with renal involvement, may cause a primary defect in the secretion of potassium. The exact mechanism of the defect is not certain but may involve reduced tubular sensitivity to aldosterone as well as an increased tubular absorption of chloride ion.

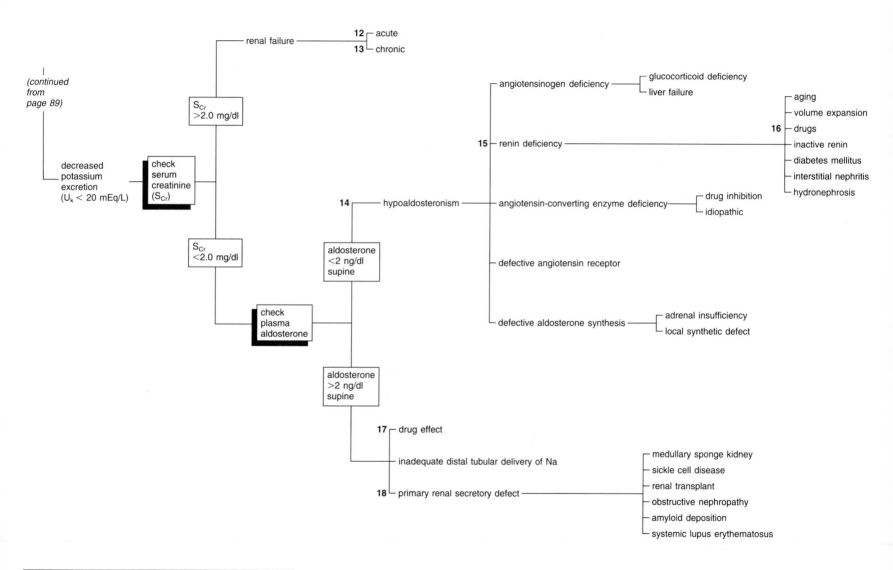

(continued from page 89)

decreased potassium excretion ($U_k < 20$ mEq/L)

check serum creatinine (S_{Cr})

S_{Cr} >2.0 mg/dl

S_{Cr} <2.0 mg/dl

renal failure

12 ┌ acute
13 └ chronic

check plasma aldosterone

aldosterone <2 ng/dl supine

aldosterone >2 ng/dl supine

14 hypoaldosteronism

angiotensinogen deficiency ┌ glucocorticoid deficiency
└ liver failure

15 renin deficiency

┌ aging
├ volume expansion
16 ├ drugs
├ inactive renin
├ diabetes mellitus
├ interstitial nephritis
└ hydronephrosis

angiotensin-converting enzyme deficiency ┌ drug inhibition
└ idiopathic

defective angiotensin receptor

defective aldosterone synthesis ┌ adrenal insufficiency
└ local synthetic defect

17 ┌ drug effect

├ inadequate distal tubular delivery of Na

18 └ primary renal secretory defect

┌ medullary sponge kidney
├ sickle cell disease
├ renal transplant
├ obstructive nephropathy
├ amyloid deposition
└ systemic lupus erythematosus

Cecil Chapter	**75**
Harrison Chapter	**50**

Hypocalcemia

1 Approximately 40 per cent of the total calcium (Ca) in the serum is bound to proteins, with 80 to 90 per cent of this Ca bound to albumin. A decrease in serum albumin will decrease the amount of protein-bound Ca and therefore the total Ca. An approximation of this effect can be obtained by assuming a 0.8-mg/dl change in serum Ca for each 1-gm/dl change in albumin concentration. Globulins have a much smaller effect. A change of 1 gm/dl in globulin concentration will change serum Ca concentration by approximately 0.12 mg/dl. Changes in pH can also affect protein binding by Ca. A change of 0.1 pH unit will change protein-bound Ca by 0.12 mg/dl.

2 Ionized hypocalcemia is most commonly seen in the setting of resuscitation of trauma patients in the Emergency Department. The etiology is multifactorial and includes administration of large volumes of crystalloids and citrated blood products, as well as iodinated contrast dye and hyperventilation therapy for severe head injury. The incidence of ionized hypocalcemia in this setting is unclear, but it should be suspected when refractory hypotension or electromechanical dissociation occurs. Ionized hypocalcemia may also be seen during blood component pheresis procedures when the donor is given too little calcium to counteract the effects of citrate used during the procedure.

3 Parathyroid hormone (PTH) is a single-chain polypeptide of 84 amino acids with a molecular weight of 9500. Biologic activity resides in the N-terminal portion consisting of the amino acid sequence 1–34. The PTH effect on kidney and bone is mediated through the activation of adenylcyclase, with the subsequent formation of cyclic adenosine 3',5'-monophosphate (cyclic AMP). Several radioimmunoassays are available to measure PTH. These include assays for the N-terminal and carboxy or C-terminal, as well as the whole molecule. Measurement of the C-terminal portion or the whole molecule appears to be best correlated with clinical disorders of PTH except in renal failure. With renal failure, the C-terminal, or inactive fragments, accumulate, and measurement of the N-terminal is necessary for an accurate measurement of active PTH.

4 The most common cause of hypoparathyroidism is the surgical removal of one or more parathyroid glands because of an adenoma or hyperplasia. Damage to the glands can also occur during thyroid or other extensive neck surgery. The usual postoperative fall in serum Ca is temporary if it is related to suppression of the parathyroid glands from the previous long-standing hypercalcemia, or if rapid remineralization of bone occurs, as with the hungry bone syndrome (see No. 17). In these cases, serum Ca usually will not fall below 8.5 mg/dl, and the hypocalcemia does not last for more than 7 to 10 days. Prolonged hypocalcemia or a more profound decrease in serum Ca is indicative of possible permanent hypoparathyroidism, and appropriate treatment should be started. Infiltrative diseases of the parathyroid glands such as amyloidosis, hemochromatosis related to thalassemia or Wilson's disease, and metastatic cancer may also cause hypoparathyroidism. Idiopathic hypoparathyroidism begins either in childhood as a sex-linked recessive disorder or in adolescence as an autosomal recessive disorder. Hypoparathyroidism has also been associated with adrenal insufficiency and has been described in association with pernicious anemia. Aminoglycoside antibiotics and certain cytotoxic agents may also directly suppress production of PTH.

5 Vitamin D (vit D) is present in many plants and as 7-dehydrocholesterol in the skin of humans. Skin exposure to ultraviolet radiation converts the 7-dehydrocholesterol to cholecalciferol (vit D_3), the primary endogenous source of vit D. Vit D_3 is then metabolized to 25(OH)-vit D_3 (calcifediol) in the liver. The calcifediol undergoes enterohepatic circulation and is further metabolized in the kidney to 1,25-dihydroxy vit D_3 (calcitriol) via the enzyme 1-hydroxylase. Calcitriol is the most biologically active form of vit D. Biochemical properties of vit D include increased absorption of Ca and PO_4 in the intestine and possibly increased mineralization of bone. Production of calcitriol is increased by PTH, a low Ca diet, and hypophosphatemia. There is a marked reduction in the production of calcitriol in advanced renal failure. Calcitriol also exists in the 24,25-dihydroxy form, but its significance is unclear.

6 Malabsorption of vit D may be a result of a reduction of intraluminal bile salts, rapid intestinal transit time, or mucosal disease in the gastrointestinal (GI) tract. In each of these cases there is decreased vit D absorption, and increased fecal loss of the 25(OH)-vit D derived from enterohepatic circulation. Clinical conditions associated with malabsorption of vit D include gastrectomy, tropical and nontropical sprue, chronic pancreatitis, biliary cirrhosis, laxative abuse, and intestinal bypass.

7 Increased metabolism with a shortened half-life of vit D_3 and 25(OH)-vit D_3 is thought to be the result of microsomal enzyme induction in the liver secondary to the use of anticonvulsant drugs. Increased metabolism causes a more rapid turnover of vit D along with production of certain inactive forms of vit D.

8 Ethanol (ETOH) may act to reduce vit D levels via poor nutrition and hepatic dysfunction.

9 The decreased levels of vit D in nephrotic syndrome have been attributed to the loss of vit D–binding globulin in the urine. The clinical significance of hypocalcemia in this setting is unclear.

10 Decreased production of vit D and subsequent hypocalcemia are common in liver disease, because the liver is the site of the conversion of vit D into one of its active forms.

11 Advanced renal failure with GFR less than 25 ml/min is associated with decreased production of the 1,25-dihydroxy form of vit D. The exact mechanism of this decreased production is not well understood but is probably related to the decrease in renal mass. The availability of oral 1,25-dihydroxy vit D has helped to prevent much of the bone disease associated with renal failure.

12 The bone disease seen with vit D–dependent rickets is a result of a deficiency in the 1-hydroxylase enzyme that metabolizes 25(OH)-vit D_3 to the more active form 1,25-dihydroxy vit D_3. Pharmacologic doses of vit D or small doses of the 1,25-dihydroxy form of vit D are effective in treating this disorder.

13 In pseudo–idiopathic hypoparathyroidism, hypocalcemia is thought to be due to production of an abnormal PTH molecule or cleavage of the PTH prohormone at an incorrect site. The hypocalcemia responds to the administration of exogenous PTH. The elevated levels of PTH in this disorder are secondary to the hypocalcemia.

14 Pseudohypoparathyroidism is a rare inheritable disease consisting of the somatic manifestations of mental retardation, short stature, brachydactyly, exostosis, and "expressionless face." Biochemical abnormalities include hypocalcemia and hyperphosphatemia. The disorder can take two forms. Type 1A has both the somatic and biochemical abnormalities, whereas type 1B

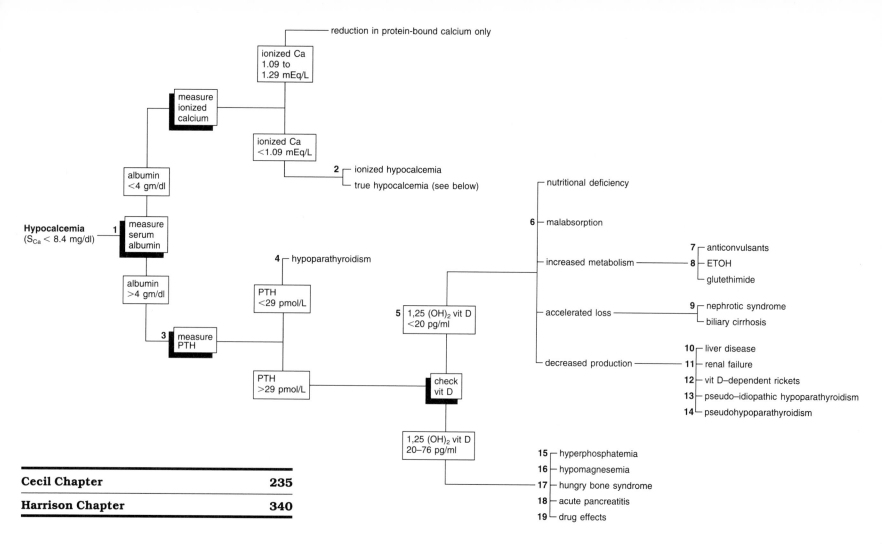

reduction in protein-bound calcium only

ionized Ca
1.09 to
1.29 mEq/L

measure
ionized
calcium

ionized Ca
<1.09 mEq/L

2 ┌ ionized hypocalcemia
  └ true hypocalcemia (see below)

nutritional deficiency

albumin
<4 gm/dl

6 ─ malabsorption

Hypocalcemia
(S_{Ca} < 8.4 mg/dl)

1 │ measure
    serum
    albumin

4 ─ hypoparathyroidism

increased metabolism ───── 7 ┌ anticonvulsants
                            8 ├ ETOH
                              └ glutethimide

albumin
>4 gm/dl

PTH
<29 pmol/L

accelerated loss ───── 9 ┌ nephrotic syndrome
                         └ biliary cirrhosis

5 │ 1,25 (OH)$_2$ vit D
    <20 pg/ml

3 │ measure
    PTH

decreased production ───── 10 ┌ liver disease
                           11 ├ renal failure
                           12 ├ vit D–dependent rickets
                           13 ├ pseudo–idiopathic hypoparathyroidism
                           14 └ pseudohypoparathyroidism

PTH
>29 pmol/L

check
vit D

1,25 (OH)$_2$ vit D
20–76 pg/ml

15 ┌ hyperphosphatemia
16 ├ hypomagnesemia
17 ├ hungry bone syndrome
18 ├ acute pancreatitis
19 └ drug effects

presents with only the biochemical abnormalities. The mechanism of the biochemical abnormalities is thought to be due to end-organ unresponsiveness to PTH secondary to a presumed failure of renal and bone adenyl cyclase stimulation. There is no response to exogenous PTH administration. PTH levels are again increased owing to hypocalcemia.

15 The mechanism for the reduction in serum Ca with hyperphosphatemia is unknown but is possibly deposition of $CaPO_4$ in bone and soft tissue. Either the endogenous release or the increased intake of PO_4 can be associated with decreases in serum Ca. A product of serum Ca and PO_4 greater than 70 is associated with an increased risk for the precipitation of $CaPO_4$ in the tissues.

16 The hypocalcemia associated with hypomagnesemia arises from a combination of PTH suppression and skeletal resistance to the effects of PTH. The hypocalcemia will usually not respond to treatment until the Mg level has been restored to normal.

17 The mechanism of the hypocalcemia seen in the hungry bone syndrome is the same as that described in the section on hypophosphatemia (see page 96).

18 Both the precipitation of intra-abdominal Ca soaps and the suppression of PTH are thought to be responsible for the hypocalcemia, at times profound, seen in acute pancreatitis.

19 Several drugs including colchicine and estrogen have been associated with hypocalcemia. Both mithramycin and calcitonin have been used therapeutically for their calcium-lowering effects. A decreased ionized Ca may be seen following transfusion of large amounts of citrated blood.

Hypercalcemia

1 Average dietary intake of Ca is 900 mg, with only 30 to 35 per cent of this Ca absorbed in the small bowel. There are both active and passive components to absorption; the active component requires vit D. Between 150 and 200 mg of Ca are absorbed from the GI tract. This absorption presents the extracellular fluid with 150 to 200 mg of Ca per day. Because there is no net gain or loss of bone Ca under normal circumstances, renal excretion is approximately 150 to 200 mg/day. Ninety-eight per cent of the filtered load of Ca is reabsorbed. Sixty to 70 per cent of Ca is reabsorbed in the proximal tubule, 20 to 25 per cent in the loop of Henle, and 5 to 10 per cent in the distal tubule, where absorption is influenced by PTH. Ca reabsorption by the renal tubule is enhanced by PTH and metabolic alkalosis and inhibited by metabolic acidosis and phosphate depletion.

2 The effects of albumin concentration on serum Ca are described on page 92. In diseases with increased paraprotein production, such as multiple myeloma, there may be sufficient elevation in the Ca-binding protein to produce an increase in the total serum Ca, although ionized Ca is normal.

3 Primary hyperparathyroidism is seen most commonly in women over 60 years of age. Eighty per cent of patients have a single parathyroid adenoma. Hyperplasia, multiple adenomas, and the rare parathyroid carcinoma account for the remainder of cases. Apart from the multiple endocrine neoplasia (MEN) syndromes described below, several disorders, including sarcoidosis, Hashimoto's disease, some malignancies, medullary sponge kidney, and Cushing's syndrome, have been associated with primary hyperparathyroidism. Laboratory findings in primary hyperparathyroidism may include hypercalciuria, low or normal inorganic phosphate level, normal alkaline phosphatase (in the absence of overt bone disease), a PTH level inappropriately high for the level of serum Ca, and elevated urinary cyclic AMP (cAMP) excretion.

4 Ninety per cent of patients with MEN 1 have hyperparathyroidism secondary to parathyroid hyperplasia. MEN 1 is also associated with pituitary and pancreatic islet tumors, including Zollinger-Ellison syndrome. MEN 1 is inherited as an autosomal dominant trait.

5 In MEN 2, parathyroid hyperplasia is associated with medullary carcinoma of the thyroid, and pheochromocytoma. MEN 2 is also inherited as an autosomal dominant trait.

6 Isolated adult hyperparathyroidism is a rare disorder with poorly understood inheritance. MEN syndromes must first be eliminated before the diagnosis can be made.

7 Familial hypocalciuric hyperparathyroidism is an autosomal dominant disorder with onset at an early age, hypocalciuria, occasional hypermagnesemia, and a benign course.

8 Lithium-induced hypercalcemia is a benign condition with hypercalcemia thought to be due to decreased entry of Ca into the parathyroid cells, thereby altering the set point for PTH release. It is reversible by discontinuing the drug.

9 Increased PTH with subsequent hypercalcemia can be seen in the recovery phase of acute renal failure due to rhabdomyolysis.

10 Tertiary hyperparathyroidism describes the development of autonomous hyperparathyroidism following a prolonged period of secondary hyperparathyroidism with its associated parathyroid hyperplasia. Several cases have been described in celiac disease. Far more common is the secondary hyperparathyroidism seen in chronic renal failure. This hyperparathyroidism is probably a result of hypocalcemia, hyperphosphatemia, and altered vit D metabolism. Hypercalcemia may occur for varying periods of time following correction of the renal failure with recovery or renal transplant. The persistent hypercalcemia of tertiary hyperparathyroidism is due to the now autonomous function of the parathyroid glands.

11 The effects of vit D intoxication may last for months after the discontinuation of the vit D. The effect probably results from high levels of 25(OH)-vit D, which has a half-life of 10 to 20 days.

12 Up to 25 per cent of patients with sarcoidosis have hypercalcemia. Etiologies of the hypercalcemia include intestinal hyperabsorption of Ca as well as elevated levels of 1,25(OH)$_2$-vit D, probably of nonrenal origin. The granulomatous tissue itself is the most likely source of the increased vit D. The same increase in vit D has been seen in other granulomatous disorders such as tuberculosis, berylliosis, histoplasmosis, and coccidioidomycosis.

13 In hyperthyroidism, hypercalcemia is common and PTH is suppressed. The cause of the hypercalcemia is thought to be increased bone resorption secondary to the effect of thyroid hormone.

14 The hypercalcemia associated with adrenal insufficiency is partially attributable to volume contraction and increased Ca-binding protein. There may also be enhanced renal tubular and GI absorption of calcium due to the loss of the suppressive effect of glucocorticoids on vit D.

15 Although the hypercalcemia associated with pheochromocytoma is usually seen with MEN 2, isolated hypercalcemia and pheochromocytoma have also been described. Tumor production of PTH and stimulation of PTH secretion are the probable mechanisms.

16 The hypercalcemia associated with immobilization occurs in patients with high bone turnover, usually children and patients with Paget's disease. Immobilization may also contribute to the hypercalcemia associated with malignancy and the osteomalacia of renal failure. The mechanism of the hypercalcemia is not clear, but the PTH is usually low.

17 Etiologies of malignancy-associated hypercalcemia include ectopic PTH production; direct bone invasion by tumor; immobilization; prostaglandin effects; osteoclast-activating factor; and the release of vit D–like substances.

18 Hypervitaminosis A is associated with increased bone resorption, nephrocalcinosis, and renal failure. Vitamin A doses of 50,000 to 100,000 units/day have been reported as causing this syndrome.

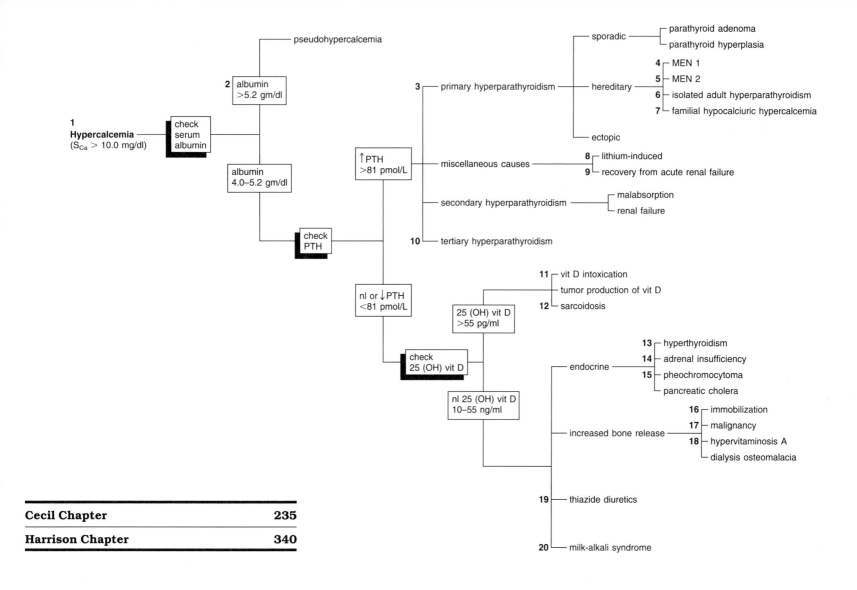

1
Hypercalcemia
(S_{Ca} > 10.0 mg/dl)

check serum albumin

pseudohypercalcemia

2 albumin >5.2 gm/dl

albumin 4.0–5.2 gm/dl

check PTH

↑PTH >81 pmol/L

nl or ↓PTH <81 pmol/L

3 primary hyperparathyroidism

sporadic
parathyroid adenoma
parathyroid hyperplasia

hereditary
4 MEN 1
5 MEN 2
6 isolated adult hyperparathyroidism
7 familial hypocalciuric hypercalcemia

ectopic

miscellaneous causes
8 lithium-induced
9 recovery from acute renal failure

secondary hyperparathyroidism
malabsorption
renal failure

10 tertiary hyperparathyroidism

check 25 (OH) vit D

25 (OH) vit D >55 pg/ml
11 vit D intoxication
tumor production of vit D
12 sarcoidosis

nl 25 (OH) vit D 10–55 ng/ml

endocrine
13 hyperthyroidism
14 adrenal insufficiency
15 pheochromocytoma
pancreatic cholera

increased bone release
16 immobilization
17 malignancy
18 hypervitaminosis A
dialysis osteomalacia

19 thiazide diuretics

20 milk-alkali syndrome

19 The hypercalcemia seen with the administration of thiazide diuretics is partially due to volume contraction with an increase in Ca-binding protein, but increased renal tubular reabsorption of calcium is also a factor. Patients with hyperparathyroidism or patients undergoing vit D therapy are particularly at risk for the development of severe hypercalcemia with the administration of thiazide diuretics.

20 The milk-alkali syndrome, consisting of hypercalcemia, alkalosis, and renal insufficiency, can occur in both acute and chronic forms. The intake of milk and absorbable alkali or the ingestion of large quantities of $CaCO_3$ is needed to produce the syndrome. The alkalosis reduces the renal Ca excretion so that a combination of increased intake and decreased excretion produces the disorder.

Hypophosphatemia

1 Hypophosphatemia is defined as serum phosphate (PO_4) below 2.5 mg/dl. Approximately 1000 mg of phosphate are consumed daily, with 75 to 90 per cent of the dietary phosphate retained by the kidney. Eighty-five per cent of the total body PO_4 resides in the skeleton, 9 per cent in muscle, and only 0.08 per cent in the extracellular space. Hypophosphatemia may be divided into two classes: moderate hypophosphatemia, with levels between 1.0 and 2.5 mg/dl, and severe hypophosphatemia, with levels below 1.0 mg/dl. The degree of hypophosphatemia may help to differentiate between etiologies.

2 The fractional excretion of PO_4, or $FePO_4$, is the amount of filtered PO_4 that is not reabsorbed. $FePO_4$ is calculated using the formula

$$FePO_4 = \frac{\text{Unfiltered } PO_4 \text{ mg/day}}{\text{filtered } PO_4 \text{ or } GFR \times 0.95(\text{serum } PO_4)}$$

Renal reabsorption of PO_4 is nearly complete unless tubular function is altered.

3 PTH is the most potent inhibitor of PO_4 transport in the kidney. PTH inhibits proximal tubular reabsorption of PO_4 by the stimulation of adenylate cyclase and the production of cAMP. Alterations in both the active and passive transport mechanisms for PO_4 have been found with increased intracellular levels of cAMP, although the exact mechanism of PTH inhibition of PO_4 transport is still unclear.

4 Ninety per cent of filtered PO_4 is reabsorbed in the proximal tubule. Any condition affecting proximal tubular function may decrease reabsorption of PO_4. The most common disorder reducing PO_4 reabsorption is Fanconi's syndrome, which is associated with multiple myeloma, heavy metal poisoning, systemic lupus erythematosus, and cystinosis.

5 Phosphate clearance is increased in almost all conditions associated with extracellular volume expansion. Included among these conditions are hyperaldosteronism, high-salt diets, SIADH, and saline infusions. The mechanism of the increased PO_4 excretion is thought to be a direct decrease in the maximum PO_4 reabsorption rate and stimulation of PTH release.

6 Vit D–resistant rickets is a rare sex-linked dominant disorder in which an isolated defect in PO_4 reabsorption is present. Small mesenchymal tumors have been frequently associated with this disorder and have been shown to alter $1,25(OH)$-vit D_3 synthesis or to produce a circulating PTH-like substance. Patients with this disorder develop severe rickets in childhood.

7 Severe hypophosphatemia frequently develops in the setting of uncontrolled diabetes mellitus, most commonly when ketoacidosis is present. Acidosis causes the breakdown of compounds within the cells and allows the liberated inorganic PO_4 to move into the plasma. The increased plasma PO_4 is then excreted in the urine. Renal PO_4 excretion is enhanced by the osmotic diuresis caused by the glycosuria and ketonuria. Owing to the shift of PO_4 into the plasma, initial serum PO_4 levels may appear normal and not reflect the underlying PO_4 depletion. If the initial serum PO_4 is low, severe hypophosphatemia must be suspected.

8 Severe hypophosphatemia can result from the use of large quantities of PO_4-binding antacids in the treatment of peptic ulcer disease or chronic renal failure. These antacids include both magnesium hydroxide and aluminum hydroxide. When PO_4 intake is also inadequate, serum PO_4 levels may fall below 1 mg/dl and symptoms appear.

9 Vit D and its metabolites play a major role in PO_4 absorption in the jejunum. Deficiency of vit D usually results from dietary deficiency, lack of sun exposure, malabsorption, or a decrease in the 25-hydroxylation of vit D, as may occur in liver disease. The most potent stimulator of PO_4 absorption is $1,25(OH)_2$-vit D_3. Vit D_3 production may be decreased by inadequate delivery of $25(OH)$-vit D to the kidney or by renal disease.

10 The severe hypophosphatemia seen in up to 50 per cent of patients hospitalized for alcoholism is multifactorial. Poor oral intake and chronic vomiting result in decreased intake of PO_4. Magnesium deficiency is commonly seen in alcoholism and may be responsible for the renal PO_4 wasting. Ketonuria and occasional ketoacidosis cause PO_4 losses similar to those seen in diabetic ketoacidosis (see No. 7). Initially serum PO_4 may be normal, increased, or low, but the hypophosphatemia will become apparent once treatment for acidosis is instituted.

11 Prolonged respiratory alkalosis may cause severe hypophosphatemia, with serum PO_4 falling as low as 0.3 mg/dl. Respiratory alkalosis produces a rise in intracellular pH because of the preferential diffusibility of CO_2 over bicarbonate. The rise in pH in turn activates phosphofructokinase, increasing phosphorylation of glucose. This process utilizes extracellular PO_4 as the source of the phosphorus. The serum PO_4 falls and renal excretion of PO_4 decreases to zero. Metabolic alkalosis is associated with a much smaller rise in intracellular pH. Glycolysis is not accelerated, and severe hypophosphatemia does not usually occur.

12 The administration of glucose may cause a moderate decrease in serum PO_4 levels. Glucose causes an increase in insulin secretion, which in turn increases cellular uptake of PO_4. Cellular uptake increases primarily in skeletal muscle and in the liver. Serum PO_4 rarely falls by more than 0.5 mg/dl except in malnourished patients or patients with severe hepatic cirrhosis.

13 Hyperalimentation in malnourished patients may result in severe hypophosphatemia when adequate PO_4 replacement is not provided. Malnutrition alone does not cause hypophosphatemia, but refeeding with a high-calorie substance may force PO_4 into the cells. In this setting, muscle PO_4 as well as serum PO_4 may fall dramatically in order to provide adequate PO_4 for vital organs such as the brain and the heart.

14 In nutritional recovery syndrome, severe hypophosphatemia can occur during refeeding with only the normally required calories. The syndrome can occur in any patient with underlying protein-calorie malnutrition. Included in this group are alcoholics, patients with anorexia nervosa, surreptitious vomiters, and patients with malabsorption syndromes.

15 A marked period of diuresis occurs during recovery from severe burns. This diuresis may lead in turn to renal PO_4 wasting. The change from a catabolic to an anabolic state may also shift large amounts of PO_4 into the cells.

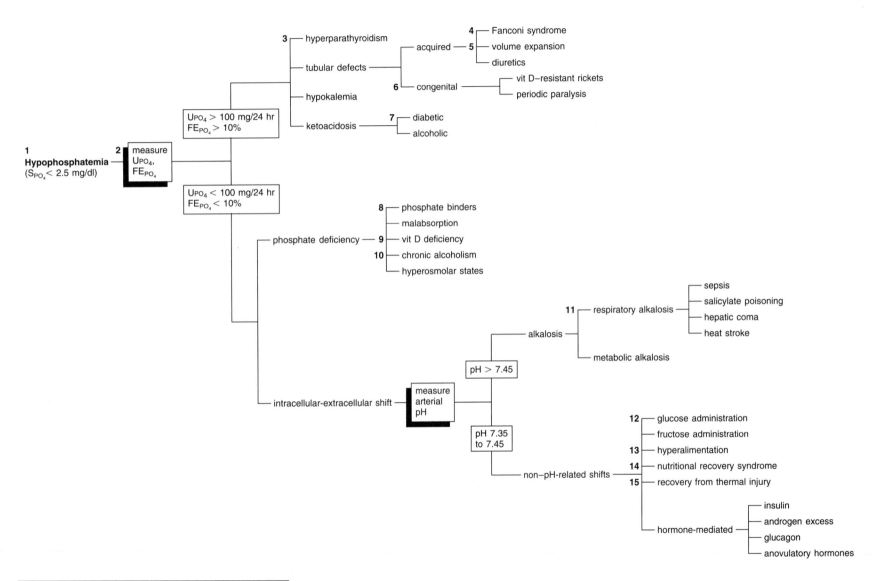

| 1 **Hypophosphatemia** ($S_{PO_4} < 2.5$ mg/dl) | 2 measure U_{PO_4}, FE_{PO_4} |

$U_{PO_4} > 100$ mg/24 hr
$FE_{PO_4} > 10\%$

3 — hyperparathyroidism

tubular defects
- acquired
  - 4 — Fanconi syndrome
  - 5 — volume expansion
  - diuretics
- 6 — congenital
  - vit D–resistant rickets
  - periodic paralysis

hypokalemia

ketoacidosis
- 7 — diabetic
- alcoholic

$U_{PO_4} < 100$ mg/24 hr
$FE_{PO_4} < 10\%$

phosphate deficiency
- 8 — phosphate binders
- malabsorption
- 9 — vit D deficiency
- 10 — chronic alcoholism
- hyperosmolar states

intracellular–extracellular shift — measure arterial pH

pH > 7.45

alkalosis
- 11 — respiratory alkalosis
  - sepsis
  - salicylate poisoning
  - hepatic coma
  - heat stroke
- metabolic alkalosis

pH 7.35 to 7.45

non–pH-related shifts
- 12 — glucose administration
- fructose administration
- 13 — hyperalimentation
- 14 — nutritional recovery syndrome
- 15 — recovery from thermal injury

hormone-mediated
- insulin
- androgen excess
- glucagon
- anovulatory hormones

Cecil Chapter	194
Harrison Chapter	342

Hyperphosphatemia

1 Hyperphosphatemia, although less common than hypophosphatemia, can cause a number of serious clinical problems. Hyperphosphatemia may contribute to acute renal failure, metastatic extravascular calcification, and cardiac failure.

2 Neoplasms with extremely high cell turnover rates or with a large necrotic tumor mass can release large quantities of PO_4 into the circulation. Hyperphosphatemia most commonly occurs in the early phases of chemotherapy or radiation therapy (see No. 3).

3 Tumor lysis syndrome occurs after the treatment of certain tumors with radiotherapy or chemotherapy. Acute leukemia, most commonly the lymphocytic type, and several of the lymphomas, most notably the Burkitt's variety, can release large quantities of PO_4, uric acid, and potassium when treated. Acute renal failure, metastatic calcification, and life-threatening hyperkalemia may result.

4 Normally renal reabsorption of filtered PO_4 is nearly complete. Small increases in serum PO_4 or in the quantity of PO_4 ingested can be excreted by small decreases in the fraction of PO_4 reabsorbed. For hyperphosphatemia to develop when PO_4 intake is increased, a decrease in renal function with decreased PO_4 excretion is usually necessary.

5 Renal excretion of PO_4 may occasionally be overwhelmed when large oral or intravenous loads of PO_4 are administered, as in the treatment of hypercalcemia or hypophosphatemia.

6 Several laxatives and PO_4-containing enemas have been shown to cause hyperphosphatemia. Children taking laxatives have a higher incidence of severe hyperphosphatemia, with reported serum PO_4 levels as high as 15 mg/dl.

7 Acidosis of any type may cause a shift of dissociated PO_4 from the intracellular to the extracellular space. The rise in serum PO_4 is partially offset by increased excretion of PO_4 because of the decreased pH in the renal tubular lumen.

8 Diabetic ketoacidosis is a rare cause of hyperphosphatemia. The serum PO_4 may appear normal or slightly elevated when the acidosis is most severe, but treatment may uncover severe hypophosphatemia owing to prolonged renal losses. Assuming that the PO_4 is normal or elevated may lead to profound hypophosphatemia if it is left untreated. Subsequent hemolysis and decreased tissue oxygenation caused by decreased red cell 2,3-DPG (2,3-diphosphoglycerate) may occur.

9 Serum phosphorus will increase moderately when glomerular filtration rate falls below 25 ml/min, provided that intake remains constant. In acute oliguric renal failure, PO_4 may rise to 8 to 10 mg/dl. When serum PO_4 is above 12 mg/dl, tissue breakdown or cell lysis must be suspected. Crush injury with myoglobin-associated renal failure and tumor lysis syndrome are the most common etiologies of a serum PO_4 greater than 12 mg/dl.

10 Chronic renal failure is the most common cause of hyperphosphatemia. In the absence of PO_4 binders, serum PO_4 may increase to 8 to 10 mg/dl. Metastatic calcification is common in patients with hyperphosphatemia when the product of Ca and PO_4 is greater than 70. Increased serum PO_4 with its concomitant decrease in serum Ca is the major contributor to the secondary hyperparathyroidism and consequent renal osteodystrophy seen in chronic renal failure. Control of hyperphosphatemia with oral PO_4 binders such as aluminum hydroxide and $CaCO_3$, as well as vit D supplementation, is effective in decreasing the incidence and severity of osteodystrophy in these patients.

11 Hypoparathyroidism decreases the renal excretion of PO_4. Normally parathyroid hormone inhibits the reabsorption of PO_4 in both the proximal and distal tubule. In hypoparathyroidism this inhibitory mechanism is lost and PO_4 reabsorption increases.

12 Hyperthyroidism significantly increases PO_4 absorption in the kidney. Thyroid hormone increases the sodium gradient–dependent uptake of PO_4 by the brush border of the proximal tubule.

13 An excess of growth hormone may cause hyperphosphatemia by increasing PO_4 absorption in the intestine and increasing renal absorption by a mechanism similar to that of thyroid hormone (see No. 12).

14 Hyperthermia may cause hyperphosphatemia by increasing the reabsorption of PO_4 in the kidney via increased generation of cAMP as well as by PO_4 release from tissue breakdown.

15 Tumor calcinosis is the exact reverse of vit D–resistant rickets. In this disorder there is a tubular defect causing increased reabsorption of PO_4.

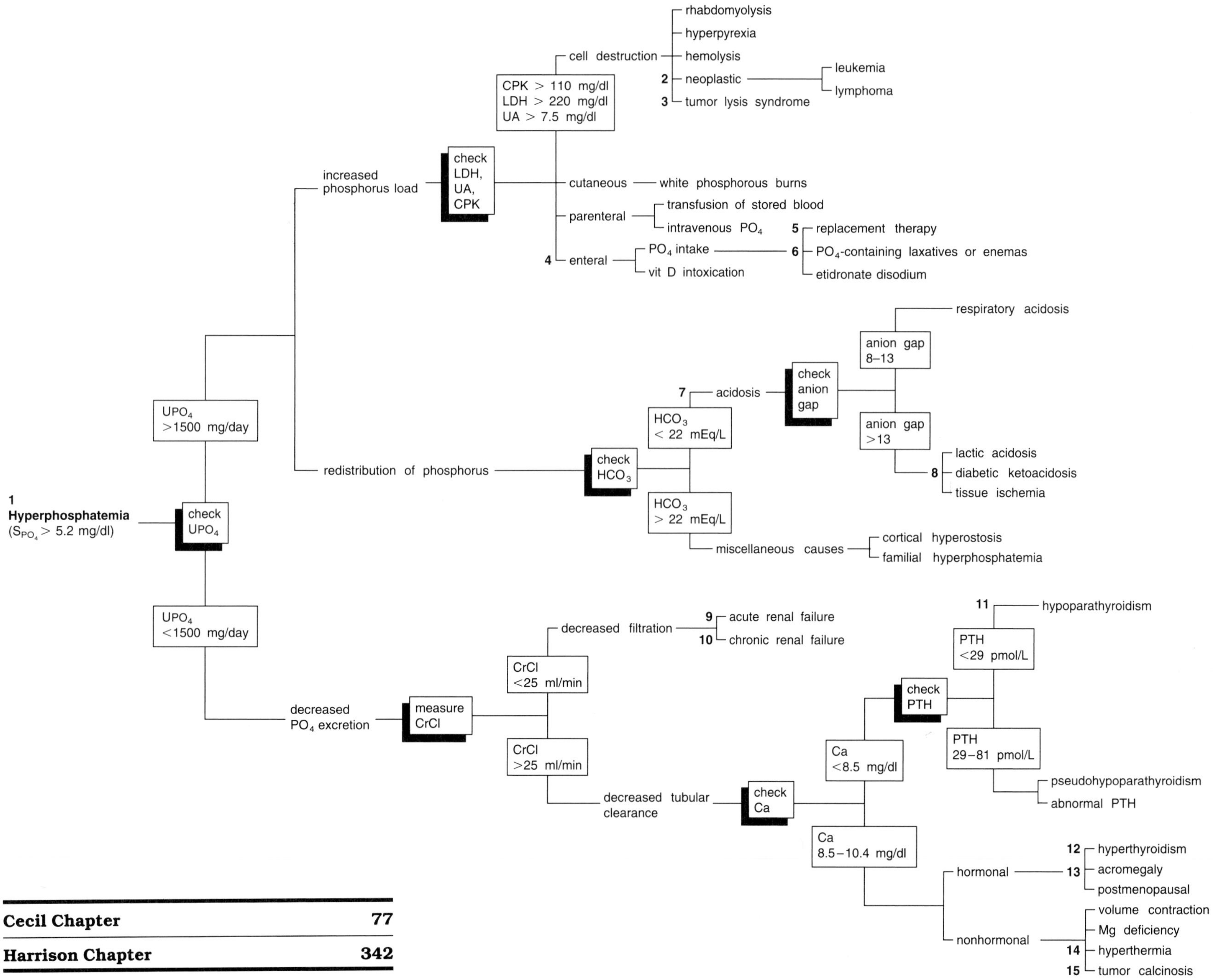
1
Hyperphosphatemia
(S_{PO_4} > 5.2 mg/dl)
check UPO_4
UPO_4 >1500 mg/day
increased phosphorus load
check LDH, UA, CPK
CPK > 110 mg/dl
LDH > 220 mg/dl
UA > 7.5 mg/dl
cell destruction
rhabdomyolysis
hyperpyrexia
hemolysis
2 neoplastic
leukemia
lymphoma
3 tumor lysis syndrome
cutaneous
white phosphorous burns
parenteral
transfusion of stored blood
intravenous PO_4
4 enteral
PO_4 intake
vit D intoxication
5 replacement therapy
6 PO_4-containing laxatives or enemas
etidronate disodium
redistribution of phosphorus
check HCO_3
HCO_3 < 22 mEq/L
7 acidosis
check anion gap
anion gap 8–13
respiratory acidosis
anion gap >13
lactic acidosis
8 diabetic ketoacidosis
tissue ischemia
HCO_3 > 22 mEq/L
miscellaneous causes
cortical hyperostosis
familial hyperphosphatemia
UPO_4 <1500 mg/day
decreased PO_4 excretion
measure CrCl
CrCl <25 ml/min
decreased filtration
9 acute renal failure
10 chronic renal failure
CrCl >25 ml/min
decreased tubular clearance
check Ca
Ca <8.5 mg/dl
check PTH
PTH <29 pmol/L
11 hypoparathyroidism
PTH 29–81 pmol/L
pseudohypoparathyroidism
abnormal PTH
Ca 8.5–10.4 mg/dl
hormonal
12 hyperthyroidism
13 acromegaly
postmenopausal
nonhormonal
volume contraction
Mg deficiency
14 hyperthermia
15 tumor calcinosis

Cecil Chapter	**77**
Harrison Chapter	**342**

Hypomagnesemia

1 Normally, 30 to 40 per cent of dietary magnesium (Mg) is absorbed in the GI tract. Absorption can increase to as much as 80 per cent when dietary Mg is restricted. Poor intake alone is a rare cause of significant hypomagnesemia, owing to this inverse relationship between dietary Mg and the absorption of Mg.

2 When protein-calorie malnutrition occurs, the hypomagnesia is probably a result of decreased intake as well as increased GI loss of Mg secondary to vomiting and diarrhea.

3 Selective Mg malabsorption is a rare, probably X-linked disorder that can cause profound hypomagnesemia on normal diets. Increasing the Mg intake can overcome the defect and prevent the clinical consequences.

4 Approximately 30 per cent of patients with disorders associated with fat malabsorption develop hypomagnesemia. The serum Mg level roughly parallels the degree of steatorrhea. Magnesium probably forms soaps in the intestinal lumen and is lost in the stool. Decreasing the dietary intake of fat can help to alleviate this problem.

5 Oral calcium competes with magnesium in the intestine for transport into the extracellular space.

6 The Mg concentration of pancreatic fluid, gastric secretions, and biliary fluid is between 0.4 and 1.1 mEq/L. Because the amount of Mg loss needed to produce significant hypomagnesemia is 1 to 2 mEq/kg of body weight, Mg lost in the colon accounts for most of the extrarenal causes of hypomagnesemia.

7 The Mg concentration of stool water is 5 to 6 mEq/L but can increase to 14 to 15 mEq/L in severe diarrhea.

8 Internal redistribution of Mg is usually seen when the underlying disorder has also caused Mg wasting. Causes of redistribution can include both cellular and skeletal Mg mobilization, allowing the serum Mg to appear normal or slightly elevated. When treatment of the underlying abnormality is undertaken, Mg shifts back into its various storage pools, causing a rapid fall in the serum Mg. This situation is worsened when there is inadequate Mg replacement during treatment of the underlying disorder.

9 Hungry bone syndrome usually occurs following the removal of a parathyroid adenoma or hyperplastic parathyroid glands. Mg, like Ca, may rapidly shift out of the extracellular fluid into newly formed bone salts.

10 The mechanism of hypomagnesemia in the setting of acute pancreatitis is unclear but may be the formation of Mg-fat salts similar to those formed with Ca in this disorder.

11 Alcoholism and its treatment are the most common causes of significant hypomagnesemia. The etiology is multifactorial, with each of the major contributors—including extrarenal losses, renal losses, and redistribution of magnesium—playing a role. Decreased intake, alcohol-induced Mg malabsorption, liver disease, and diarrhea contribute to the extrarenal causes of the hypomagnesemia. Secondary hyperaldosteronism and ketoacidosis can cause severe renal Mg wasting. Alcohol itself may cause decreased tubular reabsorption of Mg. Treatment of the decompensated alcoholic usually includes refeeding with high-calorie, high-protein supplements. This refeeding may cause a rapid shift of Mg from the extracellular to the intracellular space, causing severe hypomagnesemia.

12 Selective magnesium wasting can occur in both congenital and acquired forms. Congenital Mg wasting is extremely rare and is associated with nephrocalcinosis, hypokalemia, and hypocalcemia. The acquired form is usually drug related (see No. 15).

13 Hypercalciuric states of any etiology are associated with increased Mg excretion. Ca competes with Mg for reabsorption in both the proximal tubule and the loop of Henle. Any syndrome that increases serum calcium, and therefore urinary calcium excretion, can be associated with Mg wasting. Malignancy, sarcoidosis, hyperparathyroidism, and vit D therapy are most commonly associated with this form of renal Mg wasting.

14 Chronic renal tubular acidosis causes increased bone demineralization and the consequent hypercalciuria. This hypercalciuria may cause increased renal Mg excretion (see No. 13).

15 The drug most commonly associated with renal Mg wasting is cisplatin. As many as 50 per cent of patients receiving this drug develop hypomagnesemia. The effect appears to be a direct one on the renal tubule and may persist for several months after the drug is discontinued. Antibiotic-induced nephropathy, most commonly seen with the aminoglycosides and amphotericin, is also associated with renal Mg wasting.

16 Interstitial nephritis is usually associated with administration of synthetic penicillins, but drug-induced interstitial nephritis of any etiology can be associated with renal Mg wasting.

17 Increased Mg excretion in hyperaldosteronism is probably secondary to the extracellular volume expansion (see No. 21).

18 Increased PTH is occasionally associated with hypomagnesemia, but it is unclear whether this is due to a direct effect of the hormone or secondary to the associated hypercalciuria.

19 Thiazide diuretics may cause acute, mild hypomagnesemia, but loop-acting diuretics may have a profound effect on renal Mg reabsorption and are the most common cause of hypomagnesemia. Passive Mg reabsorption is reduced owing to the direct inhibition of the sodium-potassium-chloride transport system. Osmotic diuretics like mannitol or urea decrease Mg reabsorption at the loop in direct proportion to the osmotic load. Decreased reabsorption in the loop, coupled with increased delivery of Mg to this portion of the tubule, enhances excretion of Mg. Potassium-sparing diuretics may also have a significant Mg-sparing effect.

20 PO_4 depletion has been associated with mild hypomagnesemia and is probably related to defective tubular Mg reabsorption.

21 An immediate increase in Mg excretion is seen with volume expansion. There is a marked reduction in proximal tubular reabsorption and a more modest reduction of reabsorption at the loop of Henle. The reduced reabsorption is probably due to an increased flow rate past these portions of the nephron.

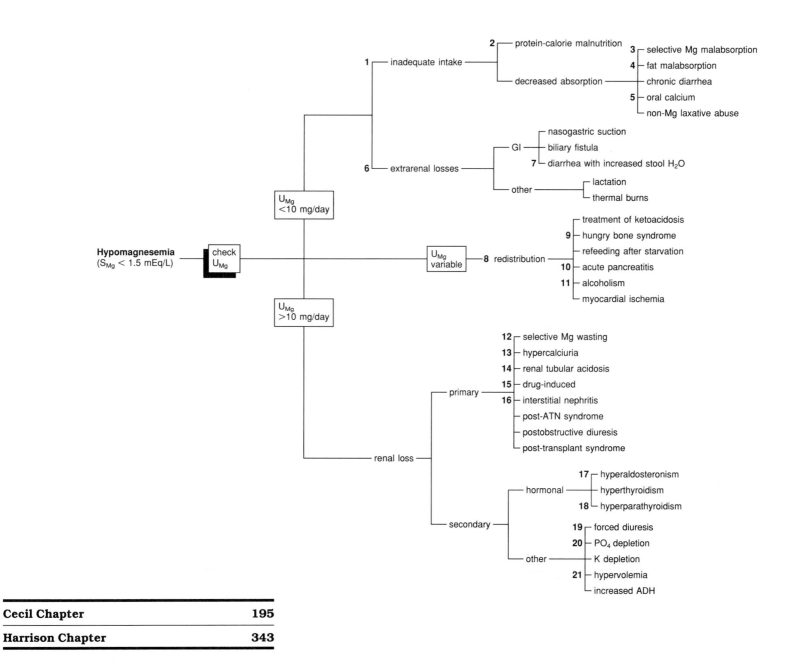

Hypomagnesemia
($S_{Mg} < 1.5$ mEq/L)

check U_{Mg}

U_{Mg} <10 mg/day

U_{Mg} variable

U_{Mg} >10 mg/day

1 inadequate intake
  2 — protein-calorie malnutrition
  decreased absorption
    3 — selective Mg malabsorption
    4 — fat malabsorption
    chronic diarrhea
    5 — oral calcium
    non-Mg laxative abuse

6 extrarenal losses
  GI
    nasogastric suction
    biliary fistula
    7 — diarrhea with increased stool H_2O
  other
    lactation
    thermal burns

8 redistribution
  treatment of ketoacidosis
  9 — hungry bone syndrome
  refeeding after starvation
  10 — acute pancreatitis
  11 — alcoholism
  myocardial ischemia

renal loss
  primary
    12 — selective Mg wasting
    13 — hypercalciuria
    14 — renal tubular acidosis
    15 — drug-induced
    16 — interstitial nephritis
    post-ATN syndrome
    postobstructive diuresis
    post-transplant syndrome
  secondary
    hormonal
      17 — hyperaldosteronism
      hyperthyroidism
      18 — hyperparathyroidism
    other
      19 — forced diuresis
      20 — PO_4 depletion
      K depletion
      21 — hypervolemia
      increased ADH

Hypermagnesemia

1 Mg excretion is dependent upon both GFR and tubular reabsorption. Seventy to 80 per cent of plasma Mg is ultrafilterable. Twenty to 40 per cent of the filtered Mg is then reabsorbed in the proximal tubule, with the remainder reabsorbed in the thick ascending loop of Henle and the distal tubule.

2 With normal dietary intake, urinary Mg excretion is usually between 100 and 150 mg/24 hr. Excretion can be increased to 500 to 600 mg/24 hr if the intake of Mg is increased. Conversely, a normal kidney can decrease excretion to as little as 6 to 12 mg/24 hr within a few days after Mg intake has been decreased.

3 Normal renal excretion of Mg can increase rapidly, so that hypermagnesemia from excessive intake usually requires some concurrent decrease in renal function.

4 The hypermagnesemia associated with $MgSO_4$ ingestion is caused by the combination of a large Mg load plus third spacing of intravascular fluid into the intestine. The mechanisms of the hypermagnesemia are therefore both increased absorption and decreased excretion secondary to intravascular volume depletion (see No. 9).

5 Hypermagnesemia due to increased GI absorption rarely occurs if the GFR is greater than 15 ml/min. Marked hypermagnesemia is possible when the GFR is less than 5 ml/min (see No. 8).

6 The mechanism for hypermagnesemia in ketoacidosis is not well understood. Exchange of Mg ions for hydrogen ions in the distal tubule is one possible cause. Another cause may be the decreased Mg excretion seen with the intravascular volume depletion common in this disorder.

7 Hypermagnesemia in acute renal failure usually occurs when excessive intake is not corrected. The most common sources of increased intake are Mg-containing antacids, laxatives, and additives to hyperalimentation solutions.

8 Hypermagnesemia rarely occurs in chronic renal failure until GFR is less than 15 ml/min. This is due to the kidney's ability to increase Mg excretion to up to 30 to 60 per cent of the filtered load. The dietary restrictions usually placed on patients with chronic renal failure may also protect against excessive Mg intake. Oral intake of Mg-containing products in this setting, however, can cause severe hypermagnesemia.

9 In hypoaldosteronism, enhanced tubular reabsorption in addition to the decreased intravascular volume is the mechanism of hypermagnesemia.

10 In hyperparathyroidism, PTH may act directly on the distal tubule to increase Mg absorption. This cause of hypermagnesemia is unusual because the increased calcium concentration in the serum and urine can increase renal Mg excretion, thereby preventing hypermagnesemia.

11 Decreased intravascular volume is associated with an increase in Mg reabsorption in the proximal tubule.

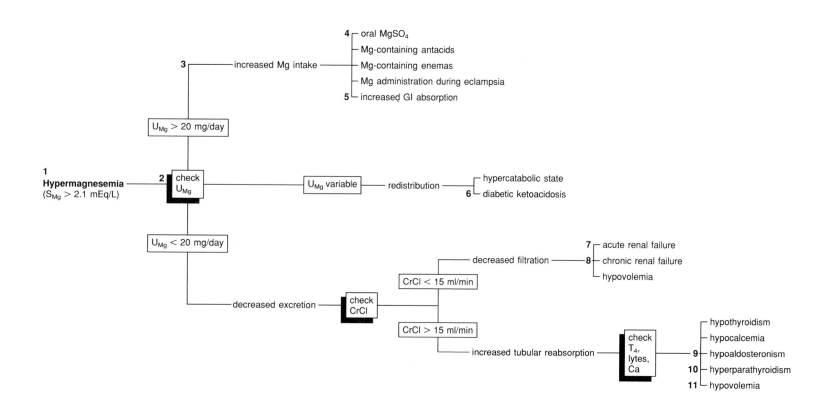

Acidosis

1 Acidosis is the result of the net addition of hydrogen ion (H^+) to the extracellular space or loss of bicarbonate (HCO_3) from that space. Hydrogen ion may be added by the increased production of strong acids, an increase in CO_2 concentration, or the addition of exogenous acid. The equation

$$CO_2 + H_2O \leftrightarrow H_2CO_3 \leftrightarrow H^+ + HCO_3^-$$

demonstrates how H^+ concentration increases as CO_2 increases. Both respiratory and metabolic acidosis may also occur as part of a mixed acid-base disturbance, or as a compensatory mechanism for a primary alkalosis (see page 106). The loss of HCO_3 may occur both renally and extrarenally.

2 The anion gap is the most useful measurement for differentiating between the forms of metabolic acidosis. The anion gap is composed of those unmeasured anions liberated into the extracellular fluid when a strong acid is produced and buffered by HCO_3^-. The anion gap (AG) is calculated by using the formula $AG = Na^+ - (Cl^- + HCO_3)$. Organic anions, sulfate, and phosphate are the most common contributors to the AG. The normal AG is 10 to 14 mEq/L. Any increase above 14 represents the abnormal accumulation of unmeasured anions in the extracellular fluid.

3 The severe acidosis seen with nonketotic hyperosmolar coma is thought to be due to the accumulation of as yet unknown organic acids. The measured quantities of lactate and ketones in the serum do not account for all of the unmeasured anions usually seen in this syndrome.

4 In diabetic ketoacidosis the lack of insulin causes the overproduction and underutilization of both glucose and the fatty ketoacids beta-hydroxybutyrate and acetoacetate. These strong acids dissociate in the extracellular fluid to form H^+ and ketoanions. The degree of acidosis may be severe, with HCO_3^- falling as low as 5 to 10 mEq/L. Elevated glucose concentrations are not always present, with approximately 15 per cent of patients having a serum glucose of less than 350 mg/dl.

5 Alcohol-induced acidosis is usually associated with binge drinking, poor nutrition, and vomiting. Ketoacids are the most prominent organic acid pro-

duced, but lactic acid may also contribute to the acidosis and the increased AG. Serum glucose is usually normal or low. Thirteen per cent of patients present with a serum glucose of less than 50 mg/dl.

6 Starvation leads to the production of ketoacids by the same mechanism as diabetic ketoacidosis (see No. 4). There is also increased hepatic ketogenesis and decreased tissue breakdown of the ketoacids. The acidosis is usually mild. Serum HCO_3^- is rarely less than 18 mEq/L.

7 Methanol intoxication is one of the few causes of an AG greater than 50 mEq/L. The methanol is metabolized by alcohol dehydrogenase into formic acid. Formic acid interferes with oxidative metabolism, leading to the accumulation of large quantities of lactic acid.

8 Ethylene glycol ingestion may cause an AG greater than 50 mEq/L. Metabolism of ethylene glycol to glycolic acid and finally to glyoxylic acid and oxalic acid results in a high AG acidosis.

9 Lactic acid is the end-product of the anaerobic metabolism of glucose. The major sites of lactic acid production are skeletal muscle and the small intestine. When cells receive inadequate oxygen delivery or oxygen utilization is impaired, lactic acid is produced in quantities that cannot be completely metabolized in the liver. Shock, severe hypoxia ($PaO_2 < 35$ mm Hg), seizures, hepatic failure, phenformin, and carbon monoxide intoxication are the most common causes of lactic acidosis.

10 Aspirin or other salicylates in large doses may cause a severe metabolic acidosis. Respiratory alkalosis is the most common presenting sign in adults (see No. 3, Alkalosis Algorithm), but an AG acidosis supervenes in more than 50 per cent of the patients.

11 In acute renal failure, the acidosis results from the kidney's failure to excrete the entire daily production of endogenous acid. The body normally produces about 1 mmol/kg/day of acid from the breakdown of foods and body protein. Acid production may increase owing to infection, increased catabolism, or tissue injury. In chronic renal failure, titratable acid excretion is impaired and the AG is increased by the accumulation of sulfate, phosphate, and other organic acids.

12 Several other drugs and chemicals can be associated with AG acidosis. These include phenformin, isoniazid in high dosage, chloramphenicol, sodium azide poisoning, hydrofluoric acid exposure, and inorganic sulfur sometimes used in certain folk remedies.

13 The accurate measurement of urinary pH requires that the sample be taken in the early morning when urine is maximally acidified. The sample should be placed under oil to prevent the loss of dissolved CO_2 and the resultant increase in pH.

14 RTA may involve defects in either the proximal or distal tubule. In the proximal tubular form (type 2), the proximal tubule is unable to reabsorb the filtered HCO_3^-. Increased HCO_3^- is delivered to the distal tubule, where much of the HCO_3^- can be reabsorbed. Serum HCO_3^- rarely falls below 15 mEq/L. In the distal tubular form (type 1), the distal tubule is unable to secrete H^+ ions. The HCO_3^- may fall to extremely low levels, often below 15 mEq/L. Both of these forms of RTA are commonly associated with other tubular defects. Proximal RTA is most commonly associated with cystinosis, multiple myeloma, amyloidosis, medullary cystic disease, and heavy metal toxicity. Distal RTA is most commonly associated with hypercalcemia, lupus nephritis, medullary sponge kidney, renal transplant rejection, and toxicity from amphotericin B and lithium. There are also idiopathic forms of both proximal and distal RTA.

15 Diarrhea is the most common form of normal AG metabolic acidosis. The concentration of HCO_3^- in diarrheal fluid is usually higher than in serum. Patients with inflammatory or infectious colitis may lose up to 20 liters of fluid per day. Each liter of fluid may contain up to 50 mmol of HCO_3^-.

16 Hypoaldosteronism may cause an acidosis similar to that of distal RTA (see No. 14). Both hydrogen ion and potassium secretion are reduced, leading to a hyperkalemic metabolic acidosis. Patients with hypoaldosteronism may, however, achieve a urine pH of less than 5.5. A form of this syndrome associated with hyporeninism is commonly seen in diabetes mellitus.

17 Amino acid solutions commonly used for intravenous hyperalimentation may contain organic cations in excess over organic anions. Metabolism of these cations produces H^+. The H^+ is buffered by HCO_3^- and a hyperchloremic metabolic acidosis develops.

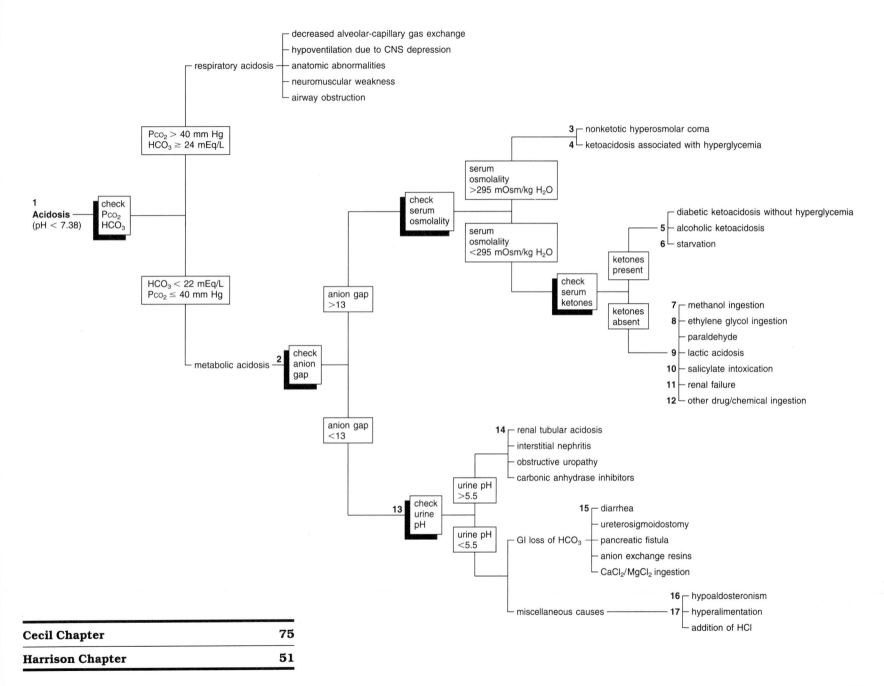

decreased alveolar-capillary gas exchange

hypoventilation due to CNS depression

respiratory acidosis — anatomic abnormalities

neuromuscular weakness

airway obstruction

Pco₂ > 40 mm Hg
HCO₃ ≥ 24 mEq/L

3 — nonketotic hyperosmolar coma

4 — ketoacidosis associated with hyperglycemia

serum osmolality
>295 mOsm/kg H₂O

1
Acidosis — check Pco₂ HCO₃
(pH < 7.38)

check serum osmolality

diabetic ketoacidosis without hyperglycemia

5 — alcoholic ketoacidosis

6 — starvation

serum osmolality
<295 mOsm/kg H₂O

ketones present

HCO₃ < 22 mEq/L
Pco₂ ≤ 40 mm Hg

anion gap >13

check serum ketones

ketones absent

7 — methanol ingestion

8 — ethylene glycol ingestion

paraldehyde

9 — lactic acidosis

10 — salicylate intoxication

11 — renal failure

12 — other drug/chemical ingestion

metabolic acidosis — **2** check anion gap

anion gap <13

14 — renal tubular acidosis

interstitial nephritis

obstructive uropathy

carbonic anhydrase inhibitors

urine pH >5.5

13 check urine pH

15 — diarrhea

ureterosigmoidostomy

urine pH <5.5

GI loss of HCO₃ — pancreatic fistula

anion exchange resins

CaCl₂/MgCl₂ ingestion

16 — hypoaldosteronism

miscellaneous causes — **17** — hyperalimentation

addition of HCl

Alkalosis

1 Alkalosis is defined as an excess of total body bicarbonate (HCO_3) or a deficit of total body hydrogen ion (H^+). Alkalemia is defined as a serum pH greater than 7.45. Although this algorithm will deal with the differential diagnosis of primary alkalosis, alkalosis may also be one of the body's compensatory mechanisms in the setting of acidosis or may be part of mixed acid-base disorder.

2 Acute decreases in PCO_2 will be accompanied by simultaneous decreases in the HCO_3 concentration. The HCO_3 will fall approximately 1 to 3 mEq/L for each 10-mm Hg fall in PCO_2 in accordance with the laws of mass action. In more chronic forms of decreased PCO_2, the HCO_3 concentration will fall approximately 2 to 5 mEq/L for each 10-mm Hg fall in PCO_2 but will rarely fall below 14 mEq/L.

3 Salicylates stimulate the medullary respiratory centers directly, causing increased respiratory drive. Respiratory alkalosis is usually the earliest clinical sign. Metabolic acidosis will eventually supervene as the intoxication becomes more severe (see No. 10, Acidosis Algorithm). Respiratory alkalosis is a more common presenting sign in adults than in children.

4 A variety of mechanisms contribute to the respiratory alkalosis that commonly occurs with hepatic failure. These mechanisms include hypoxemia related to pulmonary shunts, increased progesterone levels (see No. 6), increased ammonium levels, and increased intra-abdominal pressure due to ascites.

5 With sepsis, endotoxins liberated by many gram-negative organisms probably cause respiratory alkalosis by direct stimulation of the medullary respiratory centers.

6 An increased progesterone level may directly stimulate the medullary respiratory center, causing respiratory alkalosis. Increased progesterone levels may be the result of increased production occurring in pregnancy or decreased metabolism as occurs with hepatic insufficiency (see No. 4).

7 Acute mountain sickness may be seen following ascent to altitudes above 8000 feet by persons usually residing at sea level. The resultant hypoxemia stimulates hyperventilation and respiratory alkalosis. Pulmonary and cerebral edema may also occur with this syndrome.

8 The respiratory alkalosis that occurs following a pulmonary embolus is due to hypoxemia, bronchospasm, and the stimulation of intrapulmonary stretch receptors.

9 If serum HCO_3 rises above 28 mEq/L, the PCO_2 will rise 0.25 to 1 mm Hg for each 1-mEq/L increase in HCO_3 concentration.

10 Metabolic alkalosis requires two phases. The alkalosis must be generated by either the net addition of HCO_3 (or its metabolic precursors such as citrate, acetate, or lactate) or the net loss of H^+. These events can occur either intra- or extrarenally. The resultant pH increase is rapidly corrected unless other factors allow the second phase or maintenance of the alkalosis to occur. Factors that maintain the alkalosis include volume depletion, potassium depletion, and mineralocorticoid excess. Each of these factors inhibits the kidney's ability to either excrete HCO_3 or retain H^+.

11 Loss of gastric acid as a result of vomiting or gastric suction is the prototype of the generation and maintenance of metabolic alkalosis. Hydrogen ion and chloride are lost in the gastric fluid. These losses lead to generation of increased HCO_3 in the serum and generation of the alkalosis. The consequent volume depletion causes increased aldosterone production and the avid reabsorption of sodium by the kidney. The lack of reabsorbable chloride, resulting from its previous loss from the stomach, allows HCO_3 to be reabsorbed with the Na^+, thus maintaining the alkalosis even after GI losses have stopped.

12 The administration of large quantities of nonreabsorbable anions, usually in the form of sodium salts of penicillin or carbenicillin, can lead to metabolic alkalosis by enhancing distal tubular acid and potassium secretion. Increased secretion is due to delivery of large quantities of sodium past the distal secretory sites. Delivery of large quantities of sodium to the distal tubule without chloride will, in addition, enhance distal tubular reabsorption of HCO_3.

13 Bartter's syndrome is a rare disorder usually seen in children associated with increased renin and aldosterone production, hypokalemia, hypertrophy of the juxtaglomerular apparatus, and nonresponsiveness of the vascular system to angiotensin II. The metabolic alkalosis is probably due to the hypokalemia (see No. 14) and the hyperaldosteronism (see No. 16).

14 Although metabolic alkalosis is almost always present with potassium depletion, the mechanism is unclear. There is some evidence that potassium depletion directly increases distal tubular HCO_3 reabsorption.

15 Diuretics lead to metabolic alkalosis by causing volume depletion and loss of chloride (see No. 11).

16 Hyperaldosteronism, or an excess of any other mineralocorticoid, generates metabolic alkalosis by enhancing distal tubular H^+ secretion. The alkalosis is maintained by increased reabsorption and generation of HCO_3 resulting from the increased exchange of sodium for secreted potassium and hydrogen ion.

17 Ingestion of substances with potent mineralocorticoid activity may cause metabolic alkalosis via the mechanisms described above (see No. 16). These substances include certain forms of licorice, carbenoxolone, chewing tobacco, and some nasal sprays. Liddle's syndrome is a rare disease in which an unidentified mineralocorticoid is produced.

18 Renal artery stenosis may cause metabolic alkalosis by increasing renin and aldosterone production (see No. 16).

BIBLIOGRAPHY

Brenner BM, Rector FC: The Kidney, Philadelphia, W. B. Saunders Company, 1986.

Glassock RJ: Current Therapy in Nephrology and Hypertension 1984–1985. St. Louis, C. V. Mosby Company, 1984.

Kurtzman NA, Batlle DC: Acid-base disorders. Med Clin North Am 67:4, 1983.

Lieu TA, Grasmeder HM, Kaplan BS: An approach to the evaluation and treatment of microscopic hematuria. Pediatr Clin North Am 38(3)579–589, 1991.

Narins RG, Jones ER, et al.: Diagnostic strategies in disorders of fluid, electrolyte, and acid-base homeostasis. Am J Med 72:496–520, 1982.

Schrier RW: Renal and Electrolyte Disorders. Boston, Little, Brown and Company, 1986.

Schrier RW, Briner VA: The differential diagnosis of hyponatremia. Hosp Practice 29:32–38, 1990.

Stein JH: Nephrology: The Science and Practice of Clinical Medicine. Vol. 7. New York, Grune and Stratton, 1980.

Taylor RB: Difficult Diagnosis. Philadelphia, W. B. Saunders Company, 1985.

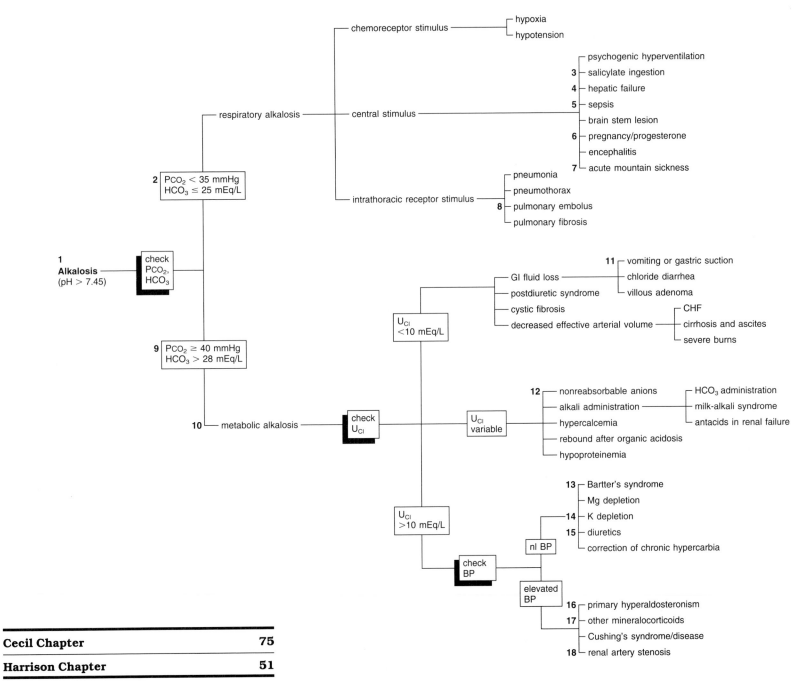

chemoreceptor stimulus ─┬─ hypoxia
                        └─ hypotension

respiratory alkalosis ─┬─ chemoreceptor stimulus

central stimulus ─┬─ psychogenic hyperventilation
                  3├─ salicylate ingestion
                  4├─ hepatic failure
                  5├─ sepsis
                   ├─ brain stem lesion
                  6├─ pregnancy/progesterone
                   ├─ encephalitis
                  7└─ acute mountain sickness

intrathoracic receptor stimulus ─┬─ pneumonia
                                  ├─ pneumothorax
                                8├─ pulmonary embolus
                                  └─ pulmonary fibrosis

2 | PCO$_2$ < 35 mmHg
       HCO$_3$ ≤ 25 mEq/L

1
Alkalosis
(pH > 7.45) ─ check PCO$_2$, HCO$_3$

GI fluid loss ─┬─ **11** vomiting or gastric suction
               ├─ chloride diarrhea
               └─ villous adenoma

U$_{Cl}$ <10 mEq/L ─┬─ GI fluid loss
                    ├─ postdiuretic syndrome
                    ├─ cystic fibrosis
                    └─ decreased effective arterial volume ─┬─ CHF
                                                            ├─ cirrhosis and ascites
                                                            └─ severe burns

9 | PCO$_2$ ≥ 40 mmHg
       HCO$_3$ > 28 mEq/L

10 ─ metabolic alkalosis ─ check U$_{Cl}$

U$_{Cl}$ variable ─┬─ **12** nonreabsorbable anions
                   ├─ alkali administration ─┬─ HCO$_3$ administration
                   │   ├─ milk-alkali syndrome
                   │   └─ antacids in renal failure
                   ├─ hypercalcemia
                   ├─ rebound after organic acidosis
                   └─ hypoproteinemia

U$_{Cl}$ >10 mEq/L ─ check BP

nl BP ─┬─ **13** Bartter's syndrome
       ├─ Mg depletion
     14├─ K depletion
     15├─ diuretics
       └─ correction of chronic hypercarbia

elevated BP ─┬─ **16** primary hyperaldosteronism
           17├─ other mineralocorticoids
             ├─ Cushing's syndrome/disease
           18└─ renal artery stenosis

7 · Hematologic Disorders

Signs and symptoms:
Bleeding
Lymphadenopathy
Splenomegaly
Labs:
Anemia
Microcytic anemia
Normocytic anemia
　Hemolytic anemia
　　Immune hemolytic
　　anemia
Aplastic anemia
Macrocytic anemia
　Vitamin B₁₂ deficiency

Folic acid deficiency
Myelodysplastic syndromes
　(MDS) (refractory
　anemia)
Polycythemia
Pancytopenia
Neutropenia
Neutrophilia
Monocytosis
Lymphocytosis
Eosinophilia
Thrombocytosis
Thrombocytopenia
Dysproteinemia

Bleeding

1 Bleeding occurring spontaneously or for a prolonged period following trauma indicates abnormal hemostatic mechanisms. A history of the type of bleeding experienced is the most helpful clue to the diagnosis of the source of a bleeding problem. Delayed, prolonged bleeding or significant deep tissue bleeding (muscle and soft tissue hematomas, hemarthroses) suggests a coagulation cascade abnormality. Skin and mucosal bleeding manifested as petechiae and purpura suggest a platelet abnormality. A thorough medication history as well as a family history of abnormal bleeding may also provide important information regarding platelet dysfunction or coagulation defects.

2 Initial tests of coagulation include a platelet count, prothrombin time (PT), and partial thromboplastin time (PTT).

3 The bleeding time measures the speed of platelet plug formation and does not require clotting factors. Bleeding time can be prolonged because of decreased number of platelets or platelet dysfunction.

4 If all tests of the hemostatic mechanism are normal, the most likely source of abnormal bleeding is a vessel defect or nonthrombocytopenic bleeding. Vascular defects, although common, usually do not result in serious bleeding problems.

5 In hereditary hemorrhagic telangiectasia (Osler–Weber–Rendu disease), multiple fragile telangiectases appear on the skin, mucosae, and gastrointestinal tract. The telangiectases are responsible for abnormal bleeding. The disorder is transmitted as an autosomal dominant trait.

6 The nonallergic purpuras are a mixed group of disorders in which vascular abnormalities result in purpura. Many are due to the poor dermal vascular support, as in senile purpura, Cushing's disease, drug-induced purpura (treatment with corticosteroids), scurvy, and the inherited connective tissue disorders. Many mechanisms have been proposed to explain the bleeding abnormality that accompanies the dysproteinemias. Proposed mechanisms include perivascular deposition of paraproteins or interference of clotting proteins owing to hyperviscosity. In the latter case, platelet and clotting tests may be altered. Infections are well established as a source of nonthrombocytopenic purpura, especially meningococcemia and subacute bacterial endocarditis. Infection-related purpura is thought to be due to vasculitis secondary to vascular microemboli.

7 Allergic purpura, also known as Henoch-Schönlein purpura, is a nonthrombocytopenic purpura in which a vasculitis is the cause of the purpura. Renal failure may be a serious sequela of the disorder. This condition is primarily a disease of children. The etiology is unknown but is thought to be an allergic response to a foreign antigen.

8 Platelet dysfunction can be congenital or acquired. The acquired disorders are by far more common. The two categories can most easily be differentiated by history. The cause of abnormal platelet function in uremia is unclear. It is thought a dialyzable low-molecular-weight inhibitor of platelet function is present in uremic plasma. Drug-induced platelet dysfunction is probably the most commonly seen abnormality clinically. The most commonly implicated drugs are aspirin and prostaglandin inhibitors. Other drugs responsible for platelet dysfunction include anesthetics, carbenicillin, dextran and hydroxyethyl starch (plasma expanders), dipyridamole, ethanol, and sulfinpyrazone.

9 Bleeding disorders associated with abnormal coagulation are accompanied by abnormalities of the PT and PTT. The PT measures clot formation via the extrinsic pathway and tests for Factors VII, X, V, II, and I. The PTT measures clot formation via the intrinsic pathway and tests for all factors except Factor VII. These tests often overlap, because an isolated deficiency of Factor VII is rare. If the PT is prolonged but all other tests are normal, Factor VII deficiency is implicated. The hereditary form of Factor VII deficiency is a rare autosomal dominant condition. A prolonged PT is more commonly due to deficiency of the vitamin K–dependent synthesis of Factor VII. The vitamin K–dependent factors are synthesized in the liver and include Factors II, VII, IX, and X. Vitamin K deficiency, severe liver disease, or vitamin K antagonists (warfarin) will result in a decreased level of these factors. In these conditions there is usually a prolongation of both the PT and PTT.

10 Circulating anticoagulants are antibodies to specific clotting factors. Although circulating anticoagulants are not usually associated with bleeding, they can cause a prolongation of the PTT. Antibodies to Factors I, V, VIII, IX, X, XI, and XIII have been found. Antibodies can be found in patients with a normal coagulation system, in patients with a congenital factor deficiency (with a history of multiple transfusions), or as part of an autoimmune disease such as systemic lupus erythematosus (SLE). Antibodies to Factor VIII are the most common, occurring in up to 10 per cent of patients with hemophilia A as well as in patients with SLE.

11 Disseminated intravascular coagulation (DIC) is a complex interaction of the blood coagulation system in which thrombin is activated and fibrinogen and other clotting factors are consumed. Fibrin degradation products act as anticoagulants. Although the exact mechanism initiating DIC is unknown, gram-negative septicemia, subacute bacterial endocarditis, certain neoplasms, anaphylaxis, liver failure (with resulting impaired clearance of activated anticoagulant factors), shock, snake venoms, burns, and obstetric complications have all been associated with DIC.

12 The vitamin K–dependent factors (II, VII, IX, X) are synthesized in the liver. Vitamin K is a fat-soluble vitamin produced by the normal gut flora. Only very small stores of vitamin K are normally present in the body. Any interference with the absorption or action of

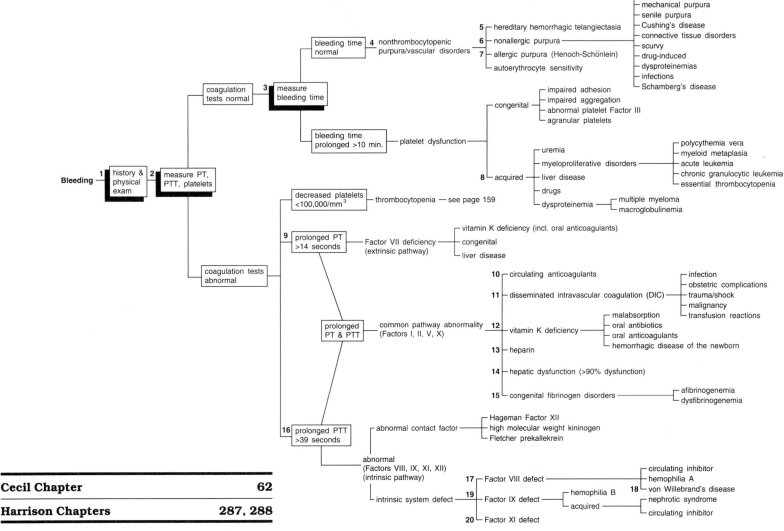

Cecil Chapter	62
Harrison Chapters	**287, 288**

vitamin K will result in decreased synthesis of its dependent clotting factors. Malabsorption, prolonged use of oral antibiotics, liver failure, or the use of vitamin K antagonists (coumarins) may result in prolonged PT and PTT.

13 Heparin inactivates thrombin (Factor IIa), and, to a lesser degree, Factors IX, X, XI, and XII. Both the PT and PTT are affected by heparin, although the PTT is the best measure of heparin effect in normal therapeutic use.

14 Liver disease results in impaired coagulation, not only by decreased hepatic protein synthesis but also by increased plasma proteolytic activity. The latter is probably due to the decreased clearance of proteases from the circulation by the liver.

15 Fibrinogen (Factor I) levels can be specifically assayed to determine the presence of a congenital fibrinogen disorder. Both afibrinogenemia and dysfibrinogenemia are inherited as autosomal recessive disorders.

Dysfibrinogenemia refers specifically to the fact that the fibrinogen functions abnormally in these patients, and the fibrinogen level may be normal or low. Acquired disorders in which fibrinogen functions inadequately include hepatic insufficiency, DIC, and heparin administration.

16 If the PTT is prolonged and the PT normal, there is an abnormality of one of the factors of the intrinsic pathway (XII, XI, IX, VIII). An abnormality of a contact factor (Hageman, Fletcher, or Fitzgerald factor) is

Bleeding (Continued)

usually inherited and is manifested only as abnormal laboratory results without an associated bleeding tendency. Specific contact factors can be assayed to help distinguish among the diagnostic categories. Deficiencies of Factors VIII, IX, and XI account for the majority of inherited bleeding disorders.

17 Factor VIII deficiency is the most common clotting factor deficiency and can be diagnosed with a Factor VIII assay. Hemophilia A (Factor VIII deficiency) is inherited as a sex-linked recessive disorder (70 per cent) or may occur as a spontaneous mutation (30 per cent).

18 Von Willebrand's disease is a Factor VIII deficiency, although it presents clinically like a platelet disorder. The basic defect is the lack of the von Willebrand component of Factor VIII, which results in decreased platelet adhesiveness. Most cases of von Willebrand's disease are autosomal dominant with variable penetrance, although there is a rare autosomal recessive type.

19 Hemophilia B, or Christmas disease, is only 20 per cent as prevalent as hemophilia A. If the Factor VIII assay is normal, the likely diagnosis is deficiency of Factor IX. Factor IX can also be assayed. In the nephrotic syndrome, Factor IX can be lost in the urine, causing an acquired Factor IX deficiency.

20 Deficiency of Factor XI is less common than Factor IX deficiency and causes a mild to moderate hemophilia. It is an autosomal dominant disorder occurring most commonly in people of Jewish origin.

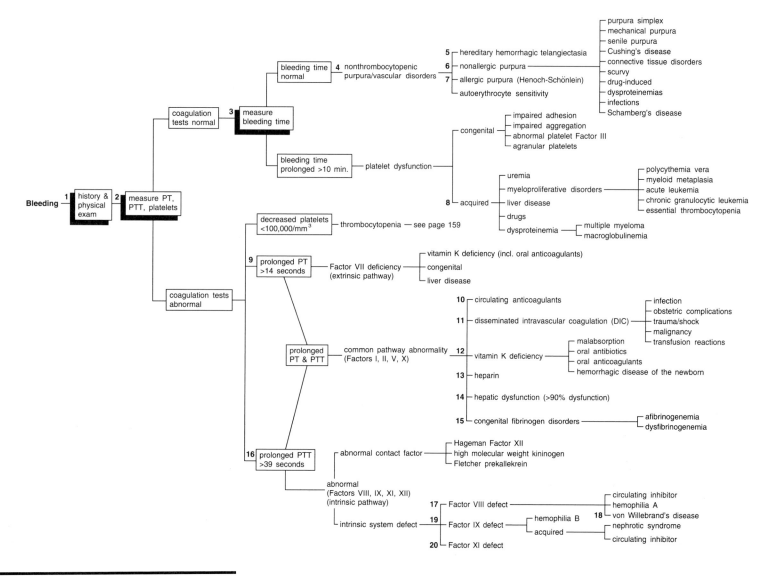

Bleeding

1 history & physical exam

2 measure PT, PTT, platelets

coagulation tests normal

3 measure bleeding time

bleeding time normal

4 nonthrombocytopenic purpura/vascular disorders

5 hereditary hemorrhagic telangiectasia
6 nonallergic purpura
7 allergic purpura (Henoch-Schönlein)
autoerythrocyte sensitivity

- purpura simplex
- mechanical purpura
- senile purpura
- Cushing's disease
- connective tissue disorders
- scurvy
- drug-induced
- dysproteinemias
- infections
- Schamberg's disease

bleeding time prolonged >10 min.

platelet dysfunction

congenital
- impaired adhesion
- impaired aggregation
- abnormal platelet Factor III
- agranular platelets

8 acquired
- uremia
- myeloproliferative disorders
  - polycythemia vera
  - myeloid metaplasia
  - acute leukemia
  - chronic granulocytic leukemia
  - essential thrombocythemia
- liver disease
- drugs
- dysproteinemia
  - multiple myeloma
  - macroglobulinemia

coagulation tests abnormal

decreased platelets <100,000/mm^3 — thrombocytopenia — see page 159

9 prolonged PT >14 seconds

Factor VII deficiency (extrinsic pathway)
- vitamin K deficiency (incl. oral anticoagulants)
- congenital
- liver disease

prolonged PT & PTT

common pathway abnormality (Factors I, II, V, X)

10 circulating anticoagulants
11 disseminated intravascular coagulation (DIC)
- infection
- obstetric complications
- trauma/shock
- malignancy
- transfusion reactions
12 vitamin K deficiency
- malabsorption
- oral antibiotics
- oral anticoagulants
- hemorrhagic disease of the newborn
13 heparin
14 hepatic dysfunction (>90% dysfunction)
15 congenital fibrinogen disorders
- afibrinogenemia
- dysfibrinogenemia

16 prolonged PTT >39 seconds

abnormal (Factors VIII, IX, XI, XII) (intrinsic pathway)

abnormal contact factor
- Hageman Factor XII
- high molecular weight kininogen
- Fletcher prekallekrein

intrinsic system defect
17 Factor VIII defect
- circulating inhibitor
- hemophilia A
- von Willebrand's disease 18
19 Factor IX defect
- hemophilia B
- acquired
  - nephrotic syndrome
  - circulating inhibitor
20 Factor XI defect

Cecil Chapter	62
Harrison Chapters	287, 288

Lymphadenopathy

1 The etiology of lymphadenopathy depends on whether an enlarged lymph node is an isolated finding or generalized adenopathy exists. There is, however, overlap among diseases causing localized and generalized lymphadenopathy. Lymphadenopathy is considered generalized if there is enlargement of the cervical, axillary, and inguinal nodes. Painful adenopathy is more likely due to an inflammatory condition, whereas non-painful adenopathy is more likely due to infiltration of the node with tumor.

2 If generalized adenopathy is present, a thorough history and physical examination are crucial to diagnosis. Further laboratory studies are obtained based on the clinical indications. A complete blood count (CBC), including a peripheral blood smear, is one of the most useful initial tests. The presence of atypical lymphocytes may indicate a viral illness, e.g., mononucleosis. Immature leukocytes present on CBC point toward leukemia, and leukocytosis indicates infection. Anemia often accompanies connective tissue diseases, e.g., SLE. Ultimately, excisional biopsy of a lymph node (for histologic exam and culture) may be necessary if the tests performed as indicated by history and physical examination are non-diagnostic. Lymph node excision is the standard for diagnosis (see No. 11).

3 Malignant cells may rarely be found in the circulation in patients with lymphoma.

4 Hypersensitivity reactions can result in lymph node enlargement. Hypersensitivity to drugs, such as the hydantoins (e.g., phenytoin), may result in a generalized lymphadenopathy known as "pseudolymphoma." Anemia, mild leukocytosis, and occasionally eosinophilia can occur in serum sickness.

5 The most common cause of generalized adenopathy is infection. Acquired immunodeficiency syndrome (AIDS) is a common cause of generalized adenopathy and should be a strong diagnostic consideration in any patient with generalized adenopathy and risk factors for AIDS. Common communicable diseases such as measles, rubella, mumps, and chickenpox are frequently associated with generalized lymphadenopathy. Other common infectious etiologies of generalized adenopathy include infectious mononucleosis (both Epstein-Barr virus and cytomegalovirus), toxoplasmosis, and bacterial, rickettsial, fungal, and other viral diseases. Clues to diagnosis include the presence of fever, skin rash, and atypical lymphocytes on CBC. Depending on the clinical situation, further testing, including appropriate cultures, a serologic test for syphilis, a mono spot test, antibody tests for toxoplasmosis, a chest radiograph, and skin tests, may reveal the source of infection.

6 Hyperthyroidism may be accompanied by generalized lymphadenopathy, splenomegaly, and lymphocytosis. The changes revert to normal when the euthyroid state is attained.

7 Generalized lymphadenopathy is commonly found with sarcoidosis, although mediastinal and hilar nodes are most frequently involved. Although bilateral hilar adenopathy is characteristic of sarcoidosis, tuberculosis and coccidioidomycosis should also be considered. Asymmetric hilar adenopathy is more commonly seen with metastatic carcinoma, non-Hodgkin's lymphoma, and nodular sclerosing Hodgkin's lymphoma. Hilar adenopathy is rarely seen with bacterial or viral pulmonary infections.

8 Localized adenopathy is common in both infection and malignancy. Localized adenopathy owing to metastatic disease is usually firm or hard on palpation, whereas adenopathy owing to infection is commonly tender. Again, careful review of the history and thorough physical examination are critical to diagnosis. Adenopathy that is seemingly localized may truly be generalized but have one prominent group of nodes.

9 Localized lymph node enlargement may be due to lymphoma or metastatic disease. The location of the enlarged node is critical to the diagnosis of metastatic disease. For example, an isolated supraclavicular node on the left (Virchow node) may be the only clue to an intra-abdominal neoplasm. Isolated axillary nodes would indicate breast carcinoma, and cervical nodes indicate carcinoma of the head and neck. With isolated node enlargement and no evidence for local inflammation or infection, an excisional biopsy of the entire node is important for diagnosis. A lymph node biopsy should also be performed in both localized and generalized lymphadenopathy if the diagnosis is in doubt.

10 Any group of lymph nodes that provides drainage to an area of recurrent trauma, skin inflammation, or vaccination is subject to inflammation and enlargement. For example, epitrochlear nodes can be enlarged in a patient who does manual labor.

11 In 40 to 60 per cent of patients who undergo lymph node biopsy, the biopsy is not diagnostic and only a reactive hyperplasia is found. If the biopsy is nondiagnostic and other nodes are palpable, repeat biopsy should be performed. If repeat biopsy is nondiagnostic and lymphoma is a strong consideration, abdominal laparotomy may be necessary. Several studies have shown that 25 to 60 per cent of patients with initially nondiagnostic lymph node biopsies were found to have lymphoma, carcinoma, connective tissue diseases, or infection on close follow-up and rebiopsy.

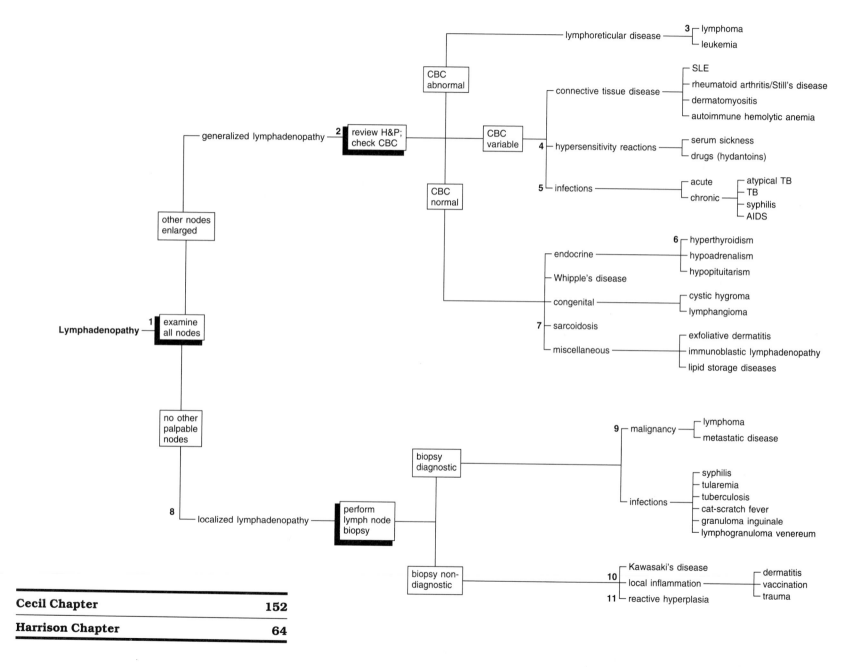

Lymphadenopathy

1 examine all nodes

other nodes enlarged

generalized lymphadenopathy

2 review H&P; check CBC

CBC abnormal

CBC variable

CBC normal

lymphoreticular disease
3 ┌ lymphoma
  └ leukemia

connective tissue disease
┌ SLE
├ rheumatoid arthritis/Still's disease
├ dermatomyositis
└ autoimmune hemolytic anemia

4 hypersensitivity reactions
┌ serum sickness
└ drugs (hydantoins)

5 infections
┌ acute
└ chronic ┌ atypical TB
          ├ TB
          ├ syphilis
          └ AIDS

endocrine
6 ┌ hyperthyroidism
  ├ hypoadrenalism
  └ hypopituitarism

Whipple's disease

congenital ┌ cystic hygroma
           └ lymphangioma

7 sarcoidosis

miscellaneous ┌ exfoliative dermatitis
              ├ immunoblastic lymphadenopathy
              └ lipid storage diseases

no other palpable nodes

8 localized lymphadenopathy

perform lymph node biopsy

biopsy diagnostic

9 malignancy ┌ lymphoma
            └ metastatic disease

infections ┌ syphilis
           ├ tularemia
           ├ tuberculosis
           ├ cat-scratch fever
           ├ granuloma inguinale
           └ lymphogranuloma venereum

biopsy non-diagnostic

Kawasaki's disease
10 local inflammation ┌ dermatitis
                      ├ vaccination
                      └ trauma

11 reactive hyperplasia

| Cecil Chapter | 152 |
| Harrison Chapter | 64 |

Splenomegaly

1 Although splenomegaly may be the first sign of disease, an enlarged spleen may not be clinically significant. A palpable spleen is not always an enlarged spleen. Several studies have revealed a 2 to 6 per cent prevalence of a palpable spleen in large series of healthy patients, although no etiology could be discovered in 25 to 41 per cent of those patients. In a large series of normal college students, spleens were palpable in approximately 3 per cent of those examined. A third of these patients continued to have palpable spleens at 3 years' follow-up examination without associated disease.

2 If a young individual with a palpable spleen has an otherwise normal history and physical examination and a normal CBC, it is likely that the spleen is normal and the splenomegaly is idiopathic (see No. 1 above). Splenic imaging (see No. 3) may not confirm splenic enlargement or may show a displaced spleen. If splenomegaly is confirmed but the etiology is uncertain, the patient should be followed closely and re-examined periodically, with further testing as indicated by changes in the patient's history or physical examination.

3 Spleen size can be evaluated by a variety of methods, including computed tomography (CT) scan, radionuclide spleen scan, ultrasonography, and magnetic resonance imaging (MRI). Ultrasonography is probably the most accurate, low-cost, noninvasive technique available to image the spleen. If splenic imaging is normal, the spleen is probably normal. Splenic imaging is useful to confirm splenic enlargement but will also uncover causes of splenic displacement or space-occupying splenic lesions.

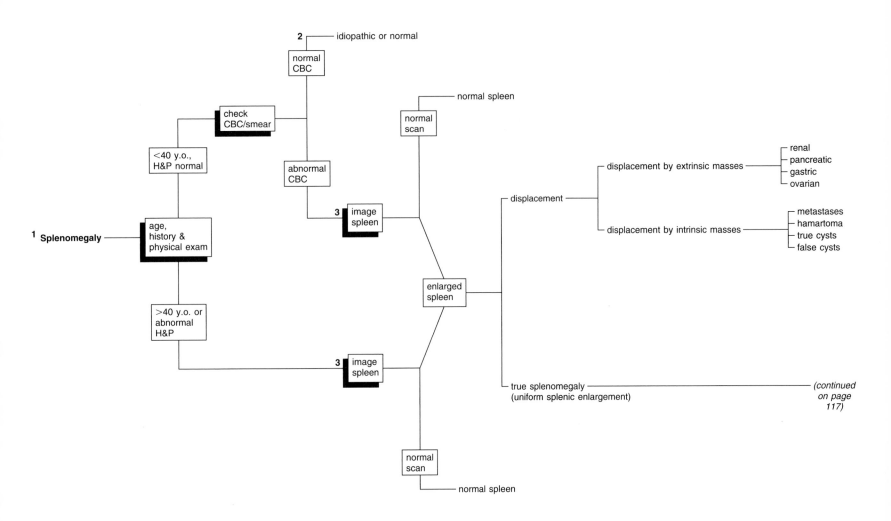

1 Splenomegaly

age, history & physical exam

<40 y.o., H&P normal

check CBC/smear

2 idiopathic or normal

normal CBC

abnormal CBC

3 image spleen

normal scan — normal spleen

>40 y.o. or abnormal H&P

3 image spleen

normal scan — normal spleen

enlarged spleen

displacement

displacement by extrinsic masses
- renal
- pancreatic
- gastric
- ovarian

displacement by intrinsic masses
- metastases
- hamartoma
- true cysts
- false cysts

true splenomegaly (uniform splenic enlargement)

(continued on page 117)

Cecil Chapter	152
Harrison Chapter	64

Splenomegaly (Continued)

4 The term hypersplenism has been used to designate the concept that the spleen is producing hematologic abnormalities via an exaggeration of its normal activities. Hematologic abnormalities owing to hypersplenism include anemia, leukopenia, and thrombocytopenia. In many cases of splenomegaly, a "pseudoanemia" is a result of increased total plasma volume and a normal red cell mass that is sequestered in the enlarged spleen. Primary hypersplenism refers to a state in which no underlying disease can be discovered.

5 Chronic congestive splenomegaly, known as Banti's syndrome, consists of splenomegaly, pancytopenia, portal hypertension, and gastrointestinal bleeding. Any condition that causes portal hypertension can cause Banti's syndrome. Underlying causes of portal hypertension include portal or splenic vein thrombosis or compression, as well as intrahepatic processes such as Laënnec's cirrhosis. The portal hypertension is responsible for the increased incidence of gastrointestinal bleeding and splenomegaly. The enlarged spleen, in turn, may cause pancytopenia.

6 Splenic hyperplasia is thought to be due to an increase in workload placed on the spleen. The spleen hypertrophies in response to increased work of removal of abnormal blood cells from the circulation. The abnormal cells may have intrinsic defects or may be cells coated with antibody. The chief causes of splenic hyperplasia include various forms of anemia and many autoimmune disorders. In some cases, splenic hyperplasia is a result of extramedullary hematopoiesis. Diagnosis is apparent upon appropriate hematologic testing.

7 A benign generalized lymphoid hyperplasia is the source of splenomegaly that may be seen in Graves' disease.

8 Splenomegaly is often the result of infiltrative diseases including Gaucher's disease, Niemann-Pick disease, and amyloidosis. The spleen can be infiltrated by leukemic cells and lymphoma. Occasionally, the enlarged spleen may be the presenting site of lymphoma. In Hodgkin's disease, palpable splenomegaly is usually indicative of more advanced disease. Histologic confirmation of suspected splenic disease may ultimately require fine needle biopsy or splenectomy for diagnosis.

9 Splenomegaly is commonly associated with acute inflammatory processes, usually in response to an increase in the activity of the immune functions of the spleen. Chronic infections causing splenomegaly may mimic a primary hematologic disorder. The clinician must have a high suspicion of infection in order to make an accurate diagnosis. Blood cultures and appropriate serologic testing for infectious agents will aid in diagnosis.

10 Felty's syndrome is defined as splenomegaly and leukopenia associated with rheumatoid arthritis in adults. Splenomegaly may precede the development of leukopenia by many years.

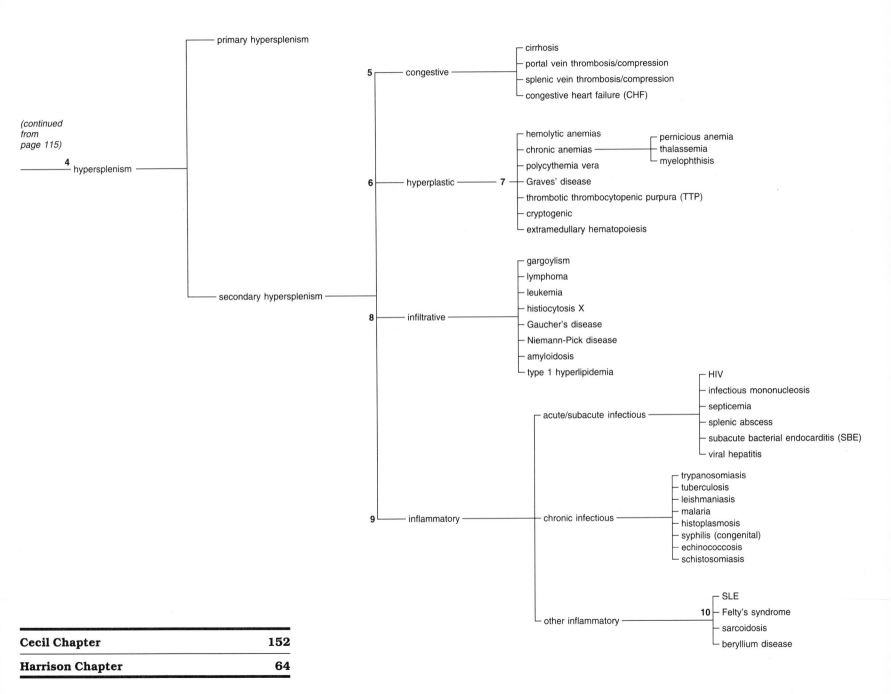

(continued from page 115)

4 hypersplenism

primary hypersplenism

secondary hypersplenism

5 congestive
- cirrhosis
- portal vein thrombosis/compression
- splenic vein thrombosis/compression
- congestive heart failure (CHF)

6 hyperplastic
- hemolytic anemias
- chronic anemias **7**
  - pernicious anemia
  - thalassemia
  - myelophthisis
- polycythemia vera
- Graves' disease
- thrombotic thrombocytopenic purpura (TTP)
- cryptogenic
- extramedullary hematopoiesis

8 infiltrative
- gargoylism
- lymphoma
- leukemia
- histiocytosis X
- Gaucher's disease
- Niemann-Pick disease
- amyloidosis
- type 1 hyperlipidemia

9 inflammatory
- acute/subacute infectious
  - HIV
  - infectious mononucleosis
  - septicemia
  - splenic abscess
  - subacute bacterial endocarditis (SBE)
  - viral hepatitis
- chronic infectious
  - trypanosomiasis
  - tuberculosis
  - leishmaniasis
  - malaria
  - histoplasmosis
  - syphilis (congenital)
  - echinococcosis
  - schistosomiasis
- other inflammatory **10**
  - SLE
  - Felty's syndrome
  - sarcoidosis
  - beryllium disease

Cecil Chapter	152
Harrison Chapter	**64**

Anemia

1 Red cell indices are calculated with automated equipment and include the following:

MCV = mean corpuscular volume. The MCV represents the average size of the red blood cell. To calculate:

$$MCV = Hct/RBC$$

where Hct is hematocrit and RBC is red blood cells ($\times\ 10^6/\mu l$). Normal range MCV = 82 to 98 fl. The red blood cells are microcytic if the MCV is low and macrocytic if the MCV is high.

MCHC = mean corpuscular hemoglobin concentration. The MCHC calculates the weight of hemoglobin per volume of red cells. To calculate:

$$MCHC = Hgb/Hct$$

where Hgb is hemoglobin and Hct is hematocrit. Normal range MCHC = 32 to 34 gm/dl. Cells are hypochromic if the MCHC is low and hyperchromic if the MCHC is high.

MCH = mean corpuscular hemoglobin. The MCH represents the average weight of hemoglobin in the red blood cell. To calculate:

$$MCH = Hgb/RBC$$

where Hgb is hemoglobin and RBC is red blood cells ($\times\ 10^6/\mu l$). Normal range MCH = 27 to 34 pg/cell. MCH reflects both the size and hemoglobin concentration of the red blood cells. Low MCH indicates hypochromia, microcytosis, or both.

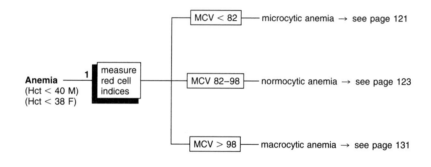

Anemia
(Hct < 40 M)
(Hct < 38 F)

1 — measure red cell indices

MCV < 82 —— microcytic anemia → see page 121

MCV 82–98 —— normocytic anemia → see page 123

MCV > 98 —— macrocytic anemia → see page 131

MICROCYTIC ANEMIA

1 In hereditary spherocytosis, the MCV is usually normal (normocytic) or slightly decreased (microcytic), and the MCHC is increased to 35 to 40 gm/dl. Hereditary spherocytosis is usually classified as a normocytic hemolytic anemia. Almost all other hemolytic anemias are normocytic, normochromic.

2 Iron deficiency is the most common cause of microcytic, hypochromic anemia. Iron deficiency anemia may not be hypochromic until the hemoglobin level is very low.

3 Total iron binding capacity (TIBC) is a measure of serum transferrin content. Serum iron is decreased in both iron deficiency anemia and in anemia associated with chronic disease. In iron deficiency, TIBC is usually increased. The anemia of chronic disease is usually associated with a decreased TIBC. The relationship between iron and TIBC can be expressed as per cent transferrin saturation such that normally approximately 30 per cent transferrin is saturated with iron. In iron deficiency, the transferrin saturation is usually less than 15 per cent.

4 Measurement of serum ferritin also provides a reliable estimate of iron stores. In normal persons, ferritin reflects the size of body iron stores. A decrease in plasma ferritin to less than 10 ng/ml is strongly indicative of iron deficiency. Some individuals with iron deficiency anemia, however, may have serum ferritin levels up to 50 ng/ml.

5 Dietary deficiency is a rare cause of iron deficiency anemia. However, dietary iron absorption can be decreased owing to dietary calcium and phytates (in cereals), which complex with iron and decrease its absorption. Vitamin C promotes iron absorption, probably by allowing reduction of ferric iron to the ferrous form, which is more readily absorbed.

6 Cow's milk is a poor source of iron. Infants fed primarily cow's milk are prone to iron deficiency anemia.

7 Frequent pregnancies increase iron requirement. Frequent blood donation may also deplete iron stores.

8 Except in infants and rapidly growing children, iron deficiency anemia is most commonly caused by chronic blood loss.

9 Iron deficiency may result from hemoglobinuria and hemosiderinuria resulting from severe intravascular hemolysis. Serum lactate dehydrogenase (LDH) is usually increased in iron deficiency anemia associated with hemolysis.

10 Examination of the stool for occult blood is critical in the investigation of iron deficiency anemia. Gastrointestinal (GI) blood loss may be intermittent, requiring the testing of several stool specimens for occult blood over a prolonged period of time. In the absence of another source of bleeding, the GI tract may require evaluation even when stool tests for occult blood are negative. Iron deficiency in men and postmenopausal women is most often due to GI blood loss.

11 Iron deficiency anemia associated with hemodialysis may be due to treatment-related blood loss (e.g., trapping of blood in the dialyzing equipment).

12 An increase in plasma ferritin may indicate increased iron stores. Various other conditions can result in increased plasma ferritin without coexistent iron overload. These other conditions include increased metabolism, inflammation, liver or kidney disease, tissue damage, and neoplastic disease. In order to diagnose iron overload based on increased plasma ferritin, these other causes must first be excluded.

13 Plumbism, or lead poisoning, causes anemia primarily by inhibiting several enzymes important to heme synthesis. Lead may also cause hemolysis. Examination of the blood smear characteristically reveals basophilic stippling of the red cells. Plumbism usually results in a normocytic, hypochromic anemia, although it may also cause a microcytic anemia.

14 Sideroblastic anemias are a heterogeneous group of disorders with the common feature of ringed sideroblasts in the bone marrow. The anemia is caused by an enzymatic defect in the synthesis of heme. Sideroblasts are red blood cell precursors that contain non-heme iron granules. With sideroblastic anemia, hypochromic cells can be found among relatively normal cells so that a "partial hypochromia" exists. Diagnosis requires examination of bone marrow aspirate stained for iron.

15 Isoniazid is an inhibitor of pyridoxal kinase and may cause a pyridoxine-responsive sideroblastic anemia.

16 Anemia associated with chronic inflammatory conditions is usually normocytic, normochromic, but the smear may have a mixed population of cells—including hypochromic red cells.

17 Hemoglobinopathies can be classified broadly into two categories: (1) Inherited structural alteration in one of the globin chains. This category includes sickle cell anemia and related disorders. The hemoglobinopathies in this group may also be microcytic anemias but are usually normocytic. Electrophoresis is the test of choice to define globin chain abnormality. (2) Inherited defects in the rate of synthesis of one or more of the globin chains. This category includes the thalassemias. Thalassemia minor is 90 per cent probable if significant microcytosis is found to accompany minimal anemia. Over 350 different abnormal human hemoglobins have been described.

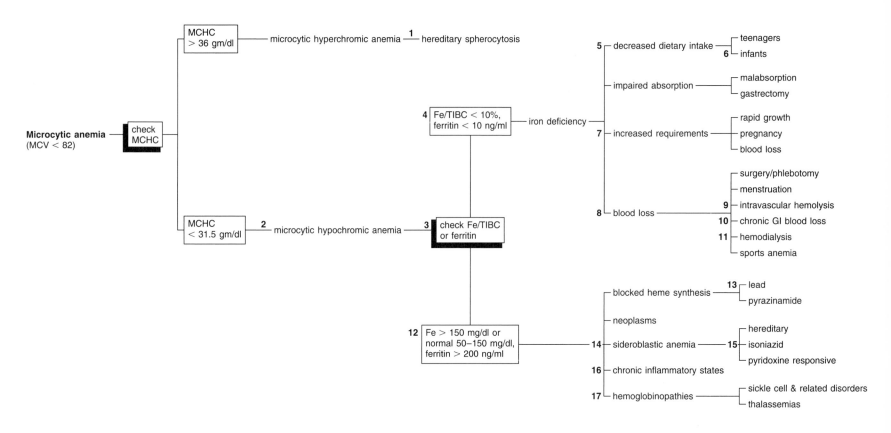

Microcytic anemia (MCV < 82) — check MCHC

- MCHC > 36 gm/dl — microcytic hyperchromic anemia — **1** hereditary spherocytosis
- MCHC < 31.5 gm/dl — **2** microcytic hypochromic anemia — **3** check Fe/TIBC or ferritin

4 Fe/TIBC < 10%, ferritin < 10 ng/ml — iron deficiency
- **5** decreased dietary intake — teenagers — **6** infants
- impaired absorption — malabsorption — gastrectomy
- **7** increased requirements — rapid growth — pregnancy — blood loss
- **8** blood loss — surgery/phlebotomy — menstruation — **9** intravascular hemolysis — **10** chronic GI blood loss — **11** hemodialysis — sports anemia

12 Fe > 150 mg/dl or normal 50–150 mg/dl, ferritin > 200 ng/ml
- blocked heme synthesis — **13** lead — pyrazinamide
- neoplasms
- **14** sideroblastic anemia — **15** hereditary — isoniazid — pyridoxine responsive
- **16** chronic inflammatory states
- **17** hemoglobinopathies — sickle cell & related disorders — thalassemias

Cecil Chapter	**131**
Harrison Chapter	**291**

NORMOCYTIC ANEMIA

1 Reticulocytes are red cells newly released from the bone marrow. The reticulocyte count is obtained by noting the number of reticulocytes per thousand red cells—expressed as per cent reticulocytes. Normal values are 0.5 to 1.5 per cent. The reticulocyte count is dependent upon the total number of red cells in circulation; therefore, the total number of reticulocytes varies with different hematocrits. A correction factor based on a normal hematocrit of 45 per cent can be used to calculate the corrected reticulocyte count:

Per cent corrected reticulocyte count
= per cent reticulocyte count × patient hematocrit/45

2 An elevated reticulocyte count anemia indicates increased marrow production of red blood cells. The reticulocyte count is a good indicator of adequate marrow function.

3 Visual examination of a smear of the peripheral blood quickly reveals whether increased marrow activity is due to destruction of red cells by hemolysis or to blood loss.

4 There are a number of laboratory tests useful in establishing or confirming the presence of hemolysis: (1) Examine the blood smear. Review of the smear may reveal red cell fragments or the characteristic shape of cells found in some hereditary membrane abnormalities. Spherocytes, fragmented RBCs, and spiculated red cells are important findings. (2) Unconjugated or indirect bilirubin is elevated in patients with hemolysis. The serum level of conjugated bilirubin remains within normal limits, unless there is coexistent liver disease. (3) Haptoglobin, an alpha globulin that binds to the protein (globin) in hemoglobin, is decreased or absent owing to the release of globin from the lysed red cells. (4) Urine hemoglobin is found when the absorptive capacity of the renal tubule has been exceeded. Normally, the hemoglobin is bound to haptoglobin and is not filtered by the kidney, but once the haptoglobin-binding capacity has been exceeded, hemoglobinuria occurs. These abnormalities usually occur only with severe hemolysis.

5 A normal or decreased reticulocyte count may indicate inadequate bone marrow response to anemia, although a reduced reticulocyte count is not always due to a primary marrow disturbance.

6 Causes of a dilutional anemia include rapid infusion of intravenous fluids and venipucture proximal to the site of infusion of intravenous fluids.

7 Myelophthisic marrow refers to bone marrow that has been infiltrated—usually by tumor or granuloma, although marrow infiltration can also occur with lipid storage diseases. Tumor infiltration may be by metastatic solid tumor or by cells indigenous to the marrow such as myeloma or leukemia. Invasion of bone marrow by metastatic tumor inhibits erythropoiesis and thrombopoiesis, but neutrophil production may be normal or increased.

8 Aplastic anemia refers to a bone marrow that is acellular or hypocellular, resulting in a pancytopenia—i.e., anemia, neutropenia, and thrombocytopenia.

9 In red cell aplasia, a cytotoxic antibody is directed against an early red cell antigen, causing a selective failure of the production of the erythroid elements of the bone marrow although other marrow cell lines are normal. Red cell aplasia is associated with autoimmune diseases such as rheumatoid arthritis and SLE.

10 Anemia of chronic liver disease is associated with any advanced liver disease, commonly alcoholic liver disease. Alcohol directly suppresses erythropoiesis, and blood loss is common in alcoholics. Inadequate intake and impaired utilization of folate and a shortened red cell life span also contribute to the anemia in alcoholics.

11 In anemia associated with chronic inflammation, the extent of the anemia is roughly proportional to the duration and severity of the inflammatory process. Chronic infections, collagen-vascular diseases, and neoplasms are all classified in this group. Neoplastic disorders alone can cause anemia, but commonly anemia develops via a variety of other mechanisms with neoplasms—e.g., blood loss (colon cancer), invasion of bone marrow (myelophthisis), and suppression of hematopoiesis by chemotherapy or radiation therapy.

12 The low red cell production associated with uremia is due to inadequate secretion of erythropoietin. Other factors that may contribute to the anemia associated with renal failure include hemolysis, dialysis-related blood loss, and GI bleeding.

13 Thyroxine, glucocorticoids, testosterone, and growth hormone all affect hematopoiesis. Patients with myxedema have an increased incidence of pernicious anemia. Hypothyroid patients also often develop iron deficiency anemia. Anemia associated with endocrine failure may be corrected with hormone replacement.

14 In early iron deficiency anemia, the peripheral red cells may remain normocytic (MCV is usually in the low normal range), but examination of the bone marrow reveals moderate erythroid hyperplasia. Marrow stains for iron are decreased or absent.

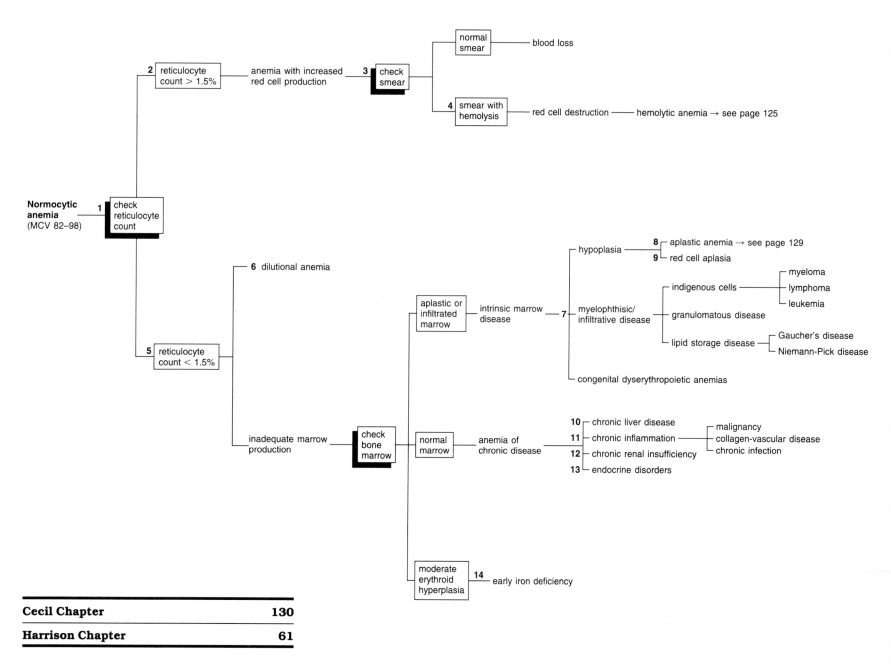

Normocytic anemia (MCV 82–98)

1 check reticulocyte count

2 reticulocyte count > 1.5% — anemia with increased red cell production — **3** check smear

- normal smear — blood loss
- **4** smear with hemolysis — red cell destruction — hemolytic anemia → see page 125

5 reticulocyte count < 1.5%

- **6** dilutional anemia
- inadequate marrow production — check bone marrow

  - aplastic or infiltrated marrow — intrinsic marrow disease — **7** myelophthisic/infiltrative disease
    - hypoplasia
      - **8** aplastic anemia → see page 129
      - **9** red cell aplasia
    - myelophthisic/infiltrative disease
      - indigenous cells
        - myeloma
        - lymphoma
        - leukemia
      - granulomatous disease
      - lipid storage disease
        - Gaucher's disease
        - Niemann-Pick disease
    - congenital dyserythropoietic anemias

  - normal marrow — anemia of chronic disease
    - **10** chronic liver disease
    - **11** chronic inflammation
      - malignancy
      - collagen-vascular disease
      - chronic infection
    - **12** chronic renal insufficiency
    - **13** endocrine disorders

  - moderate erythroid hyperplasia — **14** early iron deficiency

Hemolytic Anemia

1 A direct Coombs' test is used to determine whether the red cell destruction is due to the presence of antibodies and complement coating the red cell surface. The presence of these antibodies leads to increased clearance and destruction of these cells by the macrophages in the reticuloendothelial system.

2 A positive direct Coombs' test indicates the presence of antibodies in the patient's serum directed against his own red cells.

3 A negative direct Coombs' test indicates that hemolysis is usually unrelated to an immune mechanism, although about 5 to 10 per cent of patients with autoimmune hemolytic anemia have a negative direct Coombs' test. Nonimmune causes of hemolytic anemia include agents that physically damage red cells and abnormalities intrinsic to red cells resulting in hemolysis.

4 Fibrin deposition is the primary cause of the red cell fragmentation that occurs in microangiopathic hemolytic anemia.

5 A variety of infectious agents may be associated with severe hemolysis, some by parasitization of the red cell, others by indirect action as is seen with clostridial infections.

6 Chemical agents such as benzene and copper can have a direct hemolytic effect on the red blood cell. The hemolysis seen in Wilson's disease is thought to be due to copper toxicity.

7 Hypersplenism may result in hemolysis of otherwise normal red blood cells.

8 The shape of the red cells in spur-cell anemia accounts for their entrapment and destruction by the reticuloendothelial system. Spur cells occur most commonly in patients with severe cirrhosis.

9 Paroxysmal nocturnal hemoglobinuria (PNH) is an acquired intracorpuscular red cell defect with a markedly increased sensitivity to complement-mediated hemolysis. Clues to diagnosis include decreased leukocyte alkaline phosphatase and hemosiderinuria. Either a Ham's test or a sucrose hemolysis test can be used to diagnose PNH. Ham's test is too insensitive to detect all patients with PNH. The sucrose hemolysis test is more sensitive but is less specific (see No. 5, page 140).

10 Hereditary spherocytosis, elliptocytosis, and stomatocytosis are all autosomal dominant disorders in which the poor deformability of the red cell membrane allows for red blood cell destruction by a normal spleen.

11 Internal red cell disorders are caused by red cell enzyme defects and hemoglobinopathies. Both result in premature red cell destruction.

12 Glucose-6-phosphate dehydrogenase (G-6-PD) is an important enzyme employed by the red cell to protect itself against oxidant stress. G-6-PD deficiency is inherited as an X-linked trait and is found in 10 to 15 per cent of American blacks. Hemolytic anemia arises in G-6-PD deficiency only when the individual is exposed to environmental stress such as drugs or infection. Examples of drugs causing hemolysis in patients deficient in G-6-PD include the antimalarials (primaquine, chloroquine), sulfonamides (sulfanilamide, sulfisoxazole, dapsone), nitrofurans, analgesics (phenacetin), and other drugs including probenecid, nalidixic acid, quinine, quinidine, vitamin K, chloramphenicol, and fava beans. Upon oxidation, the hemoglobin tends to precipitate in the red cell, forming Heinz bodies.

13 Hemoglobinopathies, including sickle cell anemia and thalassemia, can also result in hemolytic anemia. In sickle cell anemia, the abnormally shaped cell is rapidly cleared by the reticuloendothelial system. Thalassemia is a hereditary anemia in which there is a quantitative decrease in synthesis of one or more of the globin chains, resulting in unbalanced globin chain synthesis. In the thalassemias, red cell destruction results from the precipitation of the abnormal hemoglobin (forming Heinz bodies) and the increased osmotic fragility of the red cells. The hemolysis is most severe in beta-thalassemia major.

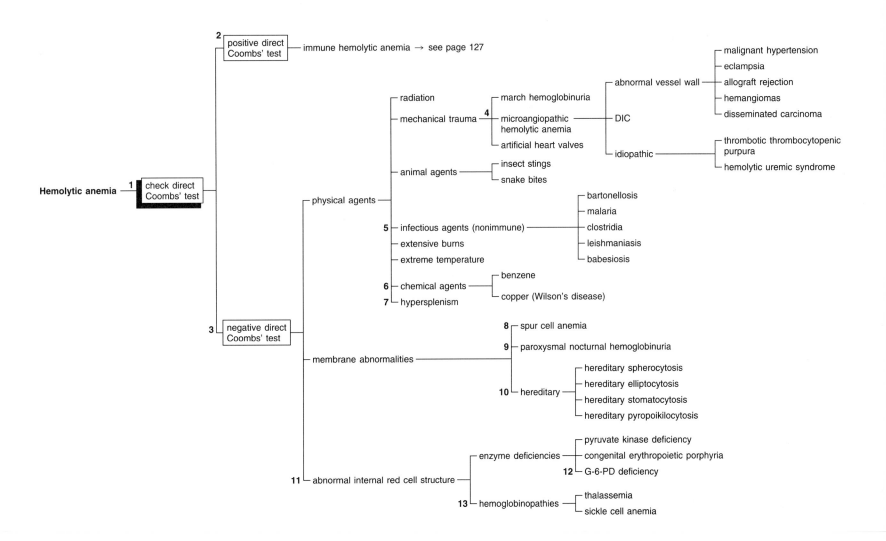

Hemolytic anemia — **1** check direct Coombs' test

2 positive direct Coombs' test — immune hemolytic anemia → see page 127

3 negative direct Coombs' test

physical agents
- radiation
- mechanical trauma — **4**
  - march hemoglobinuria
  - microangiopathic hemolytic anemia — DIC
    - abnormal vessel wall
      - malignant hypertension
      - eclampsia
      - allograft rejection
      - hemangiomas
      - disseminated carcinoma
    - idiopathic
      - thrombotic thrombocytopenic purpura
      - hemolytic uremic syndrome
  - artificial heart valves
- animal agents
  - insect stings
  - snake bites
- **5** infectious agents (nonimmune)
  - bartonellosis
  - malaria
  - clostridia
  - leishmaniasis
  - babesiosis
- extensive burns
- extreme temperature
- **6** chemical agents
  - benzene
  - copper (Wilson's disease)
- **7** hypersplenism

membrane abnormalities
- **8** spur cell anemia
- **9** paroxysmal nocturnal hemoglobinuria
- **10** hereditary
  - hereditary spherocytosis
  - hereditary elliptocytosis
  - hereditary stomatocytosis
  - hereditary pyropoikilocytosis

11 abnormal internal red cell structure
- enzyme deficiencies
  - pyruvate kinase deficiency
  - congenital erythropoietic porphyria
  - **12** G-6-PD deficiency
- **13** hemoglobinopathies
  - thalassemia
  - sickle cell anemia

Cecil Chapters	133, 135, 136
Harrison Chapters	61, 294

Immune Hemolytic Anemia

1 The indirect Coombs' test can detect alloantibodies present in a patient's serum directed against red cells that are to be transfused. It is used to detect antibodies present in maternal serum against the fetal red cells, and it is also used as a prognostic indicator in warm autoimmune hemolytic anemia. In the severe form of warm immune hemolytic anemia, antibody is found not only on the red cells but in excess in the patient's serum, and both direct and indirect Coombs' tests are positive.

2 Isoimmune hemolytic disease of the newborn, or erythroblastosis fetalis, is a hemolytic disorder caused by transplacental maternal antibodies directed against fetal red cells. Almost all cases are due to anti-Rh antibodies.

3 The division of the hemolytic anemias into warm and cold varieties is based on the optimal temperature of antibody reactivity with the red cell surface.

Warm immune hemolytic anemia is due to an IgG antibody that reacts with the red cell surface optimally at 37°C. The IgG-coated red cells are then destroyed by splenic macrophages. The majority (40 to 50 per cent) of these cases are idiopathic.

4 There are three types of drug-induced autoimmune hemolytic anemias: the hapten type, the autoimmune type, and the innocent bystander type. In the hapten type, antibody is produced against the drug, not the red cell membrane. However, the antibody-drug complex has an affinity for the red cell surface, resulting ultimately in red cell destruction. The antibody may or may not fix complement. Penicillin is an example of the hapten type of hemolytic anemia. In the autoimmune type, patients produce antibodies against their own red cells and not against the drug. The most characteristic drug in this group is Aldomet. The innocent bystander type of hemolysis is due to the generation of activated complement components by the drug-antibody complexes. Quinine, sulfonamides, and phenothiazines are examples of drugs that induce this type of hemolytic anemia.

5 Less common than warm immune hemolytic anemia, cold immune hemolytic anemia is due to an IgM complement-fixing antibody that binds to the red cell optimally at 4°C but rapidly dissociates from the red cell at increased temperatures. Cold agglutinins are present in normal serum but at such low titer that they are of no clinical concern. In certain disorders, cold agglutinin titers may range from 1:1000 to 1:100,000. Antibody attachment to red cells during transient temperature decrease (as happens when blood flows through fingertips, ears, and nose) can activate the complement sequence and cause red cell lysis. The IgM may dissociate from the red cell as the cell returns to a warmer temperature, but the complement remains bound, causing continued red cell destruction via the macrophages of the reticuloendothelial system.

6 A rare cause of cold immune hemolytic anemia is paroxysmal cold hemoglobinuria (PCH). In PCH, the antibody responsible for red cell destruction is IgG, not IgM.

Immune hemolytic anemia — check indirect Coombs' test

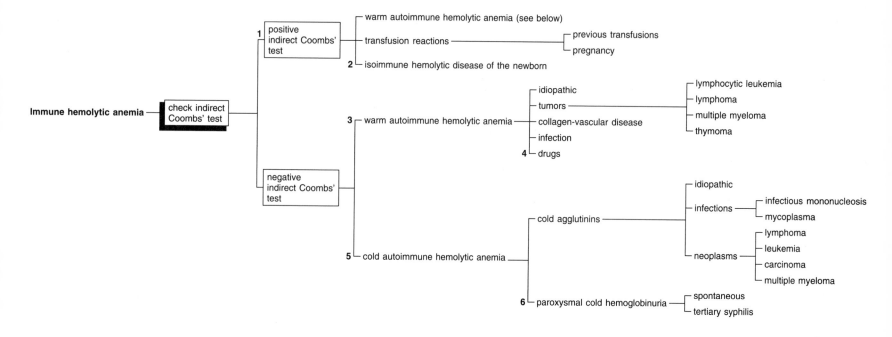

1 positive indirect Coombs' test
- warm autoimmune hemolytic anemia (see below)
- transfusion reactions
  - previous transfusions
  - pregnancy
2 isoimmune hemolytic disease of the newborn

3 warm autoimmune hemolytic anemia
- idiopathic
- tumors
  - lymphocytic leukemia
  - lymphoma
  - multiple myeloma
  - thymoma
- collagen-vascular disease
- infection
4 drugs

negative indirect Coombs' test

5 cold autoimmune hemolytic anemia
- cold agglutinins
  - idiopathic
  - infections
    - infectious mononucleosis
    - mycoplasma
  - neoplasms
    - lymphoma
    - leukemia
    - carcinoma
    - multiple myeloma
6 paroxysmal cold hemoglobinuria
  - spontaneous
  - tertiary syphilis

Cecil Chapter	**133**
Harrison Chapters	**61, 294**

Aplastic Anemia

1 Aplastic anemia refers specifically to patients with a bone marrow that is acellular or replaced with fat owing to hypoplasia of the erythroid, myeloid, and thrombopoietic cell lines. Destruction of all these cell lines is thought to be secondary to injury or destruction of a common pluripotent stem cell. The pancytopenia of aplastic anemia must be differentiated from pancytopenia owing to marrow replacement.

2 Approximately 50 per cent of all cases of aplastic anemia in the United States are of unknown etiology. Some of these cases may be due to environmental toxic exposures.

3 Approximately one fourth of patients with paroxysmal nocturnal hemoglobinuria will develop aplastic anemia during the course of their disease. Five to 10 per cent of patients with aplastic anemia are found to have hemolytic anemia with complement-sensitive red cells similar to those in paroxysmal nocturnal hemoglobinuria (see No. 9, page 124).

4 Drugs and chemicals causing marrow aplasia can do so in either a dose-related or an idiosyncratic fashion. Agents that will predictably produce marrow depression with calculated dosing include antineoplastic agents (alkylating agents and antimetabolites) and ionizing radiation. The degree of aplasia varies between individuals but in general is dose-related. Withdrawal of the drug usually allows for marrow recovery, although aplasia may at times be irreversible.

5 The most common drug causing aplastic anemia is chloramphenicol. Chloramphenicol can cause both a dose-related marrow aplasia and an idiosyncratic marrow aplasia. Idiosyncratic chloramphenicol marrow suppression may appear long after the drug has been discontinued.

6 Benzene-induced marrow aplasia is usually reversible. Pancytopenia can occur many years after actual benzene exposure, although in most cases marrow depression appears shortly after exposure and appears to be related to dose and duration of the exposure. Benzene exposure can also cause leukemia.

7 Ionizing radiation causes marrow aplasia in a dose-related manner. Patients exposed to large amounts of ionizing radiation in laboratory or nuclear reactor accidents suffer from damage to the bone marrow and intestines. If these patients can be supported for 3 to 6 weeks, the surviving stem cells may be the source of bone marrow regeneration.

8 Aplastic marrow that develops during pregnancy may recover after the fetus is born. It is thought that an inhibitor of hematopoiesis may be present during gestation.

9 Constitutional aplastic anemia is the term used to describe the group of patients with congenital marrow aplasia with or without associated visceral and bony abnormalities. The prototype is Fanconi's anemia in which a familial marrow aplasia is accompanied by multiple congenital abnormalities. There is a high incidence of late development of leukemia in those patients who survive the aplasia.

10 Aplastic anemia may appear as hepatitis resolves. It is thought that the aplasia is due to a direct effect of the virus on the bone marrow, possibly via an immune mechanism.

11 Miliary tuberculosis has been reported to cause aplastic anemia but in most cases causes bone marrow dysfunction rather than true aplasia.

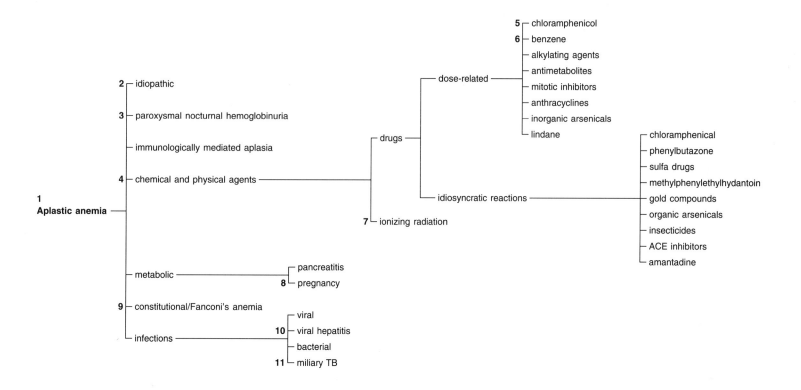

1
Aplastic anemia

2 idiopathic

3 paroxysmal nocturnal hemoglobinuria

immunologically mediated aplasia

4 chemical and physical agents

drugs

dose-related

5 chloramphenicol
6 benzene
alkylating agents
antimetabolites
mitotic inhibitors
anthracyclines
inorganic arsenicals
lindane

7 ionizing radiation

idiosyncratic reactions

chloramphenical
phenylbutazone
sulfa drugs
methylphenylethylhydantoin
gold compounds
organic arsenicals
insecticides
ACE inhibitors
amantadine

metabolic

pancreatitis
8 pregnancy

9 constitutional/Fanconi's anemia

infections

viral
10 viral hepatitis
bacterial
11 miliary TB

Cecil Chapter	129
Harrison Chapters	**61, 298**

MACROCYTIC ANEMIA

1 The term macrocytic refers to an MCV greater than 98. The term megaloblastic refers to the large red cells that result from an unbalanced growth of the cells caused by impaired DNA synthesis in the nucleus, whereas cytoplasmic RNA and protein synthesis proceed normally. Because DNA synthesis is impaired, there is more time for cell growth between cell divisions, resulting in larger cells. The terms macrocytic and megaloblastic are often interchanged because macrocytic anemias are most often associated with a megaloblastic morphology in the bone marrow. Not all macrocytic anemias are megaloblastic.

2 A low MCHC (<32) may indicate a sideroblastic anemia in which a defect in the synthesis of heme results in hypochromia. Sideroblastic anemias are most commonly microcytic, hypochromic anemias, but they can be macrocytic, with the MCHC often not decreased. Many times a "partial hypochromia" is seen in which a hypochromic population of cells is mixed with a relatively normal cell population. Bone marrow examination reveals a number of abnormalities, including erythroid hyperplasia with megaloblastic changes. The most diagnostic abnormality is the presence of ringed sideroblasts in the bone marrow, as is demonstrated with iron stains.

3 The most common causes of a macrocytic, normochromic anemia are liver disease, alcoholism, and vitamin B_{12} or folate deficiency. Both B_{12} and folate deficiencies demonstrate identical blood smears and marrow changes so that further clinical information and diagnostic studies must be undertaken to discover the cause of the macrocytic anemia. Combined deficiencies of B_{12} and folate are not uncommon. Often the underlying cause of B_{12} and folate deficiency is the same. An MCV above 110 is more predictive of vitamin deficiency, and the likelihood of a B_{12} or folate deficiency increases proportional to the MCV. An MCV greater than 130 is associated with a deficiency in B_{12}, folate, or both almost 100 per cent of the time.

4 Normal B_{12} levels are 160 to 930 pg/ml. The dietary sources of vitamin B_{12} are primarily animal protein (dairy foods, fish, meat). The average diet contains 3 to 30 μg of B_{12}, but the daily requirement is only 0.6 to 1.2 μg. Body stores are large (5000 to 11,000 μg), so that depletion is unlikely solely on a nutritional basis, except in vegetarians. Thyroid function tests should also be measured at this point because more than 50 per cent of patients with hypothyroidism demonstrate an associated macrocytic anemia.

5 B_{12} deficiency is almost always due to malabsorption, because dietary intake is usually more than adequate for the body's requirement.

6 Normal folic acid levels are 2 to 14 ng/ml. Sources of folate include fruits, vegetables, liver, kidney, and yeast. The average diet contains 200 to 700 μg, with a daily requirement of 50 μg. The body storage pool is 5 to 10 mg folate. Folate is labile and can be destroyed by cooking the foods that contain it.

7 Reticulocytes are larger than normal red cells and may raise the MCV to the macrocytic range when reticulocytosis is marked (e.g., >10 to 20 per cent).

8 If the bone marrow is megaloblastic, then deficiency of vitamin B_{12} or folate must be considered even if respective serum levels are normal.

9 Administration of vitamin B_{12} and folate and noting the clinical response of the hematocrit will help differentiate between a B_{12} or folate deficiency and a refractory anemia.

10 Lack of response to B_{12} or folate administration defines the refractory anemias.

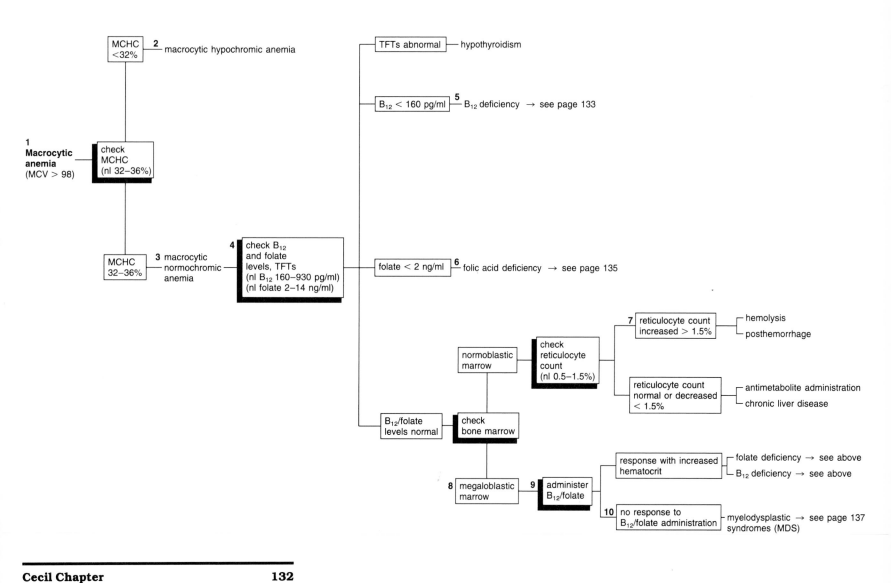

MCHC <32% — **2** macrocytic hypochromic anemia

TFTs abnormal — hypothyroidism

B₁₂ < 160 pg/ml — **5** B₁₂ deficiency → see page 133

1
Macrocytic anemia
(MCV > 98) — check MCHC (nl 32–36%)

MCHC 32–36% — **3** macrocytic normochromic anemia — **4** check B₁₂ and folate levels, TFTs (nl B₁₂ 160–930 pg/ml) (nl folate 2–14 ng/ml)

folate < 2 ng/ml — **6** folic acid deficiency → see page 135

normoblastic marrow — check reticulocyte count (nl 0.5–1.5%)

7 reticulocyte count increased > 1.5% — hemolysis / posthemorrhage

reticulocyte count normal or decreased < 1.5% — antimetabolite administration / chronic liver disease

B₁₂/folate levels normal — check bone marrow

8 megaloblastic marrow — **9** administer B₁₂/folate

response with increased hematocrit — folate deficiency → see above / B₁₂ deficiency → see above

10 no response to B₁₂/folate administration — myelodysplastic syndromes (MDS) → see page 137

Cecil Chapter	132
Harrison Chapters	61, 292

Vitamin B₁₂ Deficiency

1 Normal B_{12} absorption depends on binding to a gastric juice protein, "intrinsic factor," so that 70 per cent of dietary B_{12} is absorbed. Intrinsic factor is derived from the parietal cells of the fundus of the stomach. After binding to intrinsic factor, B_{12} is absorbed primarily from the distal ileum by attaching to specific receptor sites on the ileal mucosa. Optimal B_{12} absorption requires pancreatic enzymes as well. The pancreatic enzymes act by degrading "R proteins" that bind B_{12} and compete with the binding by intrinsic factor, thereby reducing B_{12} absorption. Once absorbed, B_{12} is carried in plasma by transcobalamins, which are B_{12}-binding proteins: TC I, II, and III. TC II binds nearly all absorbed or injected B_{12} and is therefore the true transport protein, moving B_{12} from the site of absorption to the site of storage. TC I is responsible for B_{12} transport from storage sites and is in equilibrium with tissue stores.

2 The test of choice to evaluate B_{12} absorption is the Schilling test. There are three parts to the Schilling test designed to help define the cause of malabsorption. In the first part, radioactive B_{12} in a dose of 0.5 to 2.0 µg is given orally. Two hours after oral B_{12}, 1000 µg of nonradioactive B_{12} is administered parenterally. This is a "flushing dose"; i.e., the intramuscularly administered B_{12} will block storage of orally administered B_{12} and cause any absorbed radioactive B_{12} to be excreted in the urine. The urine is then collected for the 24- to 72-hour period following the oral B_{12} dose, and the amount of radioactive B_{12} is measured. The amount of B_{12} excreted represents the amount of B_{12} absorbed. In normal individuals, 7 to 22 per cent of the initial oral radioactive B_{12} is excreted in the urine. Error can be due to inadequate collection of urine or to prolonged urinary excretion of B_{12} caused by decreased renal function. If B_{12} excretion is low, the second part of the test can be performed. Part II of the Schilling test entails giving intrinsic factor along with the oral B_{12}. Part III entails repeating the Schilling test after a course of tetracycline therapy to reduce intestinal bacterial overgrowth.

3 A normal Schilling test indicates that there is an increased requirement or inadequate dietary intake of vitamin B_{12}.

4 Inadequate dietary intake is a rare cause of B_{12} deficiency, because dietary intake usually exceeds daily requirements. Rarely a purely dietary deficiency can be seen in infants whose entire diet consists of breast milk (usually from strictly vegetarian mothers), in alcoholics with poor dietary intake of all nutrients, and in strict vegetarians who ingest no animal protein.

5 Transcobalamin II deficiency is a rare autosomal recessive trait in which B_{12} is absorbed orally but cannot be transported and stored. B_{12} is absorbed and lost to the urine owing to lack of TC II. These patients can survive when given pharmacologic but not physiologic doses of B_{12}.

6 With gastrectomy, intrinsic factor is absent because the parietal cells have been resected. However, even if B_{12} therapy has been overlooked following gastrectomy, a megaloblastic anemia will not become apparent for 5 to 6 years, because body stores are large. On the other hand, partial gastrectomy rarely results in a significant decrease in B_{12} absorption. A B_{12} deficiency after partial gastrectomy is probably due to partial excision of parietal cells as well as to atrophy of the remaining gastric mucosa.

7 The most common cause of B_{12} deficiency in adults is pernicious anemia, which is malabsorption of B_{12} owing to inadequate intrinsic factor. Pernicious anemia refers specifically to defective secretion of intrinsic factor by the gastric mucosa. Pernicious anemia occurs in two forms—a common adult type in which lack of intrinsic factor is associated with gastric atrophy and a deficiency of many other gastric secretions and a rare congenital form in which only intrinsic factor is lacking while other components of the gastric juice are normal. Pernicious anemia is usually seen in persons of northern European descent and usually occurs after the age of 40. An exception is its occurrence in young black women. The congenital form of the disease is autosomal recessive; the adult form has been found to be familial, but the pattern of inheritance remains in doubt. Parietal cell antibodies, intrinsic factor antibodies, and thyroid antibodies have all been demonstrated in the serum of some patients with pernicious anemia. If thyroid disease has not previously been investigated (see No. 1, page 190), thyroid function should be evaluated at this point. Approximately 25 per cent of patients with pernicious anemia have concomitant hypo- or hyperthyroidism.

8 Anti-intrinsic factor antibodies may also be found in patients without pernicious anemia. There is an increased frequency of anti-intrinsic factor antibodies in patients with diabetes mellitus, thyroid disease, thyrotoxicosis, Hashimoto's thyroiditis, hypogammaglobulinemia, vitiligo, rheumatoid arthritis, and gastric carcinoma.

9 A normal Schilling test following tetracycline therapy indicates that B_{12} absorption has been inhibited by bacterial overgrowth. The tetracycline decreases bacterial growth, allowing increased B_{12} absorption to normalize the Schilling test. Bacterial overgrowth can occur in several diseases, including "blind loops" created surgically and scleroderma, in which bacterial overgrowth occurs secondary to stasis.

10 Diseases involving the terminal ileum can decrease B_{12} absorption, because the terminal ileum is the site of selective B_{12} absorption.

11 B_{12} malabsorption in chronic pancreatic insufficiency is thought to be secondary to a lack of pancreatic enzymes needed to degrade the complexes of B_{12}-binding proteins ("R proteins"). These proteins are found in saliva, gastric juice, and bile and compete with intrinsic factor for the binding of B_{12}.

12 Familial selective malabsorption (the Imerslund-Gräsbeck syndrome) is a rare inherited disease in which ileal B_{12} absorption is impaired whether it is bound to intrinsic factor or not. It is characterized by the onset in childhood of a megaloblastic anemia along with persistent proteinuria thought to be due to an associated renal tubular defect.

13 Malabsorption of B_{12} observed in carriers of the fish tapeworm *Diphyllobothrium latum* is probably due to a competition between the worm and the host for dietary B_{12}. In patients with anemia, the worm has been found to lodge in the jejunum, proximal to the site of B_{12} absorption, enabling the worm to bind B_{12} before it reaches the site of normal ileal absorption. In patients without anemia, the worm has been found in the ileum. *Diphyllobothrium latum* is a common parasite of freshwater fish, and human infestation ensues after ingestion of inadequately cooked whitefish.

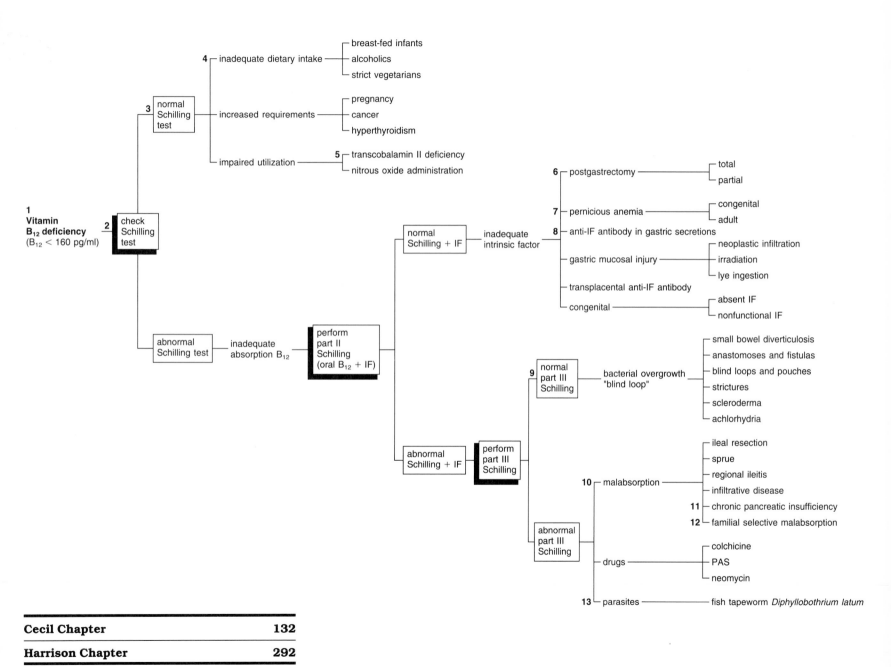

Folic Acid Deficiency

1 In patients with folate deficiency, both serum and RBC folate levels are decreased. In patients with B_{12} deficiency, serum folate levels tend to be elevated and can even be greater than the upper limits of normal, so that with combined deficiencies, serum folate levels may be normal but the RBC folate level will fall. Therefore, RBC folate levels should always be measured in addition to serum folate levels. In contrast to B_{12} stores, folate stores can be depleted within 4 to 5 months.

2 Decreased folate intake is by far the most common cause of folic acid deficiency. Folate-deficient diets are those that lack fresh, green vegetables. Folate deficiency can occasionally be seen in diets containing a large amount of vegetables when the folate has been destroyed by cooking.

3 Folate deficiency seen in alcoholics results from a combination of factors. Inadequate folate is due not only to inadequate dietary intake but also to a disordered folate metabolism seen in cirrhosis. Cirrhotic patients have impaired ability to store folate in the liver and have excessive urinary loss of folate.

4 Folate deficiency is common in patients taking oral contraceptives and the anticonvulsants phenobarbital and phenytoin. The source of this deficiency has not been determined but is thought to be due to folate malabsorption.

5 Pregnancy is a common cause of folate deficiency. Pregnancy-related folate deficiency is due to the combination of decreased folate body stores and a 5- to 10-fold increase in folate requirement, especially in the last trimester.

6 Folate deficiency seen in association with uremia is due to the loss of folate with dialysis.

7 Folate deficiency is seen as a complication of a variety of hematologic disorders characterized by rapid cellular proliferation: sickle cell anemia, paroxysmal nocturnal hemoglobinuria, acquired autoimmune hemolytic anemia, thalassemia, hereditary spherocytosis, drug-induced hemolytic anemia with G-6-PD deficiency, myelofibrosis, sideroblastic anemia, leukemia, and multiple myeloma.

8 Impaired folate utilization is caused by dihydrofolate (DHF) reductase inhibitors such as methotrexate and aminopterin. Folinic acid administration can counteract the actions of DHF reductase inhibitors by bypassing the inhibited enzyme.

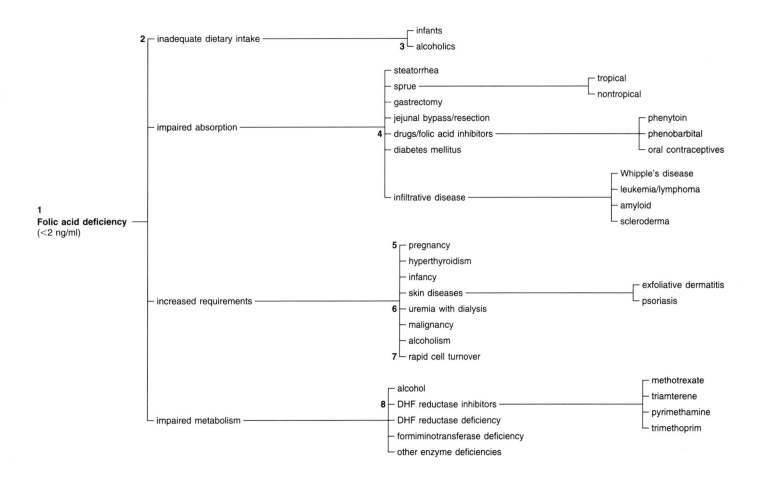

1
Folic acid deficiency
(<2 ng/ml)

2 ┬ inadequate dietary intake
  ├ infants
  3 └ alcoholics

impaired absorption
- steatorrhea
- sprue ┬ tropical
        └ nontropical
- gastrectomy
- jejunal bypass/resection
4 ─ drugs/folic acid inhibitors ┬ phenytoin
                                ├ phenobarbital
                                └ oral contraceptives
- diabetes mellitus
- infiltrative disease ┬ Whipple's disease
                       ├ leukemia/lymphoma
                       ├ amyloid
                       └ scleroderma

increased requirements
5 ┬ pregnancy
- hyperthyroidism
- infancy
- skin diseases ┬ exfoliative dermatitis
                └ psoriasis
6 ─ uremia with dialysis
- malignancy
- alcoholism
7 └ rapid cell turnover

impaired metabolism
- alcohol
8 ─ DHF reductase inhibitors ┬ methotrexate
                             ├ triamterene
                             ├ pyrimethamine
                             └ trimethoprim
- DHF reductase deficiency
- formiminotransferase deficiency
- other enzyme deficiencies

Cecil Chapter	132
Harrison Chapter	**292**

Myelodysplastic Syndromes (MDS) (Refractory Anemia)

1 Myelodysplastic syndromes (MDS), formerly known as refractory anemias, are a diverse group of hematologic disorders in which hematopoietic stem cell abnormality leads to peripheral blood cytopenia. Myelodysplastic syndromes usually present as a macrocytic anemia with a cellular bone marrow including adequate numbers of progenitor cells. An abnormality in progenitor cell differentiation leads to the anemia and varying degrees of pancytopenia.

2 Antimetabolite drugs that block DNA synthesis are commonly used in the treatment of various neoplasms and can cause a megaloblastic anemia. Included in this group are drugs that interfere with DNA synthesis without being readily reversed by simultaneously administered folic or folinic acid.

3 Hereditary orotic aciduria is a rare disease in which pyrimidine metabolism is defective, resulting in megaloblastic anemia. Associated features include growth retardation and orotic aciduria.

4 The unexplained disorders are a small group in which megaloblastic transformation of red cells occurs and the changes are unresponsive to therapy with B_{12} or folate. These disorders have not been associated with any enzyme defect or deficiency.

5 Thiamine-responsive anemia is thought to be due to a rare defect in a thiamine-dependent enzyme involved in DNA synthesis.

6 Di Guglielmo's syndrome (also known as erythremic myelosis or erythroleukemia) is a disease in which erythrocytes are primarily involved in a ''leukemic'' myeloproliferative process. Di Guglielmo's syndrome is associated with severe refractory megaloblastic anemia.

7 In a number of disorders, no underlying defect can be identified. The megaloblastic changes are unresponsive to treatment, and all current modes of therapy are considered investigational. Because an understanding of the biologic defect is lacking, this heterogeneic group of disorders has been classified into different subtypes on the basis of clinical characteristics and marrow morphology. These categories include refractory anemia without ringed sideroblasts; refractory anemia with ringed sideroblasts; refractory anemia with excess blasts; and refractory anemia in transformation.

8 Pyridoxine-responsive anemia is thought to be due to a poorly defined enzymatic defect in which pharmacologic doses of pyridoxine overcome this defect and reverse the anemia.

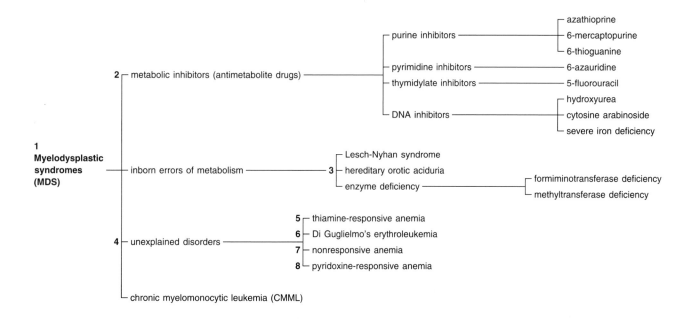

1
Myelodysplastic
syndromes
(MDS)

- **2** metabolic inhibitors (antimetabolite drugs)
  - purine inhibitors
    - azathioprine
    - 6-mercaptopurine
    - 6-thioguanine
  - pyrimidine inhibitors — 6-azauridine
  - thymidylate inhibitors — 5-fluorouracil
  - DNA inhibitors
    - hydroxyurea
    - cytosine arabinoside
    - severe iron deficiency
- inborn errors of metabolism — **3**
  - Lesch-Nyhan syndrome
  - hereditary orotic aciduria
  - enzyme deficiency
    - formiminotransferase deficiency
    - methyltransferase deficiency
- **4** unexplained disorders
  - **5** thiamine-responsive anemia
  - **6** Di Guglielmo's erythroleukemia
  - **7** nonresponsive anemia
  - **8** pyridoxine-responsive anemia
- chronic myelomonocytic leukemia (CMML)

Polycythemia

1 Polycythemia is an increase in the absolute number of circulating red blood cells, usually indicated by an elevated hematocrit. The hematocrit may be elevated without an absolute increase in the number of red blood cells in conditions in which plasma volume is decreased. Confirmation of a true increase in red cell mass is made by measuring the red cell mass with radioactive chromium (^{51}Cr). Hematocrits in the range of 60 per cent or greater almost always represent true erythrocytosis, whereas hematocrits in the 50 to 55 per cent range may be due to plasma volume contraction.

2 A normal red cell mass in the presence of an elevated hematocrit can be due to a loss of plasma volume, which may occur with diarrhea, vomiting, sweating, or diuresis. Gaisböck's syndrome, or stress erythrocytosis, is seen in active, anxious persons whose hematocrits are elevated. These patients usually are male with a high frequency of smoking, obesity, and hypertension. It is likely that the combined effects of smoking, obesity, and hypertension are the source of the red cell and volume changes that result in an apparent erythrocytosis.

3 The definitive test for diagnosing the group of diseases associated with secondary erythrocytosis is the arterial oxygen saturation test. The O_2 saturation must be interpreted with caution, however, because approximately 10 per cent of patients with polycythemia vera (PCV) will also have reduced oxygen saturation in the 88 to 92 per cent range.

4 In diseases associated with hypoxia, increased red cell mass is a compensatory response. Via this mechanism, oxygen-carrying capacity to the tissues is increased. Hypoxia associated with pulmonary diseases manifested by ventilation, perfusion, or diffusion defects can cause polycythemia. Prolonged periods at altitudes greater than 5000 feet may also cause polycythemia secondary to decreased oxygen saturation. Erythropoietin levels may be increased in this setting, but only until equilibrium is re-established.

5 Congenital heart disease associated with right-to-left shunting may produce erythrocytosis. Transposition of the great vessels, persistent truncus arteriosus, ventricular septal defect with pulmonary hypertension, and tricuspid atresia are the most common anomalies associated with right-to-left intracardiac shunting.

6 Mechanical factors may decrease pulmonary oxygenation and result in a secondary erythrocytosis. In the pickwickian syndrome, decreased alveolar oxygenation is due to massive obesity causing hypoventilation. Nonobese patients can also hypoventilate owing to decreased respiratory drive secondary to a decrease in carbon dioxide sensitivity in the respiratory center of the brain stem. The decreased ventilatory drive may be congenital, idiopathic, or a result of disease of the respiratory center such as vascular thrombosis, encephalitis, or bulbar poliomyelitis.

7 The partial pressure of oxygen at which the saturation of hemoglobin is 50 per cent, known as the P_{50}, can be measured to determine the affinity of hemoglobin for oxygen. Increased oxygen affinity of hemoglobin results in a reduced P_{50}. Abnormal hemoglobins with increased affinity for oxygen cause tissue hypoxia by failure to release adequate oxygen at the tissue level. Tissue hypoxia leads to a secondary increase in erythropoietin level and subsequent polycythemia. Arterial PO_2 and O_2 saturations are normal in this setting. At least 45 hemoglobin variants with increased oxygen affinity have been found.

8 Methemoglobinemia occurs when the heme iron is oxidized to methemoglobin and becomes incapable of binding oxygen. Less than 1 per cent methemoglobin is present in normal persons but can increase markedly with exposure to certain drugs or toxins. Hereditary methemoglobinemia is a mild disorder caused by the presence of hemoglobin M or by a deficiency of methemoglobin reductase. Acquired methemoglobinemia can be severe and can be seen in patients receiving nitrite or nitrate preparations, including sodium nitrite, amyl nitrate, nitroglycerin, nitroprusside, and silver nitrate. Other drugs capable of causing methemoglobinemia include sulfonamides, lidocaine, aniline dyes, phenacetin, and acetanilid.

9 Carboxyhemoglobinemia occurs with inhalation of carbon monoxide in cigarette smoke or after inhalation of carbon monoxide from other sources. All smokers, and nonsmokers with unexplained secondary erythrocytosis, should have their carboxyhemoglobin levels measured. Normally nonsmokers have less than 1 per cent carboxyhemoglobin, and smokers' levels range from 5 to 10 per cent. Carbon monoxide replaces oxygen in the heme molecule and increases the heme affinity for oxygen. Increased oxygen affinity by the heme molecule results in tissue hypoxia and is the source of the erythrocytosis.

10 Sulfhemoglobinemia is due to the irreversible oxidation of hemoglobin by certain drugs and chemicals. The oxidized heme is incapable of binding oxygen. The drugs most commonly causing this form of altered hemoglobin are acetanilid, phenacetin, and the sulfonamides. Sulfhemoglobinemia is uncommon despite widespread use of these drugs.

11 Polycythemia may be due to the autonomous production of erythropoietin by a neoplasm. A remission of the polycythemia has been observed after the tumor has been resected and may recur when the tumor recurs.

12 An increased erythropoietin level has been found in association with non-neoplastic renal pathology such as polycystic kidney disease and hydronephrosis. However, polycythemia is seen in less than 2 per cent of patients with non-neoplastic renal disease.

13 The polycythemia that accompanies endocrine disorders—especially endocrine tumors—is thought to be secondary to an increase in erythropoietin levels. The erythrocytosis may be due to an inappropriate secretion of erythropoietin by the tumor.

14 Hydrocortisone and other corticosteroids can cause a mild generalized stimulation of the bone marrow. The polycythemia that occurs in Cushing's disease is often accompanied by an increase in the number of granulocytes and platelets as well.

15 The erythropoietic activity of androgens is well known. Androgens can be successful in treating some forms of refractory anemia and are probably the source of the polycythemia that accompanies androgen therapy for other conditions.

16 The diagnosis of PCV is made primarily by excluding other causes for increased red cell mass, as well as utilizing the criteria for diagnosis established by the Polycythemia Vera Study Group as follows:

Polycythemia vera is diagnosed if (1), (2), and (3) are present:

(1) Red cell volume >36 ml/kg in males or >32 ml/kg in females
(2) Arterial O_2 saturation >92 per cent
(3) Splenomegaly

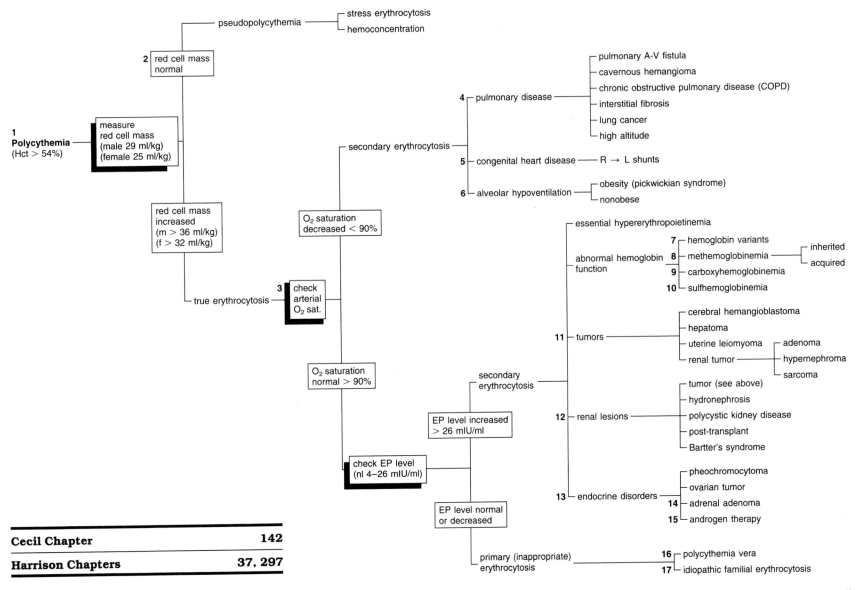

If splenomegaly is absent, then two of the following can substitute for (3):

(a) Thrombocytosis >400,000/mm³
(b) Leukocytosis >12,000/mm³ (in the absence of fever or infection)
(c) Leukocyte alkaline phosphatase >100

(d) Serum B₁₂ >900 pg/ml or serum B₁₂-binding protein >2200 pg/ml.

These criteria are more specific than sensitive, so that early cases of PCV may not meet all of the criteria. Over time a secondary cause of polycythemia may be discovered, or the disease may progress to meet these criteria.

17 Idiopathic familial erythrocytosis is a rare condition in which no hemoglobin abnormality has been found. A primary increase in erythropoietin has been found in some cases and may represent a variant of PCV.

Pancytopenia

1 Pancytopenia is defined as a pronounced reduction in the number of red cells, white cells, and platelets in the peripheral circulation. Pancytopenia is not a separate disease entity but describes a group of clinical findings that are secondary to a variety of diseases. Aplastic anemia is the most common cause of pancytopenia.

2 Bone marrow biopsy (versus aspiration alone) allows for differentiation among the disorders resulting in peripheral pancytopenia. If a hypocellular marrow is discovered, the cells must be examined carefully. Abnormal cells will be present if the marrow is infiltrated with neoplasm or granulomata or if a metabolic disorder or fibrosis is present. At times it may be difficult to distinguish between aplastic anemia and leukemia. Leukemia may be characterized by striking marrow hypocellularity and pancytopenia, making a diagnosis difficult. The presence or absence of other features such as circulating immature cells and splenomegaly may suggest a myelophthisic disorder rather than pure aplasia. Splenomegaly is absent in aplastic anemia.

3 Myelofibrosis may be primary (idiopathic) or secondary to a variety of underlying inflammatory conditions. Diseases commonly associated with marrow fibrosis include carcinomas, SLE, rheumatoid arthritis, and chronic myelogenous leukemia.

4 Miliary tuberculosis can result in marrow hypocellularity by the replacement of marrow contents with granulomata. In some patients with miliary tuberculosis, the marrow will be normocellular; therefore, bone marrow biopsy material should be routinely cultured for tuberculosis during the investigation of pancytopenia. The presence of widespread tuberculosis with pancytopenia may be coincidental to an underlying lymphoma, leukemia, or other blood dyscrasia.

5 If no abnormal cells are identified in a hypocellular bone marrow biopsy specimen, paroxysmal nocturnal hemoglobinuria (PNH) should be excluded before a diagnosis of aplastic anemia can be made. PNH is a rare acquired hemolytic anemia in which red cells, white cells, and platelets are destroyed by a complement-mediated process. The bone marrow may be profoundly hypocellular or may be hyperplastic. Ham's test is very specific for diagnosis of PNH but is too insensitive to detect all patients with PNH. The sucrose hemolysis test is much more sensitive than Ham's test but is less specific, because it may be positive in some patients with myeloproliferative disorders. Both tests depend on the detection of hemolysis of the red cell that results from activation of complement pathways. In addition, the urine should be examined for the presence of hemosiderin if the diagnosis of PNH is suspected. If hemolysis is severe, the sucrose hemolysis test may be negative and the presence of urine hemosiderin will be an important clue to the diagnosis of PNH. A decreased level of leukocyte alkaline phosphatase is a further clue to a diagnosis of PNH but is also nonspecific.

6 Hypersplenism refers to the clinical disorder in which the spleen produces hematologic abnormalities via an exaggeration of its normal activities. A hyperactive spleen can cause a peripheral pancytopenia by destroying normal circulating red cells, white cells, and platelets. The pancytopenia associated with sarcoidosis is usually a result of hypersplenism.

7 SLE is commonly associated with anemia, thrombocytopenia, and leukopenia. The leukopenia is usually mild. The simultaneous depression of red cells, white cells, and platelets is unusual, occurring in less than 5 per cent of patients with SLE.

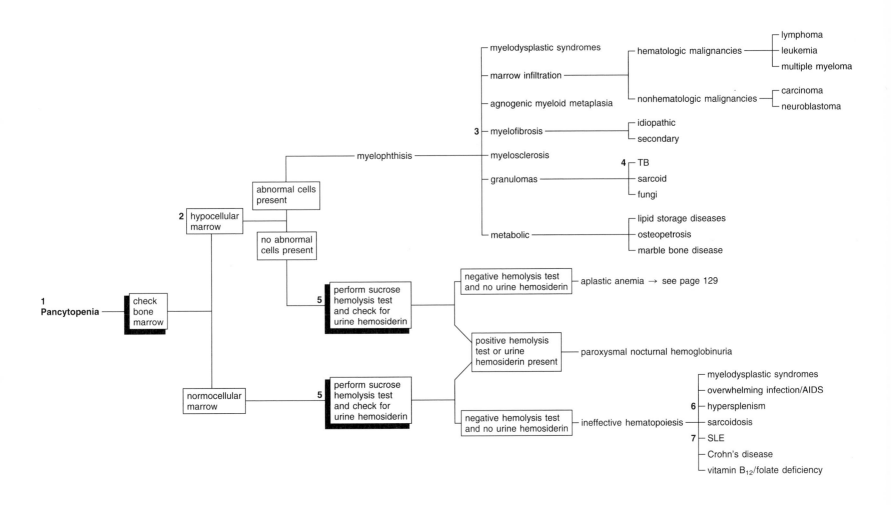

myelodysplastic syndromes

marrow infiltration ── hematologic malignancies ── lymphoma / leukemia / multiple myeloma

── nonhematologic malignancies ── carcinoma / neuroblastoma

agnogenic myeloid metaplasia

3 ├ myelofibrosis ── idiopathic / secondary

myelophthisis ── myelosclerosis

granulomas ── **4** TB / sarcoid / fungi

metabolic ── lipid storage diseases / osteopetrosis / marble bone disease

abnormal cells present

2 hypocellular marrow

no abnormal cells present

1 Pancytopenia — check bone marrow

5 perform sucrose hemolysis test and check for urine hemosiderin

negative hemolysis test and no urine hemosiderin ── aplastic anemia → see page 129

positive hemolysis test or urine hemosiderin present ── paroxysmal nocturnal hemoglobinuria

normocellular marrow

5 perform sucrose hemolysis test and check for urine hemosiderin

negative hemolysis test and no urine hemosiderin ── ineffective hematopoiesis

── myelodysplastic syndromes / overwhelming infection/AIDS / **6** hypersplenism / sarcoidosis / **7** SLE / Crohn's disease / vitamin B$_{12}$/folate deficiency

Cecil Chapters	129, 140
Harrison Chapter	**298**

Neutropenia

1 Neutropenia is defined as an absolute neutrophil count (ANC) of less than 1500/mm³. The ANC is the product of the percentage of neutrophils and the total white blood cell count. Agranulocytosis refers to a severe neutropenia, with less than 500 cells per cubic millimeter.

2 A thorough history may be the most helpful "test" in the differential diagnosis of neutropenia. Drugs and viral infections are the most common causes of acute neutropenia. The presence of splenomegaly may direct investigation toward diagnosis of diseases in which there is destruction of neutrophils.

3 Felty's syndrome is characterized by rheumatoid arthritis, splenomegaly, and neutropenia. Splenomegaly may precede the neutropenia by many years. Even after splenectomy, the neutropenia may recur (see also No. 10, page 116).

4 Many viral, bacterial, and rickettsial diseases result in neutropenia. Viral and rickettsial diseases include influenza, measles, chickenpox, rubella, infectious hepatitis, yellow fever, dengue fever, sandfly fever, and Colorado tick fever. In viral infections, there is often a lymphopenia accompanying the neutropenia. Infectious mononucleosis may be accompanied by splenomegaly and neutropenia. Most bacterial infections are accompanied by a granulocytosis. However, some bacterial infections may be associated with neutropenia. Typhoid fever, paratyphoid fever, tularemia, and occasionally brucellosis may be accompanied by a decrease in the number of neutrophils. Neutropenia can also occur in patients with overwhelming bacterial infection (septicemia), in patients with disseminated tuberculosis, and in debilitated, infected patients. Neutropenia in these settings is associated with a poor prognosis.

5 A history should reveal the ingestion or exposure to those drugs, chemotherapies, or ionizing radiation that may cause neutropenia. Some agents consistently produce marrow suppression if given in sufficient doses (dose-related), whereas other agents produce leukopenia as an idiosyncratic reaction. Examples of the former include ionizing radiation, benzene, nitrogen mustard, colchicine, the antimetabolites, and anthracyclines. Examples of the latter include phenothiazines, anticonvulsants, antithyroid drugs, sulfonamides, antihistamines, certain antimicrobial agents such as chloramphenicol and sulfa drugs, and tranquilizers.

6 Examination of the bone marrow is useful in determining whether the neutropenia is due to abnormal or decreased marrow production or to increased peripheral destruction of neutrophils.

7 If the number of neutrophils and neutrophil precursors is increased in the marrow, the neutropenia may be due to abnormal marrow release of cells or to pseudoneutropenia. Pseudoneutropenia is caused by a shift of neutrophils from the circulating pool to the marginal pool. The marginal pool of neutrophils is the group of neutrophils that are "marginated" along blood vessel walls and in the spleen. Pseudoneutropenia is rare and should not be considered until more common entities have been investigated.

8 Severe deficiencies of B₁₂ and folate cause ineffective hematopoiesis. The number of neutrophil precursors in the bone marrow is increased, but most of the precursors fail to mature. The cells that do mature and are released from the marrow are abnormally large and hypersegmented.

9 Familial neutropenia is an autosomal dominant disorder. Many patients die in early childhood as a result of infection.

10 Cyclic neutropenia is a disorder in which neutropenia recurs every 20 to 30 days and lasts for several days. During the neutropenic period, the patient may develop stomatitis and infections. There may be an accompanying monocytosis. The etiology is unknown.

11 Chronic idiopathic neutropenia, or chronic benign neutropenia, is presumed to be an acquired disorder. Patients have neutrophil counts below 1000/mm³ but tend to have few infections. The neutropenia is thought to be due either to the increased peripheral destruction of cells or to a defect in the release of neutrophils from the marrow. Myelokathexis refers to morphologically abnormal mature neutrophils that are not released from the marrow. Lazy leukocyte syndrome refers to apparently normal neutrophils with defective marrow release.

12 Severe neutropenia is observed in Kostmann's disease. The disease is thought to be recessively transmitted. Mature neutrophils are rare on marrow examination, although neutrophil precursors are increased, indicating maturation arrest or destruction of cells while still in the bone marrow. Most patients die of infection while they are young.

13 If the marrow examination is normal, an autoimmune mechanism for the neutropenia must be considered. The detection of autoimmune neutropenia is difficult because of the lack of reliable tests for antineutrophil antibodies. In a significant number of patients, neutropenia will remain unexplained. These patients must be followed closely and re-evaluated at frequent intervals in order to establish a diagnosis.

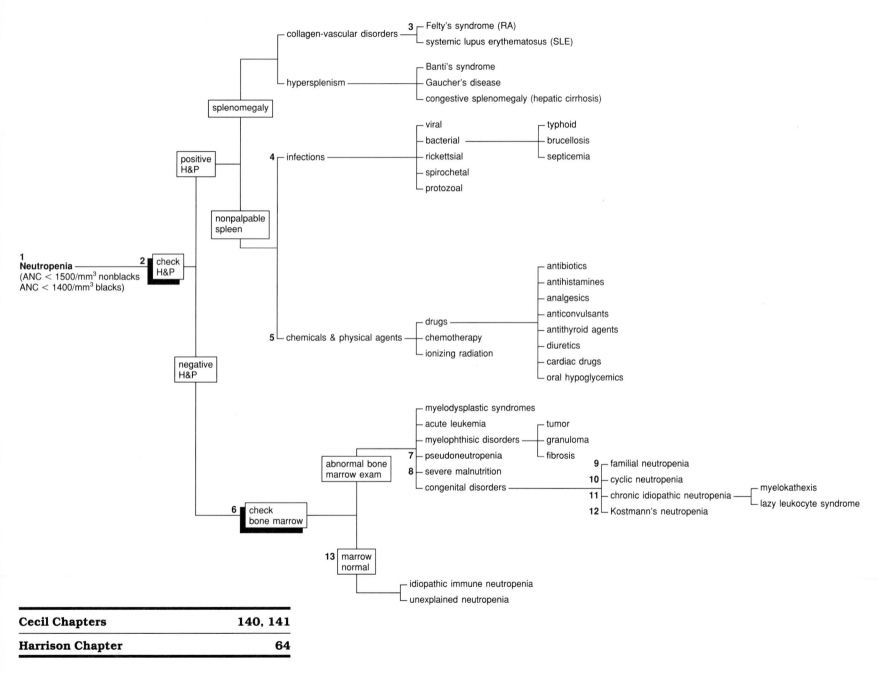

| collagen-vascular disorders | **3** ⌐ Felty's syndrome (RA) |
| | └ systemic lupus erythematosus (SLE) |

hypersplenism
- Banti's syndrome
- Gaucher's disease
- congestive splenomegaly (hepatic cirrhosis)

splenomegaly

positive H&P

4 ⌐ infections
- viral
- bacterial ─── ⌐ typhoid
- rickettsial ─── — brucellosis
- spirochetal └ septicemia
- protozoal

nonpalpable spleen

1
Neutropenia
(ANC < 1500/mm³ nonblacks
ANC < 1400/mm³ blacks)

2 check H&P

5 ⌐ chemicals & physical agents
- drugs ─────
  - antibiotics
  - antihistamines
  - analgesics
  - anticonvulsants
  - antithyroid agents
  - diuretics
  - cardiac drugs
  - oral hypoglycemics
- chemotherapy
- ionizing radiation

negative H&P

- myelodysplastic syndromes
- acute leukemia
- myelophthisic disorders ─── ⌐ tumor
- granuloma
- fibrosis

abnormal bone marrow exam

7 pseudoneutropenia
8 severe malnutrition
congenital disorders ─────
- **9** ⌐ familial neutropenia
- **10** cyclic neutropenia
- **11** chronic idiopathic neutropenia ─── ⌐ myelokathexis
- └ lazy leukocyte syndrome
- **12** └ Kostmann's neutropenia

6 check bone marrow

13 marrow normal
- idiopathic immune neutropenia
- unexplained neutropenia

Cecil Chapters	**140, 141**
Harrison Chapter	**64**

Neutrophilia

1 Neutrophilia is defined as an ANC of greater than 10,000 neutrophils per cubic millimeter. The ANC can be determined by multiplying the total white count by the per cent neutrophils.

2 Leukocytosis (increased total white count) is a normal response to many noxious stimuli. Increases in the number of neutrophils can be a physiologic response or can be an autonomous abnormal proliferation of granulocytes. The history and physical examination are the most helpful in determining whether neutrophilia is physiologic or autonomous.

3 Pseudoneutrophilia refers to the state in which the neutrophil count rises although there is no increase in granulopoiesis. The apparent neutrophil increase results when the marginal granulocyte pool quickly re-enters the circulating granulocyte pool. This granulocyte pool is made up of neutrophils that are "marginated" along the sides of small blood vessels and sequestered in the spleen. Stimuli such as epinephrine, vigorous exercise, anesthesia, paroxysmal tachycardia, and hyperthermia can cause these cells to "demarginate" and join the pool of circulating granulocytes.

4 Acute bacterial infection is the most common cause of neutrophilia. Other organisms that may cause neutrophilia include fungi, spirochetes, viruses, and parasites.

5 Elevated neutrophil counts without infection are a frequent accompaniment to inflammation. The granulocytosis that may occur with uremia or gout is secondary to inflammatory conditions associated with severe azotemia and crystal deposition. Granulocytosis that accompanies ketoacidosis should arouse suspicion of an underlying infection or inflammatory condition that may have precipitated the ketosis. The neutrophilia seen with the injection of various venoms is probably related to the severity of tissue necrosis.

6 The granulocytosis that accompanies a variety of malignant neoplasms may be due to several mechanisms. Most commonly, neutrophilia occurs when a rapidly growing neoplasm outgrows its blood supply

and undergoes necrosis. In addition, some tumors may produce a humoral substance that can cause leukocytosis. Carcinomas of the breast, lung, and kidney, as well as fibrosarcomas and liposarcomas, have been implicated in the production of a humoral neutrophilia-inducing substance. Surgical excision of the bulk of some tumors has been associated with the fall in the neutrophil count, which lends further support to the existence of a humoral neutrophil-stimulating substance.

7 A variety of drugs and toxins, including digitalis, lead, mercury, and benzene, may result in neutrophilia. Lithium has been used therapeutically to stimulate neutrophil production in the neutropenic patient.

8 The administration or overproduction of corticosteroids, as occurs in Cushing's disease, causes a granulocytosis. The neutrophilia that occurs with corticosteroid administration is due to an increase in the release of granulocytes from the bone marrow as well as a decrease of clearance of granulocytes from the circulating blood pool.

9 Neutrophilia following splenectomy is most likely due to the addition to the circulating granulocyte pool from the large marginal granulocyte pool that normally resides in the spleen (see No. 3).

10 The mechanism for granulocytosis that is seen with acute hemorrhage is unknown but is thought to be due to several factors. With hemorrhage, there is evidence for a shift of neutrophils from the marginal to the circulating pool, as well as an increase in the release of neutrophils from the bone marrow. In cases in which the hemorrhage is into a body cavity and is painful, it is thought that the neutrophilia is also due to the demargination of neutrophils resulting from epinephrine and adrenocorticosteroid release.

11 Granulocytosis is often seen, perhaps as an "overshoot" phenomenon, when the marrow is recovering from agranulocytosis. The same phenomenon is seen during treatment for megaloblastic anemia.

12 Without directly invading the bone marrow, solid tumors may cause neutrophilia by secreting neutrophil-stimulating growth factor. This phenomenon is known as a paraneoplastic syndrome (see No. 6).

13 When the history and physical examination fail to reveal a probable etiology for granulocytosis, the possibility of autonomous neutrophil production should be examined. Bone marrow examination may reveal a primary hematologic disorder such as chronic myelogenous leukemia (CML). In an early stage, CML may be difficult to diagnose without bone marrow examination.

14 The differentiation of a leukemoid reaction from a clonal myeloid neoplasm is an important, yet often difficult task. A leukemoid blood picture is one in which there is a profound neutrophilia that may suggest the diagnosis of leukemia, but the disease does not progress. A leukemoid reaction may be secondary to multiple diseases including acute and chronic infections (pneumonia, meningitis, diphtheria, tuberculosis) or due to toxins such as mercury poisoning; malignant disease including bone metastases, multiple myeloma, myelofibrosis, and Hodgkin's disease; or severe hemorrhage. A leukemoid reaction can be manifested in several ways: (1) a leukocytosis of unexpected magnitude with respect to the underlying disease; (2) immature or abnormal cells in the blood regardless of the total number of white cells; or (3) an abnormal number of immature or abnormal cells in the bone marrow.

A number of examinations may be used collectively to aid in differentiating the leukemoid reaction from clonal myeloid neoplasms, as well as distinguishing among the neoplasms themselves. The Philadelphia (Ph^1) chromosome, although not specific for CML, is present in approximately 90 per cent of patients with CML. Ph^1 is also occasionally present in patients with idiopathic myelofibrosis, acute myeloid leukemia (AML), and acute lymphoblastic leukemia (ALL). The chromosome is *not* present in patients with the leukemoid reaction. Auer rods are a useful finding for distinguishing AML from the leukemoid reaction. These granules are seen in AML and in the blast phase of CML. Down's syndrome may be associated with a unique leukemoid reaction in which the blood and bone marrow findings are indistinguishable from those of AML. The leukemoid reaction appears to resolve spontaneously in these patients. It is unclear whether these patients can truly be diagnosed with AML with long-term spontaneous remission or if the picture is consistent with a leukemoid reaction. The picture is confusing because there is a high rate of ALL and AML in Down's patients as well.

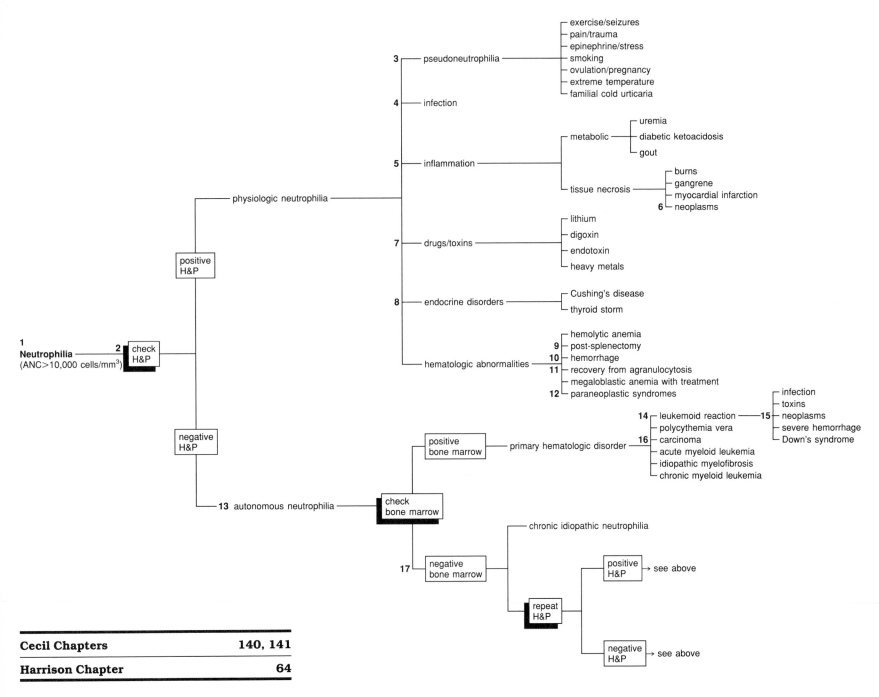

1
Neutrophilia
(ANC>10,000 cells/mm³)

2 check H&P

positive H&P

negative H&P

physiologic neutrophilia

3 — pseudoneutrophilia
- exercise/seizures
- pain/trauma
- epinephrine/stress
- smoking
- ovulation/pregnancy
- extreme temperature
- familial cold urticaria

4 — infection

5 — inflammation
- metabolic
  - uremia
  - diabetic ketoacidosis
  - gout
- tissue necrosis
  - burns
  - gangrene
  - myocardial infarction
  - 6 — neoplasms

7 — drugs/toxins
- lithium
- digoxin
- endotoxin
- heavy metals

8 — endocrine disorders
- Cushing's disease
- thyroid storm

hematologic abnormalities
- hemolytic anemia
- 9 — post-splenectomy
- 10 — hemorrhage
- 11 — recovery from agranulocytosis
- megaloblastic anemia with treatment
- 12 — paraneoplastic syndromes

13 autonomous neutrophilia

check bone marrow

positive bone marrow — primary hematologic disorder

14 — leukemoid reaction — 15
- infection
- toxins
- neoplasms
- severe hemorrhage
- Down's syndrome

- polycythemia vera
- 16 — carcinoma
- acute myeloid leukemia
- idiopathic myelofibrosis
- chronic myeloid leukemia

17 negative bone marrow

chronic idiopathic neutrophilia

repeat H&P

positive H&P → see above

negative H&P → see above

Cecil Chapters	140, 141
Harrison Chapter	64

Neutrophilia (Continued)

15 Examination of bone marrow that has been infiltrated by carcinoma cells can present a diagnostic dilemma, because the cells cannot always easily be distinguished from leukemic cells. Leukoerythroblastosis is a condition in which a large number of both mature and immature neutrophils appear in the blood along with a large number of nucleated, abnormal red cells. Metastatic cancer, fibrosis, leukemia, and granulomas are responsible for bone marrow invasion, known as myelophthisis, and a leukoerythroblastic reaction.

16 Breast and prostatic carcinomas are the two most likely tumors to infiltrate the bone marrow and result in a neutrophilia.

17 A nondiagnostic marrow examination presents a diagnostic dilemma if other sources of neutrophilia have been excluded. There have been rare reports of chronic idiopathic neutrophilia in which high neutrophil counts have been observed and have persisted without discovery of the underlying cause. It is unlikely that thorough history, physical examination, and bone marrow examination would not reveal the source of neutrophilia, but the patient without a clear diagnosis at this point should be followed closely and re-examined at intervals.

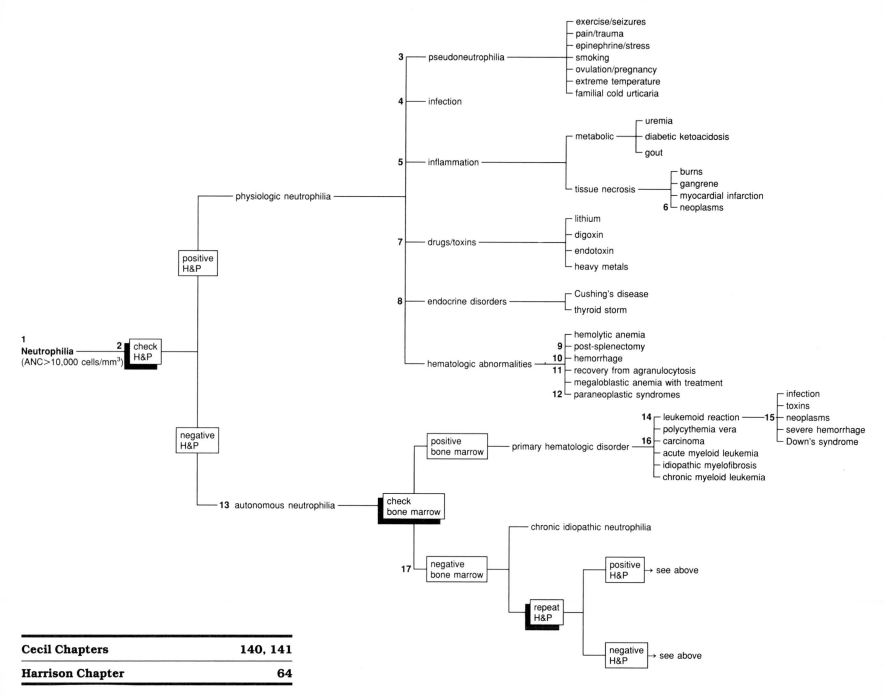

1
Neutrophilia
(ANC>10,000 cells/mm³)

2 check H&P

positive H&P

physiologic neutrophilia

3 pseudoneutrophilia
- exercise/seizures
- pain/trauma
- epinephrine/stress
- smoking
- ovulation/pregnancy
- extreme temperature
- familial cold urticaria

4 infection

5 inflammation
- metabolic
  - uremia
  - diabetic ketoacidosis
  - gout
- tissue necrosis
  - burns
  - gangrene
  - myocardial infarction
  - 6 neoplasms

7 drugs/toxins
- lithium
- digoxin
- endotoxin
- heavy metals

8 endocrine disorders
- Cushing's disease
- thyroid storm

hematologic abnormalities
- hemolytic anemia
- 9 post-splenectomy
- 10 hemorrhage
- 11 recovery from agranulocytosis
- megaloblastic anemia with treatment
- 12 paraneoplastic syndromes

negative H&P

13 autonomous neutrophilia

check bone marrow

positive bone marrow

primary hematologic disorder

14 leukemoid reaction — 15
- infection
- toxins
- neoplasms
- severe hemorrhage
- Down's syndrome

polycythemia vera
16 carcinoma
acute myeloid leukemia
idiopathic myelofibrosis
chronic myeloid leukemia

17 **negative bone marrow**

chronic idiopathic neutrophilia

repeat H&P

positive H&P → see above

negative H&P → see above

Cecil Chapters	140, 141
Harrison Chapter	64

Monocytosis

1 Monocytosis is an absolute monocyte count above 750/mm³ and is associated with a variety of hematologic and inflammatory processes. By itself, monocytosis is not diagnostic of any particular disease entity. Monocytosis is secondary to hematologic diseases in about 50 per cent of patients, collagen vascular diseases in 10 per cent of patients, and associated with malignancies in approximately 8 per cent of patients. Because monocytes and neutrophils are thought to be derived from a common progenitor cell, their regulation is closely related. Monocytosis is often accompanied by a neutrophilia.

2 A CBC may be abnormal in both hematologic diseases and inflammatory processes. The nature of the abnormality and the constellation of clinical findings will determine the need for a bone marrow examination. The CBC abnormalities may be more profound with hematologic disorders and more subtle or absent with inflammatory conditions.

3 Associated abnormalities of the CBC may provide clues to diagnosis. Because monocytosis is due most commonly to a hematologic abnormality, subsequent bone marrow aspiration and biopsy may be diagnostic. Monocytosis may be marked in patients with chronic myelogenous leukemia. Monocytosis is common in preleukemia.

4 Neutropenia is often accompanied by monocytosis. The term leukopenic infectious monocytosis has been used to refer to the condition of agranulocytosis with accompanying monocytosis. Reports have indicated that an increased number of monocytes heralds recovery from agranulocytosis.

5 Monocytosis has been observed in approximately 25 per cent of patients with Hodgkin's lymphoma.

6 A monocytosis often accompanies granulomatous diseases, because monocytes are the source of tissue macrophages. Tuberculosis is the most common infectious cause of granulomas and may be accompanied by a monocytosis. Approximately 20 per cent of patients with subacute bacterial endocarditis (SBE) have an associated monocytosis.

7 A variety of gastrointestinal disorders have been associated with monocytosis, including the granulomatous disorder, regional enteritis (see No. 6).

8 Chronic high-dose corticosteroid administration leads not only to neutrophilia but to a monocytosis as well.

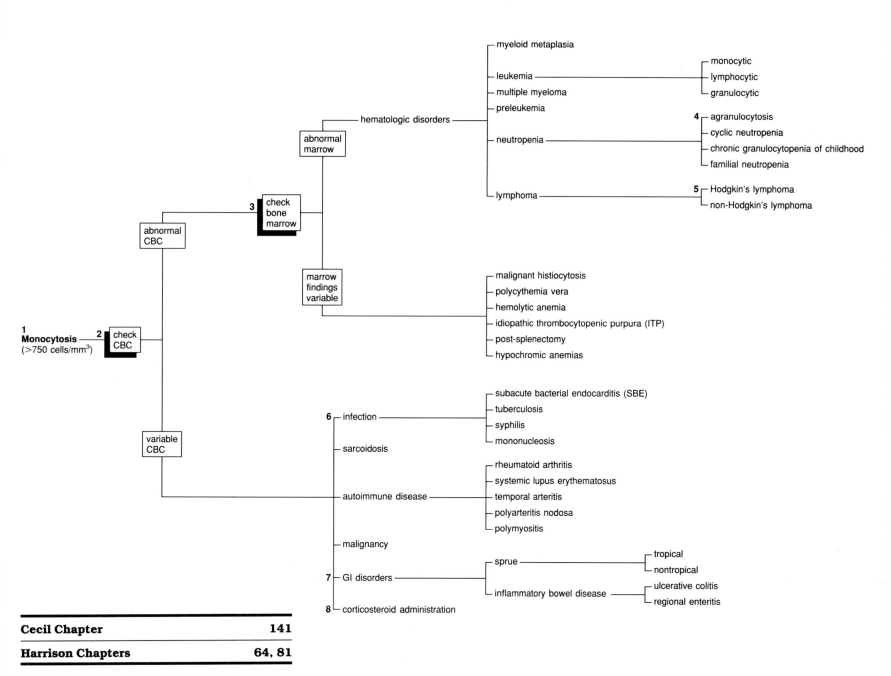

myeloid metaplasia

leukemia
- monocytic
- lymphocytic
- granulocytic

multiple myeloma

preleukemia

4 neutropenia
- agranulocytosis
- cyclic neutropenia
- chronic granulocytopenia of childhood
- familial neutropenia

5 lymphoma
- Hodgkin's lymphoma
- non-Hodgkin's lymphoma

hematologic disorders

abnormal marrow

3 check bone marrow

abnormal CBC

malignant histiocytosis
polycythemia vera
hemolytic anemia
idiopathic thrombocytopenic purpura (ITP)
post-splenectomy
hypochromic anemias

marrow findings variable

1 Monocytosis (>750 cells/mm³) — **2 check CBC**

6 infection
- subacute bacterial endocarditis (SBE)
- tuberculosis
- syphilis
- mononucleosis

sarcoidosis

variable CBC

autoimmune disease
- rheumatoid arthritis
- systemic lupus erythematosus
- temporal arteritis
- polyarteritis nodosa
- polymyositis

malignancy

7 GI disorders
- sprue
  - tropical
  - nontropical
- inflammatory bowel disease
  - ulcerative colitis
  - regional enteritis

8 corticosteroid administration

Cecil Chapter	**141**
Harrison Chapters	**64, 81**

Lymphocytosis

1 The normal lymphocyte count varies with age, but in the adult lymphocytosis is defined as an absolute lymphocyte count of greater than 4000 lymphocytes per cubic millimeter. Absolute lymphocytosis is much less common than the relative lymphocytosis that may accompany granulocytopenia and many viral infections. Lymphocytosis is due most commonly to acute viral infection and is rarely due to bacterial infection.

2 Another major clue in the differential diagnosis of lymphocytosis is the presence of atypical lymphocytes on examination of the blood smear. As many as 5 to 10 per cent of lymphocytes may appear atypical, or pleomorphic, on the normal blood smear. A marked increase in atypical lymphocytes is associated with mononucleosis (regardless of etiology), drug hypersensitivity, infectious hepatitis, transfusion, and toxoplasmosis.

3 Infectious mononucleosis is a common cause of lymphocytosis in teenagers and young adults. Symptoms may be mild or severe and include fever, fatigue, pharyngitis, lymphadenopathy, and lymphocytosis. Splenomegaly may be present in as many as 40 per cent of patients with infectious mononucleosis and may even lead to splenic rupture. Mononucleosis can be caused by several different viruses, the most common of which is Epstein-Barr virus (EBV). Other organisms implicated in infectious mononucleosis include cytomegalovirus (CMV), herpes simplex type II, rubella, *Toxoplasma gondii,* and adenovirus. Only EBV will yield a positive heterophile antibody test, although 5 per cent of EBV-induced mononucleosis may be heterophile antibody–negative.

4 The post-transfusion syndrome consists of atypical lymphocytosis in association with fever and splenomegaly. CMV has been implicated as the cause of this syndrome and appears to be transmitted via the leukocytes in the donor blood.

5 With the exception of pertussis, acute bacterial infections rarely cause lymphocytosis. Acute infectious lymphocytosis is another acute infectious cause of lymphocytosis in which no atypical lymphocytes are present, helping distinguish this entity from infectious mononucleosis. Acute infectious lymphocytosis is largely asymptomatic, occurs in children and young adults, and is thought to be virally transmitted.

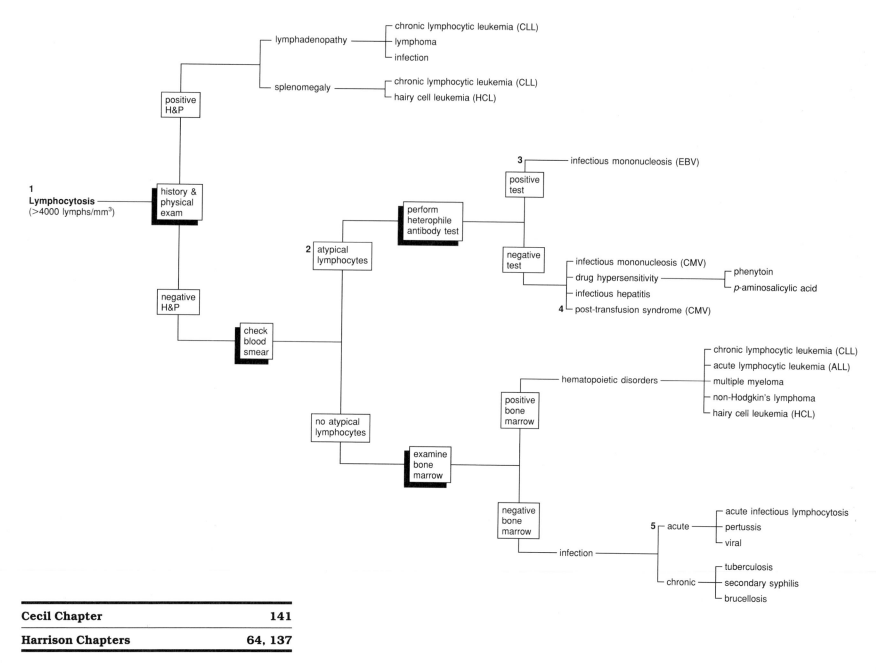

1
Lymphocytosis
(>4000 lymphs/mm³)

history & physical exam

positive H&P

lymphadenopathy
- chronic lymphocytic leukemia (CLL)
- lymphoma
- infection

splenomegaly
- chronic lymphocytic leukemia (CLL)
- hairy cell leukemia (HCL)

negative H&P

check blood smear

2 atypical lymphocytes

perform heterophile antibody test

3 positive test — infectious mononucleosis (EBV)

negative test
- infectious mononucleosis (CMV)
- drug hypersensitivity
  - phenytoin
  - p-aminosalicylic acid
- infectious hepatitis
- **4** post-transfusion syndrome (CMV)

no atypical lymphocytes

examine bone marrow

positive bone marrow — hematopoietic disorders
- chronic lymphocytic leukemia (CLL)
- acute lymphocytic leukemia (ALL)
- multiple myeloma
- non-Hodgkin's lymphoma
- hairy cell leukemia (HCL)

negative bone marrow — infection
- **5** acute
  - acute infectious lymphocytosis
  - pertussis
  - viral
- chronic
  - tuberculosis
  - secondary syphilis
  - brucellosis

Cecil Chapter   **141**

Harrison Chapters   **64, 137**

Eosinophilia

1 Eosinophilia is defined as an absolute eosinophil count greater than 500 eosinophils per cubic millimeter of blood. The absolute eosinophil count is determined by multiplying the total white count by the per cent eosinophils. As an approach to diagnosis, eosinophilia can be classified as marked, moderate, or mild, although there may be overlap between these categories. The most common causes of hypereosinophilia are allergic reactions and parasitic diseases. Hypereosinophilic syndromes are accompanied by the highest eosinophil counts, which helps distinguish these syndromes from other disorders. Most causes of eosinophilia can be uncovered with a thorough history and physical examination, with further diagnostic tests as indicated to confirm likely etiology.

2 Drug allergy is perhaps the most common source of eosinophilia. Drugs commonly causing eosinophilia include erythromycin estolate, sulfonamides, chlorpropamide, para-aminosalicylic acid, imipramine, nitrofurantoin, procarbazine, gold, iodides, and methotrexate. Asthma is commonly accompanied by an eosinophilia, ranging from 400 to 1000 eosinophils per cubic millimeter. However, if asthma is exacerbated by acute bacterial infection or complicated by infection, the eosinophilia will be absent. A characteristic of acute bacterial infection is eosinopenia, and eosinophilia has been described as a favorable prognosis in the resolution of acute infections.

3 Addison's disease may be accompanied by a mild eosinophilia. Of interest, the eosinophil count falls with the administration of corticosteroids in any patient.

4 Eosinophilia has been reported in up to 40 per cent of patients undergoing irradiation for carcinoma, most commonly in patients with intra-abdominal neoplasms.

5 A significant proportion of immune deficiency states are accompanied by eosinophilia. These disorders include Wiskott-Aldrich syndrome, hyper-IgE syndrome, Job's syndrome, and selective IgA deficiency. These syndromes may include cutaneous manifestations, primarily eczema.

6 Eosinophilia has been reported to accompany a wide variety of neoplasms. In general, eosinophilia is present when there is wide dissemination of the tumor, or if tumor necrosis is present. Eosinophilia may accompany Hodgkin's lymphoma, non-Hodgkin's lymphoma, or T-cell lymphomas (mycosis fungoides). Carcinomas of mucin-secreting epithelial cell origin are most likely to be accompanied by eosinophilia. Examples of these tumors include carcinoma of the colon, pancreas, lung, and cervix. Leukemias associated with eosinophilia include T-cell leukemia (Sézary syndrome), acute lymphoblastic leukemia, and CML. In CML, the massive increase in the number of mature white cells may increase the absolute number of eosinophils, but the percentage of eosinophils may not be increased.

7 Collagen-vascular disease is sometimes accompanied by an increase in the number of eosinophils. Eosinophilia occurs in 10 to 12 per cent of patients with rheumatoid arthritis and tends to occur primarily in patients with long-standing severe disease. Polyarteritis nodosa (PAN) had been reported to be accompanied by eosinophilia, but it appears that the eosinophilia is seen in a distinct subset of patients with PAN. The subset of patients with allergic granulomatosis, or Churg-Strauss syndrome, exhibit asthma, PAN, and hypereosinophilia. Wegener's granulomatosis has also been reported to be accompanied by hypereosinophilia.

8 A case for hereditary eosinophilia can be made if (1) there is a significant level of eosinophilia; (2) there is familial incidence with more than one generation being affected; and (3) other recognized causes of eosinophilia are absent. Hereditary hypereosinophilia is rare. Idiopathic hypereosinophilia is a diagnosis of exclusion and must be distinguished from the idiopathic hypereosinophilic syndrome. In the latter, a marked elevation of eosinophils is accompanied by organ dysfunction, presumably owing to direct deleterious effects of the eosinophil.

9 Marked eosinophilia usually accompanies invasive parasitic infections and a variety of primary skin disorders. Despite high parasite loads, the eosinophil count rarely exceeds 25,000 eosinophils per cubic millimeter and is probably the highest with trichinosis. Even if the eosinophil count is markedly elevated (i.e.,

$>50,000/mm^3$), skin diseases, parasitic infections, neoplasms, and collagen-vascular disease must still be excluded prior to the consideration of the hypereosinophilic syndrome. The hypereosinophilic syndrome is a diagnosis of exclusion (see No. 12).

10 Various skin disorders are accompanied by marked eosinophilia, most consistently urticarial pemphigoid and pemphigus vulgaris. Other skin diseases that may be accompanied by eosinophilia include exfoliative dermatitis, pityriasis rosea, leprosy, granuloma faciale, ichthyosis, and pruritus secondary to jaundice. Dermatitis herpetiformis has often been reported to be accompanied by eosinophilia, but the eosinophilia is mild and only occasionally present.

11 Dramatic and prolonged eosinophilia accompanies metazoan parasitic infections. Protozoan parasitic infections are less likely to be accompanied by a significant eosinophilia unless the parasite load is high and tissue invasion occurs. Tropical eosinophilia had been classified as a pulmonary eosinophilia, although now it is recognized to be due to filarial infestation.

12 The criteria for defining the idiopathic hypereosinophilic syndrome are as follows: (1) persistent eosinophilia of at least 1500 eosinophils per cubic millimeter for at least 6 months; (2) lack of evidence for parasitic, allergic, or other recognized causes of eosinophilia; and (3) signs and symptoms of unexplained organ system dysfunction related to the eosinophilia. It should be stressed that organ system dysfunction may also be seen in patients with other forms of eosinophilia.

13 Pulmonary infiltrates with eosinophilia (PIE) refers to a group of disorders characterized by peripheral eosinophilia and pulmonary infiltrates. The term does not imply etiology, and overlap is great. For example, tropical eosinophilia, which is now known to be due to filariae, has been classified as a pulmonary eosinophilia because the clinical features include pulmonary infiltrates and peripheral eosinophilia. The pulmonary eosinophilias comprise a diverse group of disorders and are usually secondary to other underlying abnormalities, including fungal infections, parasitic infections, neoplasms, and drugs. The pulmonary eosinophilias also include Löffler's syndrome, prolonged pulmonary eosinophilia, pulmonary

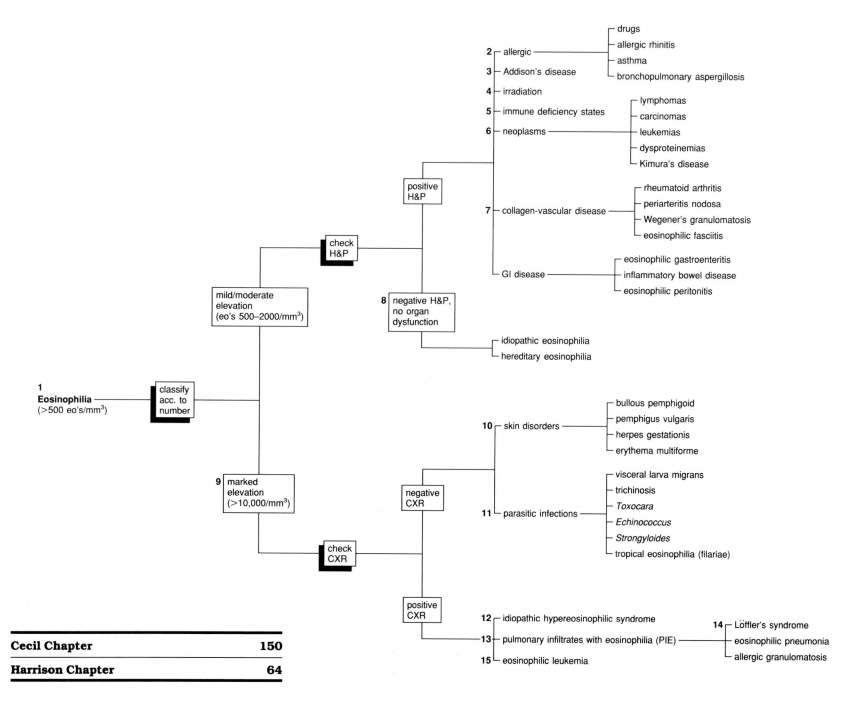

1 **Eosinophilia** (>500 eo's/mm³)

classify acc. to number

mild/moderate elevation (eo's 500–2000/mm³)

check H&P

positive H&P

2 allergic
- drugs
- allergic rhinitis
- asthma
- bronchopulmonary aspergillosis

3 Addison's disease

4 irradiation

5 immune deficiency states

6 neoplasms
- lymphomas
- carcinomas
- leukemias
- dysproteinemias
- Kimura's disease

7 collagen-vascular disease
- rheumatoid arthritis
- periarteritis nodosa
- Wegener's granulomatosis
- eosinophilic fasciitis

GI disease
- eosinophilic gastroenteritis
- inflammatory bowel disease
- eosinophilic peritonitis

8 negative H&P, no organ dysfunction
- idiopathic eosinophilia
- hereditary eosinophilia

9 marked elevation (>10,000/mm³)

check CXR

negative CXR

10 skin disorders
- bullous pemphigoid
- pemphigus vulgaris
- herpes gestationis
- erythema multiforme

11 parasitic infections
- visceral larva migrans
- trichinosis
- *Toxocara*
- *Echinococcus*
- *Strongyloides*
- tropical eosinophilia (filariae)

positive CXR

12 idiopathic hypereosinophilic syndrome

13 pulmonary infiltrates with eosinophilia (PIE)
- **14** Löffler's syndrome
- eosinophilic pneumonia
- allergic granulomatosis

15 eosinophilic leukemia

Cecil Chapter	150
Harrison Chapter	64

Eosinophilia *(Continued)*

eosinophilia with asthma, and allergic granulomatosis (Churg-Strauss).

14 Löffler's syndrome is distinguished from other pulmonary eosinophilias and the idiopathic hypereosinophilic syndrome on the basis of a short, benign clinical course. It is characterized by fleeting pulmonary infiltrates and eosinophilia, with resolution within 3 weeks.

15 The diagnostic criteria for eosinophilic leukemia include the following: (1) pronounced, persistent eosinophilia associated with immature forms either in the blood or bone marrow; (2) greater than 5 per cent blast forms in the bone marrow; (3) tissue infiltration by immature eosinophils; and (4) an acute clinical course of several months accompanied by anemia, thrombocytopenia, susceptibility to infections, or hemorrhage. Of note, a marked elevation of serum B_{12} has been found in patients with eosinophilic leukemia but is also seen in patients with the idiopathic hypereosinophilic syndrome.

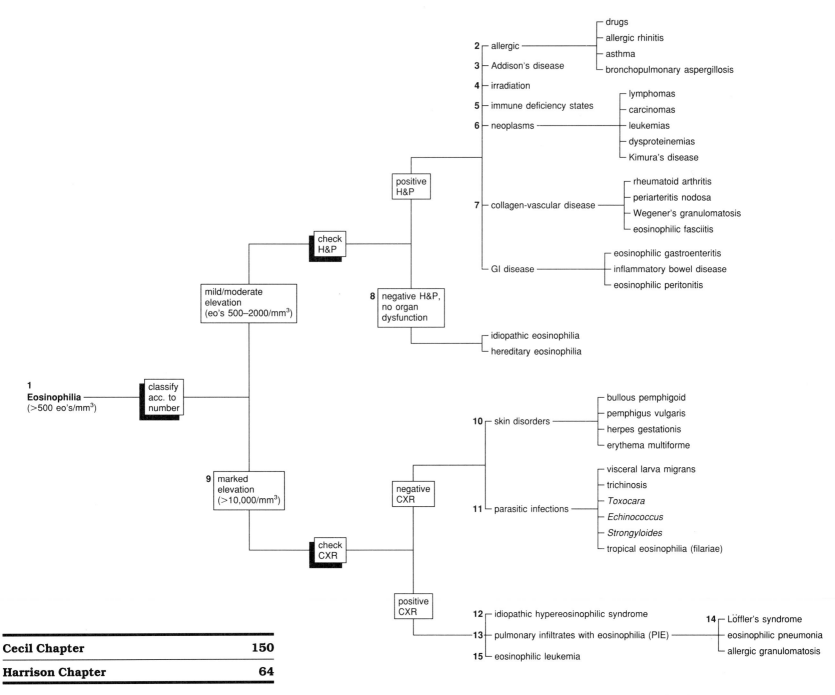

1
Eosinophilia
(>500 eo's/mm³)

classify acc. to number

mild/moderate elevation (eo's 500–2000/mm³)

check H&P

positive H&P

2 allergic
- drugs
- allergic rhinitis
- asthma
- bronchopulmonary aspergillosis

3 Addison's disease

4 irradiation

5 immune deficiency states

6 neoplasms
- lymphomas
- carcinomas
- leukemias
- dysproteinemias
- Kimura's disease

7 collagen-vascular disease
- rheumatoid arthritis
- periarteritis nodosa
- Wegener's granulomatosis
- eosinophilic fasciitis

GI disease
- eosinophilic gastroenteritis
- inflammatory bowel disease
- eosinophilic peritonitis

8 negative H&P, no organ dysfunction
- idiopathic eosinophilia
- hereditary eosinophilia

9 marked elevation (>10,000/mm³)

check CXR

negative CXR

10 skin disorders
- bullous pemphigoid
- pemphigus vulgaris
- herpes gestationis
- erythema multiforme

11 parasitic infections
- visceral larva migrans
- trichinosis
- *Toxocara*
- *Echinococcus*
- *Strongyloides*
- tropical eosinophilia (filariae)

positive CXR

12 idiopathic hypereosinophilic syndrome

13 pulmonary infiltrates with eosinophilia (PIE)

14
- Löffler's syndrome
- eosinophilic pneumonia
- allergic granulomatosis

15 eosinophilic leukemia

Cecil Chapter	**150**
Harrison Chapter	**64**

Thrombocytosis

1 Thrombocytosis is defined as a platelet count greater than 400,000/mm³ of blood. Thrombocytosis can occur in three forms: (1) autonomous or primary thrombocytosis, also known as thrombocythemia; (2) a transitory or physiologic elevation of platelets; and (3) secondary or reactive thrombocytosis. An increase in the number of platelets can translate clinically into a tendency toward bleeding or thrombosis, or the patient may remain asymptomatic. A number of other laboratory abnormalities may accompany a marked increase in the number of platelets. These abnormalities include pseudohyperkalemia (see No. 1, p. 88) as well as elevated levels of acid phosphatase, zinc, uric acid, phosphorus, and LDH.

2 Primary thrombocytosis, or thrombocythemia, is a diagnosis of exclusion. Thrombocythemia is diagnosed when there is a marked increase in the platelet count, usually exceeding 1×10^9/mm³, and no other associated disease is present. The platelet count may be elevated for months or for years. The white blood count is increased in over 90 per cent of patients with thrombocythemia, but the white count is usually normal in patients with secondary thrombocytosis. Splenomegaly, usually absent in reactive thrombocytosis, is found in up to 80 per cent of patients with thrombocythemia. Bone marrow examination will reveal a marked increase in the number of megakaryocytes. There are five diagnostic criteria for essential thrombocythemia that help distinguish this disorder from PCV and myeloid malignancies such as CML:

(1) a platelet count greater than 1×10^6/μL persisting without an indentifiable underlying cause; (2) a normal total red cell volume; (3) iron present in the bone marrow or response to oral iron therapy; (4) an absent collagen fibrosis on bone marrow biopsy; and (5) an absent Philadelphia chromosome.

3 Transitory thrombocytosis is due to the mobilization of preformed platelets, not to a true increase in platelet production. Platelets are released from a pool thought to be stored in the lung vasculature and spleen. Transitory thrombocytosis occurs most frequently following exercise, with stress, and with epinephrine release or injection.

4 An elevated platelet count is usually an isolated abnormality in transitory thrombocytosis and the remainder of the CBC is normal. An abnormal CBC would indicate that thrombocytosis is related to an underlying disorder, and the abnormality would be dependent upon the nature of the underlying disease.

5 Reactive thrombocytosis is due to a true increase in platelet production. The platelet count rarely exceeds 10^6/mm³ in secondary thrombocytosis. Reactive thrombocytosis is secondary to a variety of inflammatory and infectious diseases, although the mechanism responsible for stimulating platelet production is usually unknown. The platelet count may return to normal levels if the underlying disorder can be treated. If other components of the blood count are abnormal, the thrombocytosis may be secondary to an associated hematologic abnormality such as anemia or polycythemia vera. Plasma fibrinogen level is useful to help distinguish between myeloproliferative disorders (MPD) and reactive thrombocytosis owing to malignancy and inflammatory and infectious diseases. Plasma fibrinogen is an acute phase reactant and will be elevated with reactive thrombocytosis, usually to levels of greater than 5 gm/L, but will usually remain low in MPD. If the history, physical examination, and blood examination do not provide enough information to make a diagnosis, a bone marrow examination should be performed. Bone marrow examination may reveal leukemia or myelofibrosis.

6 Splenectomy may result in platelet counts as high as one million per cubic millimeter of blood. Increased numbers of platelets can be seen within the first few days after splenectomy but will return to normal within weeks to months postoperatively.

7 Vincristine may interfere with platelet regulation of thrombopoiesis and specifically stimulate platelet production, resulting in thrombocytosis.

8 One to 2 weeks after the withdrawal of a drug causing thrombocythemia such as methotrexate or alcohol, a rebound thrombocytosis can occur. A rebound thrombocytosis has also been observed once therapy has begun for vitamin B_{12} deficiency. Thrombocytosis has been observed, perhaps as a "rebound" phenomenon, after prednisone therapy of idiopathic thrombocytopenic purpura.

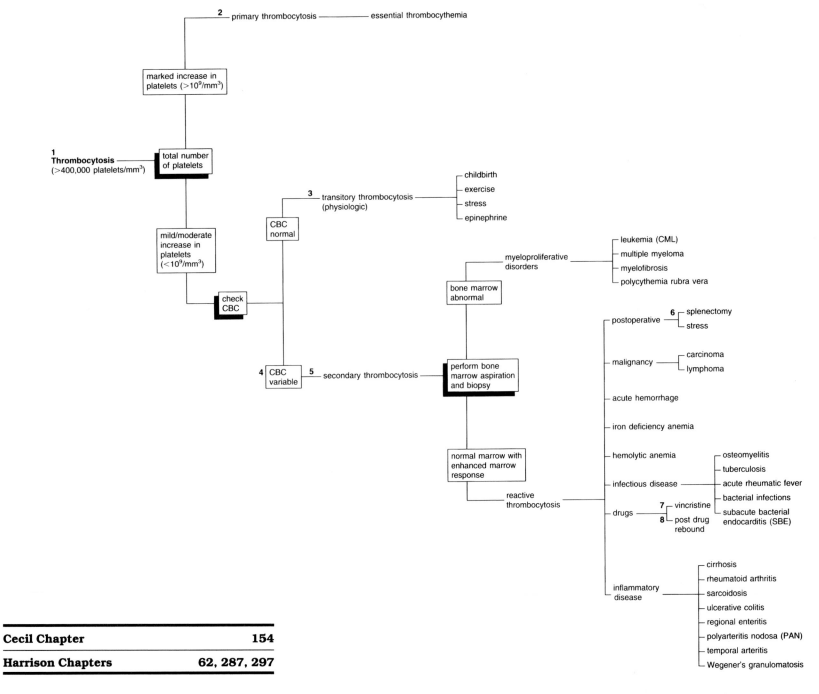

1
Thrombocytosis
(>400,000 platelets/mm³) — total number of platelets

2 primary thrombocytosis —————— essential thrombocythemia

marked increase in platelets (>10⁹/mm³)

mild/moderate increase in platelets (<10⁹/mm³)

check CBC

CBC normal

3 transitory thrombocytosis (physiologic)
- childbirth
- exercise
- stress
- epinephrine

4 CBC variable **5** secondary thrombocytosis

perform bone marrow aspiration and biopsy

bone marrow abnormal

myeloproliferative disorders
- leukemia (CML)
- multiple myeloma
- myelofibrosis
- polycythemia rubra vera

normal marrow with enhanced marrow response

reactive thrombocytosis

postoperative **6**
- splenectomy
- stress

malignancy
- carcinoma
- lymphoma

acute hemorrhage

iron deficiency anemia

hemolytic anemia

infectious disease
- osteomyelitis
- tuberculosis
- acute rheumatic fever
- bacterial infections
- subacute bacterial endocarditis (SBE)

drugs
7 vincristine
8 post drug rebound

inflammatory disease
- cirrhosis
- rheumatoid arthritis
- sarcoidosis
- ulcerative colitis
- regional enteritis
- polyarteritis nodosa (PAN)
- temporal arteritis
- Wegener's granulomatosis

Thrombocytopenia

1 The normal platelet count is 150,000 to 400,000/mm^3, usually determined by automated equipment. An estimate of the platelet count can be determined, however, by examination of the peripheral blood smear. With a normal platelet count, more than 10 platelets should be visible in each oil immersion field. Thrombocytopenia is defined as a platelet count below 150,000/mm^3. Spontaneous bleeding is uncommon with platelet counts greater than 40,000 but is often severe when the platelet count falls below 10,000/mm^3.

2 Once thrombocytopenia is confirmed, a complete history and physical examination will supply the greatest amount of information in order to discriminate among the diagnostic possibilities. In every adult patient, a drug-related etiology must be considered and an extensive drug history obtained. History of illnesses for which cytotoxic agents and ionizing radiation have been used must be known. A history of recent transfusion, blood contact with extracorporeal equipment, or recent hemorrhage with massive transfusion is also important. Splenomegaly and petechiae are the most useful physical findings.

3 Examination of the peripheral blood smear will help to diagnose pseudothrombocytopenia by demonstrating platelet aggregations or giant platelets that are not counted by automated equipment.

4 Defective maturation of megakaryocytes occurs with megaloblastic anemia (B_{12} or folate deficiency) as well as with severe iron deficiency. Bone marrow examination may reveal a normal number of megakaryocytes, but they can be decreased or absent in severe cases.

5 The administration of cytotoxic agents is a common cause of marrow injury leading to thrombocytopenia. Other drugs that can cause marrow injury resulting in thrombocytopenia include gold, sulfonamides, ethanol, thiazides, and estrogens.

6 The megakaryocyte is often a site for viral replication with subsequent decrease in megakaryocyte maturation. Viral infections associated with thrombocytopenia include measles (including measles vaccination), influenza, rubella, mononucleosis, dengue fever, and Thai hemorrhagic fever.

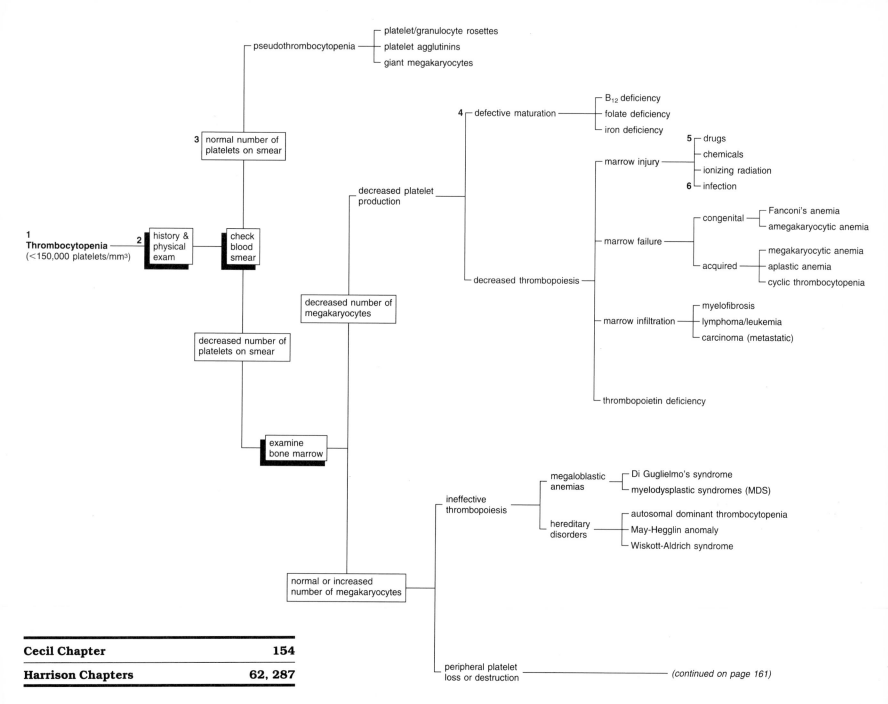

pseudothrombocytopenia
— platelet/granulocyte rosettes
— platelet agglutinins
— giant megakaryocytes

3 normal number of platelets on smear

4 defective maturation
— B$_{12}$ deficiency
— folate deficiency
— iron deficiency

decreased platelet production

marrow injury
5 — drugs
— chemicals
— ionizing radiation
6 — infection

1 **Thrombocytopenia** (<150,000 platelets/mm³)

2 history & physical exam

check blood smear

marrow failure
congenital
— Fanconi's anemia
— amegakaryocytic anemia

acquired
— megakaryocytic anemia
— aplastic anemia
— cyclic thrombocytopenia

decreased number of megakaryocytes

decreased thrombopoiesis

marrow infiltration
— myelofibrosis
— lymphoma/leukemia
— carcinoma (metastatic)

decreased number of platelets on smear

thrombopoietin deficiency

examine bone marrow

ineffective thrombopoiesis
megaloblastic anemias
— Di Guglielmo's syndrome
— myelodysplastic syndromes (MDS)

hereditary disorders
— autosomal dominant thrombocytopenia
— May-Hegglin anomaly
— Wiskott-Aldrich syndrome

normal or increased number of megakaryocytes

peripheral platelet loss or destruction ———————————— (continued on page 161)

Cecil Chapter	**154**
Harrison Chapters	**62, 287**

Thrombocytopenia (Continued)

7 In conditions associated with hypersplenism there can be splenic sequestration of platelets and decreased platelets in the peripheral circulation. Normally 70 per cent of platelets are circulating and 30 per cent are in the spleen. If splenic enlargement occurs, the balance may be altered so that up to 80 per cent of the platelets are stored in the spleen, with marked reduction in the number of circulating platelets. Platelets are stored but not destroyed by an enlarged spleen. The sequestration of platelets secondary to hypothermia is thought to be due to platelet aggregation. The platelet count returns to normal as body temperature normalizes.

8 In immune thrombocytopenia, antibodies cause platelet destruction or premature sequestration and removal from the circulation by the spleen and reticuloendothelial system. Immune destruction of the platelet may be accompanied by immune destruction of red cells as well. Examining the blood smear for evidence of hemolysis is most useful in the differential diagnosis of the immune thrombocytopenias. In isoimmune neonatal thrombocytopenia, maternal antibodies are directed against the platelet antigen (PLA 1) on the platelet surface. These antibodies are passed transplacentally to destroy fetal PLA 1 antigen-containing platelets. This disorder is very rare because 98 per cent of the population have platelets with the PLA 1 antigen on their surface.

9 Immune thrombocytopenia caused by drugs in some cases is due to the drug acting as a hapten, binding to a plasma protein to form a primary antigen. The resultant immune complexes have a high affinity for the platelet membrane and are responsible for platelet destruction. The drugs most commonly implicated in this form of thrombocytopenia include quinidine, quinine, and sulfonamides. Antilymphocyte globulin (ALG) causes thrombocytopenia because of its reactivity with platelet surface antigens. The severe thrombocytopenia that is sometimes seen with heparin therapy is due to heparin-induced antiplatelet antibodies.

10 Thrombocytopenia can occur in many autoimmune diseases. The thrombocytopenia accompanying anaphylaxis is thought to be due to immune complexes binding with platelets. The platelets are then cleared from the circulation by the spleen. Autoimmune disorders associated with platelet antibodies and thrombocytopenia include rheumatoid arthritis, Graves' disease, Hashimoto's thyroiditis, and myasthenia gravis. Lymphoreticular disorders and infections are also associated with thrombocytopenia, although the evidence for antiplatelet antibodies is less certain. Some lymphoreticular disorders associated with thrombocytopenia include tuberculosis, chronic lymphocytic leukemia (CLL), some lymphomas, sarcoidosis, and Hodgkin's disease. An important member of the group of immune thrombocytopenias is idiopathic thrombocytopenic purpura (ITP). ITP is not accompanied by hemolysis. Lack of hemolysis helps distinguish this disorder from thrombotic thrombocytopenic purpura (TTP) (see No. 14). Post-transfusion thrombocytopenia occurs in some patients who are PLA 1–negative (see No. 8). Antibodies to the PLA 1 antigen are formed by the transfused patient and are thought to result in the formation of immune complexes that aggregate on the platelet surface, resulting in platelet destruction.

11 Washout thrombocytopenia occurs when platelets are lost by massive hemorrhage. Platelet loss with extracorporeal devices is due to sequestration and consumption of platelets in the blood pump and tubing, as can occur with cardiopulmonary bypass.

12 Drugs cause a decrease in platelets by immune mechanisms (see No. 9) or by direct toxicity of the drug to platelets. Ristocetin and heparin cause a decrease in the number of circulating platelets by promoting platelet aggregation.

13 Evans' syndrome is a disease in which autoantibodies are directed against both the red cell and the platelet. Evans' syndrome is a Coombs-positive hemolytic anemia, which will distinguish Evans' syndrome from ITP. SLE is often accompanied by thrombocytopenia. Destruction of platelets in SLE is due to antiplatelet antibodies.

14 The hemolytic-uremic syndrome occurs primarily in infancy and may be a variant of TTP. This syndrome is characterized by hemolytic anemia, thrombocytopenia, and acute renal failure. In contrast to TTP, neurologic dysfunction is rare.

15 In DIC, thrombocytopenia is thought to be due to platelet consumption. In DIC, thrombin aggregates platelets and reduces the circulating platelet count. An increased amount of platelet-associated IgG is found in greater than 50 per cent of thrombocytopenic patients with DIC, however, such that platelet destruction may be partially immune-mediated.

16 TTP is characterized by the triad of thrombocytopenia, hemolytic anemia, and neurologic changes. TTP is usually accompanied by fever and renal failure. The etiology is unknown, but the thrombocytopenia is due to consumption by diffuse thrombosis. TTP has been considered the prototype of the nonimmunologic causes of thrombocytopenia, although an immunologic mechanism may be involved in its etiology.

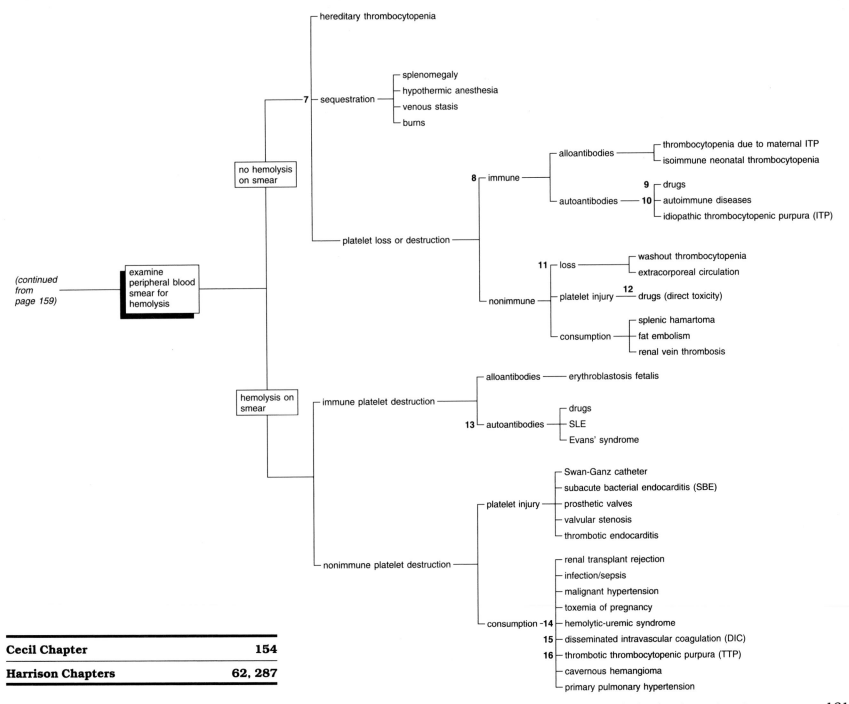

- hereditary thrombocytopenia

7 — sequestration
- splenomegaly
- hypothermic anesthesia
- venous stasis
- burns

no hemolysis on smear

platelet loss or destruction

8 — immune
- alloantibodies
  - thrombocytopenia due to maternal ITP
  - isoimmune neonatal thrombocytopenia
- autoantibodies
  - **9** — drugs
  - **10** — autoimmune diseases
  - idiopathic thrombocytopenic purpura (ITP)

nonimmune
- **11** — loss
  - washout thrombocytopenia
  - extracorporeal circulation
- platelet injury — **12** — drugs (direct toxicity)
- consumption
  - splenic hamartoma
  - fat embolism
  - renal vein thrombosis

examine peripheral blood smear for hemolysis

(continued from page 159)

hemolysis on smear

immune platelet destruction
- alloantibodies — erythroblastosis fetalis
- **13** — autoantibodies
  - drugs
  - SLE
  - Evans' syndrome

nonimmune platelet destruction
- platelet injury
  - Swan-Ganz catheter
  - subacute bacterial endocarditis (SBE)
  - prosthetic valves
  - valvular stenosis
  - thrombotic endocarditis
- consumption -**14**
  - renal transplant rejection
  - infection/sepsis
  - malignant hypertension
  - toxemia of pregnancy
  - hemolytic-uremic syndrome
  - **15** — disseminated intravascular coagulation (DIC)
  - **16** — thrombotic thrombocytopenic purpura (TTP)
  - cavernous hemangioma
  - primary pulmonary hypertension

Cecil Chapter	154
Harrison Chapters	62, 287

Hematologic Disorders—Thrombocytopenia   161

Dysproteinemia

1 Dysproteinemia refers to the group of disorders that occurs secondary to an abnormal clone of immunoglobulin-secreting cells. Other commonly used terms for dysproteinemia include plasma cell dyscrasias, gammopathies, paraproteinemias, immunoglobulinopathies, and monoclonal gammopathies. Dysproteinemia is diagnosed by the identification of a homogeneous immunoglobulin "spike" on serum protein electrophoresis (SPEP). An elevated serum globulin or a low anion gap is the usual clinical clue.

2 Examination of the bone marrow may reveal plasmacytosis with abnormal clones of plasma cells that may invade the adjacent bone. The definitive diagnosis of multiple myeloma, heavy chain disease, and Waldenström's macroglobulinemia rests on the demonstration of this plasmacytosis. Benign gammopathies are not characterized by the extensive bone marrow involvement, and the marrow is usually normal.

3 In order to identify the class of immunoglobulin responsible for the monoclonal "spike," or M-component, on the SPEP, a serum immunoelectrophoresis (IEP) must be performed. The M-component can be made up of the immunoglobulins IgG, IgM, IgD, IgA, and IgE; light chains alone; or heavy chains alone. The heavy and light chains that compose the immunoglobulins are often synthesized in unequal amounts by the neoplastic clone of cells. Usually the light chains are in excess and can be excreted in the urine owing to their low molecular weight. The monoclonal light chains that are found in the urine in association with plasma cell neoplasms are known as Bence Jones proteins. Urine dipstick analysis will not detect Bence Jones protein. Bence Jones protein can be detected only by a special technique in which the protein demonstrates certain solubility characteristics upon heating and cooling of the urine. A urine protein electrophoresis (UPEP) is perhaps the best method to demonstrate the presence of Bence Jones protein.

4 Macroglobulinemia is characterized by IgM as the M-component on IEP. Primary macroglobulinemia, or Waldenström's macroglobulinemia, is due to a primary plasma cell dyscrasia. Bence Jones proteinuria accompanies Waldenström's macroglobulinemia in approximately 10 to 30 per cent of the patients. The diagnosis of Waldenström's macroglobulinemia is made in the presence of typical clinical signs and symptoms of hyperviscosity caused by circulating IgM, an IgM concentration greater than 3 gm/dl, and evidence of a substantial number of plasma cells and plasmacytic lymphocytes on bone marrow examination. Typical clinical features of Waldenström's macroglobulinemia include fatigue and bleeding manifestations, as well as neurologic symptoms, primarily owing to hyperviscosity.

5 The diagnosis of multiple myeloma is based on the demonstration of marrow plasmacytosis, evidence of clone invasiveness (e.g., lytic bone or soft tissue lesions), and a significant M-component on SPEP. IgG is the M-component in greater than 50 per cent of the cases of myeloma. IgA is the M-component in 25 per cent of cases and free light chain in 20 per cent of cases. IgM, IgD, and IgE are the M-components in less than 5 per cent of cases of multiple myeloma.

The frequency of the class of immunoglobulin responsible for myeloma parallels the relative frequency with which the immunoglobulins are found in the blood normally. In addition, 1 per cent of patients may have plasma cell tumors that produce two or more monoclonal proteins, the so-called biclonal gammopathies. The most common biclonal gammopathy is combined IgG and IgA, which occurs in about 30 per cent of these cases.

Less than 1 per cent of the patients in whom myeloma is suspected clinically but laboratory confirmation is lacking probably have light chain myeloma with removal of the light chain by the kidney. Myeloma may be difficult to diagnose if any light chain myeloma is present because of the lack of a prominent monoclonal spike on IEP. Two thirds of the patients with IgG or IgA myeloma are also found to have Bence Jones protein in their urine. Bence Jones protein may be detected in less than 50 per cent of patients with light chain myeloma. Bence Jones protein may also be detected in the urine of patients with primary amyloidosis and in approximately 20 per cent of patients with macroglobulinemia (see No. 10).

6 Heavy chain disease is a rare condition caused by the secretion of the heavy chain, or heavy chain fragment, of an immunoglobulin by a clone of neoplastic cells. Heavy chain synthesis corresponds to the five subclasses of immunoglobulins. The presence of heavy chain protein in the urine cannot be detected by the solubility tests used to detect Bence Jones protein, but UPEP will reveal the presence of heavy chains.

7 Secondary macroglobulinemia refers to a macroglobulinemia occasionally found with lymphoma, carcinoma, and infectious and other inflammatory conditions. The IgM levels are much lower than those seen in Waldenström's macroglobulinemia.

8 Previously known as benign monoclonal gammopathy, monoclonal gammopathy of unknown significance (MGUS) denotes the presence of IgM as the M-component on IEP without the diagnostic features of macroglobulinemia, myeloma, or other plasma cell disorder. The disease may not be benign, as many of the patients develop macroglobulinemia or myeloma over time. Patients with MGUS have lower quantities of IgM in their serum than do patients with multiple myeloma, and Bence Jones protein is absent from their urine. Bone marrow examination usually demonstrates less than 5 per cent plasma cells. MGUS can be detected in approximately 1 per cent of the population over the age of 50 and in 3 per cent of the population over 70 years of age. If initial investigation of IgM M-component leads to the diagnosis of MGUS, the patient should be followed without treatment at intervals of 3 months, the IEP being repeated with each examination. If the quantity of the monoclonal IgM increases by more than 50 per cent on repeat IEP, then a complete re-evaluation, including bone marrow examination, should be performed. Previous studies of MGUS have shown that approximately 60 per cent of patients continue to have stable protein levels over a 5-year period of follow-up. Approximately 11 per cent of patients with MGUS go on to develop macroglobulinemia, myeloma, or amyloidosis.

9 Indolent myeloma occurs in about 5 per cent of patients with criteria diagnostic of myeloma but with a more indolent course. Bence Jones proteinuria is absent.

10 Amyloidosis is a complex of disorders in which kappa and lambda light chain immunoglobulin components are deposited in various body tissues. Most dysproteinemias that are associated with light chain secretion can also be accompanied by amyloid deposition. IEP detects an M-component in only about 50 per cent of patients with primary amyloidosis, but 90 per cent will have detectable Bence Jones protein in their urine. If amyloidosis is associated with myeloma, the IEP will detect an M-component in about 75 per cent of the patients. The diagnosis of amyloidosis requires the demonstration of amyloid on tissue biopsy.

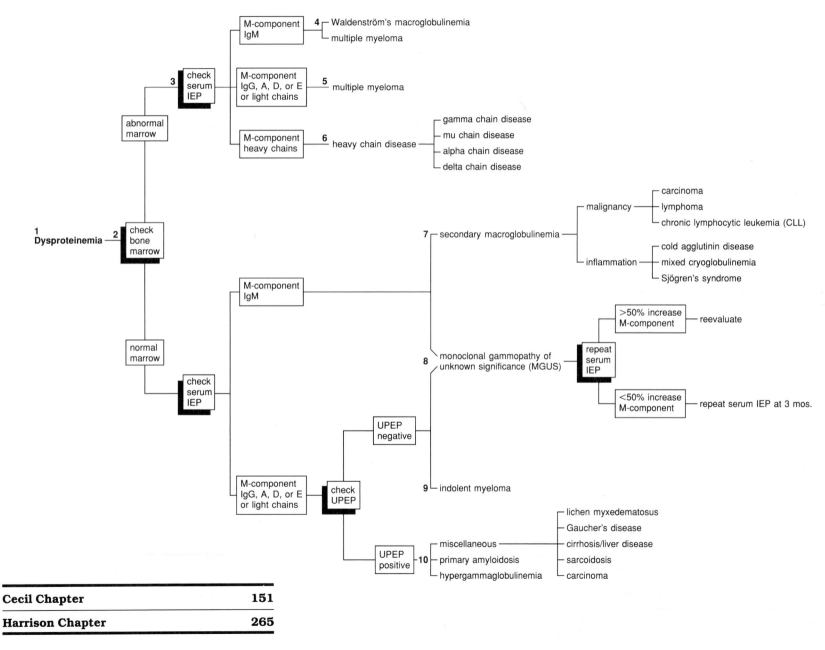

1
Dysproteinemia — **2** check bone marrow

abnormal marrow

3 check serum IEP

M-component IgM — **4** ┌ Waldenström's macroglobulinemia
└ multiple myeloma

M-component IgG, A, D, or E or light chains — **5** multiple myeloma

M-component heavy chains — **6** heavy chain disease ┌ gamma chain disease
├ mu chain disease
├ alpha chain disease
└ delta chain disease

normal marrow

check serum IEP

M-component IgM — **7** secondary macroglobulinemia ┌ malignancy ┌ carcinoma
│ ├ lymphoma
│ └ chronic lymphocytic leukemia (CLL)
└ inflammation ┌ cold agglutinin disease
├ mixed cryoglobulinemia
└ Sjögren's syndrome

8 monoclonal gammopathy of unknown significance (MGUS) — repeat serum IEP ┌ >50% increase M-component — reevaluate
└ <50% increase M-component — repeat serum IEP at 3 mos.

M-component IgG, A, D, or E or light chains — check UPEP

UPEP negative — **9** indolent myeloma

UPEP positive — **10** ┌ miscellaneous ┌ lichen myxedematosus
│ ├ Gaucher's disease
│ ├ cirrhosis/liver disease
│ ├ sarcoidosis
│ └ carcinoma
├ primary amyloidosis
└ hypergammaglobulinemia

Cecil Chapter   **151**

Harrison Chapter   **265**

BIBLIOGRAPHY

Beck WS: Diagnosis of megaloblastic anemia. Annu Rev Med 42:311–322, 1991.

Beck WS (ed): Hematology. 4th ed. Cambridge, MA, MIT Press, 1985.

Brown BA: Hematology: Principles and Procedures. Philadelphia, Lea & Febiger, 1984.

Djulbegovic B, Hadley T, Joseph G: A new algorithm for the diagnosis of polycythemia. Am Fam Physician 44(1):113–120, 1991.

Elias J, et al.: Serum beta-2-microglobulin in the differential diagnosis of monoclonal gammopathies. S Afr Med 79:650–653, 1991.

Farley PC, Foland J: Iron deficiency anemia. Postgrad Med 87(2):89, 1990.

Goerg C, Schwerk WB, Goerg K: Splenic lesions: sonographic patterns, follow-up, differential diagnosis. Eur J Radiol 13:59–66, 1991.

Goodman KI, Salt WB: Vitamin B_{12} deficiency. Postgrad Med 88(3):147, 1990.

Imbert M: Adult patients presenting with pancytopenia. Hematol Pathol 3(4):159–167, 1989.

Keisu M, Ost A: Diagnoses in patients with severe pancytopenia suspected of having aplastic anemia. Eur J Haematol 45:11–14, 1990.

Lichtman MA: Hematology for Practitioners. Boston, Little, Brown & Company, 1978.

LoBuglio AF (ed): Hematologic Disorders. Med Clin North Am 64(4), 1980.

Majer RV: Which tests are most useful in distinguishing between reactive thrombocytosis and the thrombocytosis of myeloproliferative disease? Clin Lab Haematol 13:9–15, 1991.

Meyers FJ, Welborn JL, Lewis JP: Improved approach to patients with normocytic anemia. Am Fam Physician 38(2):191–195, 1988.

Miale JB: Laboratory Medicine Hematology. St. Louis, The C. V. Mosby Company, 1977.

Murphy S: Polycythemia Vera. Disease-a-Month. 38(3). St. Louis, Mosby-Year Book, 1992.

Roskos RR, Boxer LA: Clinical disorders of neutropenia. Pediat Rev 12(7):208–212, 1991.

Ruggenenti P, Remuzzi G: Thrombotic thrombocytopenic purpura and related disorders. Hematol Oncol Clin North Am 4(1):219–231, 1990.

Spivak JL: Fundamentals of Clinical Hematology. Philadelphia, Harper & Row, 1984.

Wheby MS (ed): Anemia. Med Clin North Am 76(3), 1992.

Williams WJ, Beutler E, et al.: Hematology. 3rd ed. New York, McGraw-Hill Book Company, 1983.

Wintrobe MW (ed): Clinical Hematology. 8th ed. Philadelphia, Lea & Febiger, 1981.

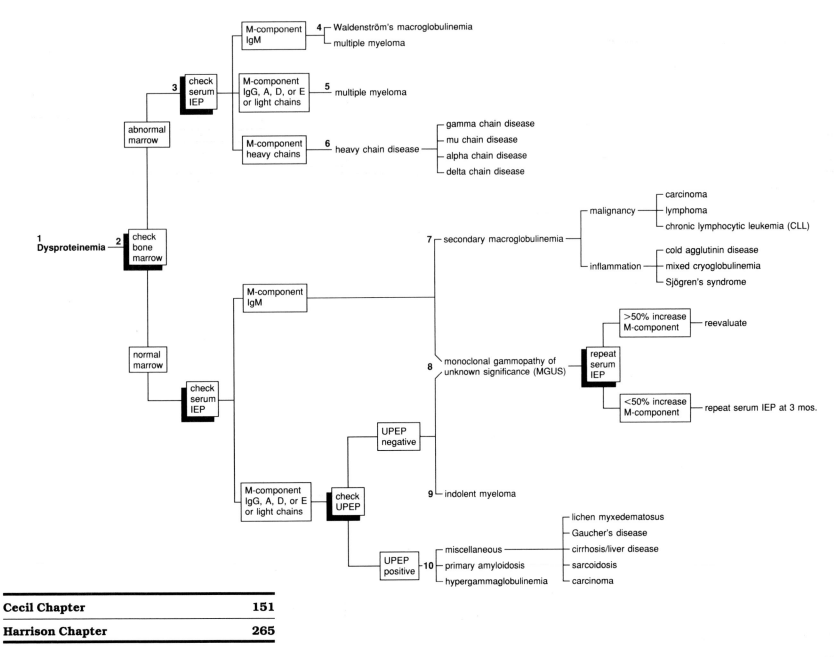

8 ▪ Neurologic Disorders

Signs and symptoms:
Headache
Vertigo

Dementia
Altered mental status
Seizure

Headache

1 Headache may be the most common of all physical symptoms. In the United States, it accounts for over 20 million physician visits per year. The severity, onset, and location of the pain may give useful clues to the diagnosis. Only the bony structure of the head and the brain parenchyma are not richly supplied with pain-sensitive nerve fibers. Headache may therefore originate from irritation to any of the other structures of the head and neck. The most severe pain originates from the arteries, cranial nerves, and dura mater.

2 Almost all of the life-threatening etiologies of headache cause sudden or rapid onset of pain. Acute-onset headache is defined as pain with an onset of less than 1 week, but often it occurs only minutes to hours prior to the patient's seeking medical care. Headaches may be also considered acute if there is a sudden change in the pattern or severity of a chronic headache. Owing to the possibly serious nature of the acute-onset headache, a thorough and often urgent evaluation should be undertaken. Even in this setting, however, less than 5 per cent of headaches have life-threatening causes, and less than 15 per cent are the result of serious neurologic disease.

3 Focal neurologic findings are signs or symptoms referable to one area of the central nervous system with relative sparing of other functions. The abnormality most commonly involves motor or sensory functions, but more subtle changes in balance, memory, and other cognitive functions must also be sought.

4 Most forms of bacterial meningitis are associated with other systemic symptoms such as fever, altered mental status, and nuchal rigidity. Viral, fungal, and certain opportunistic infections of the meninges may present with only acute-onset headache in the early stages. Although computed tomography (CT) scanning prior to lumbar puncture is desirable to rule out the possibility of increased intracranial pressure or partial herniation, lumbar puncture should never be delayed if bacterial menin-

gitis is suspected. Human immunodeficiency virus (HIV)–associated meningitis is now a well-recognized entity. It may occur in the setting of other viral or bacterial meningitides or may represent the effect of HIV itself.

5 Migraine headaches are a common form of vascular headache (see No. 11). Most are not associated with focal neurologic findings, but occasionally ocular motor palsy, as well other focal neurologic defects, may occur. A few studies have revealed ischemic changes in the involved area of the brain. A rare familial form of complex migraine is associated with aphasia, confusion, and hemiparesis or hemiplegia.

6 Thrombosis of any of the major dural sinuses may occur spontaneously or as a result of infection. Spontaneous thrombosis is usually associated with pregnancy, puerperium, collagen vascular disorders (most notably systemic lupus erythematosus), malignancy, and oral contraceptives. Infection of the dural sinuses usually occurs through direct extension of infection through a sinus wall or a draining vein or via venous embolization. Although any of the dural sinuses may be involved, the large paired lateral, cavernous, and petrosal sinuses are affected most often. Any of these conditions is potentially life-threatening and should be suspected in any person with a sudden deterioration following sinus infection.

7 Cranial arteritis occurs most commonly in patients over the age of 60. Any of the large cranial arteries may be involved, but the temporal artery is the most common site of inflammation. The pain is usually intense and localized to the temporal or fronto-occipital regions of the head. There may be tenderness to palpation as well as firmness over the affected artery. Temporal arteritis is strongly associated with polymyalgia rheumatica and, if untreated, may result in occlusion of the retinal arteries, followed by permanent blindness. The erythrocyte sedimentation rate is invariably elevated, at times to greater than 100 mm/hr. _ESR ↑_

8 The cranial neuralgias result from a sudden and excessive discharge from the involved cranial nerve. Trigeminal neuralgia or tic douloureux is the most common form of cranial neuralgia. The disorder may involve compression of the nerve by vascular structures. The syndrome has also occurred following viral infec-

tions, and rarely, secondary to a gasserian ganglion tumor. Neuralgia of other cranial nerves, including the glossopharyngeal and occular nerves, occurs occasionally.

9 Exposure to many chemicals and drugs has been associated with headache. Chemicals most frequently associated with headache include benzene, nitrates, tyramine, monosodium glutamate, carbon monoxide, insecticides, and lead. Drugs, including oral contraceptives, nitrates, indomethacin, calcium channel blockers, caffeine, and alcohol, have also been associated with headaches. Sudden withdrawal of any of these drugs may lead to headache. The etiology of the headache is usually an alteration in blood flow to cranial structures.

10 Extracranial infections are a common cause of headache. Up to 40 per cent of the acute-onset headaches may be due to extracranial infection. Generalized viral infections as well as bacterial infections involving any other areas of the body have been associated with headache. Other systemic symptoms such as fever, lethargy, and anorexia may be prominent.

11 Migraine headache is a well-defined disorder of severe headache that can be associated with generalized neurologic symptoms. These symptoms may include visual aurae, hemianoptic visual loss, vertigo, and taste and smell abnormalities. Occasionally, ataxia and generalized sensory abnormalities may also occur. At times, the symptoms may be more focal (see No. 5). Typical attacks of migraine may have up to four phases. The first phase is a prodrome lasting up to 24 hours that is associated with mood changes, drowsiness, and loss of appetite. The second phase consists of the neurologic symptoms. The third phase begins as the neurologic symptoms subside and consists of a severe headache, usually involving one of the frontotemporal regions of the head. The headache may be accompanied by photophobia, nausea, vomiting, and noise intolerance. The headache may last from 4 hours to several days if not treated. The last, or postheadache, phase consists of a feeling of exhaustion, and occasionally tenderness of the scalp. The etiology of the migraine headache is unclear, but alterations of blood flow over the cerebral cortex have been noted. The migraine attacks can mimic many other serious neurologic disorders, and these disorders must be excluded before the diagnosis can be made.

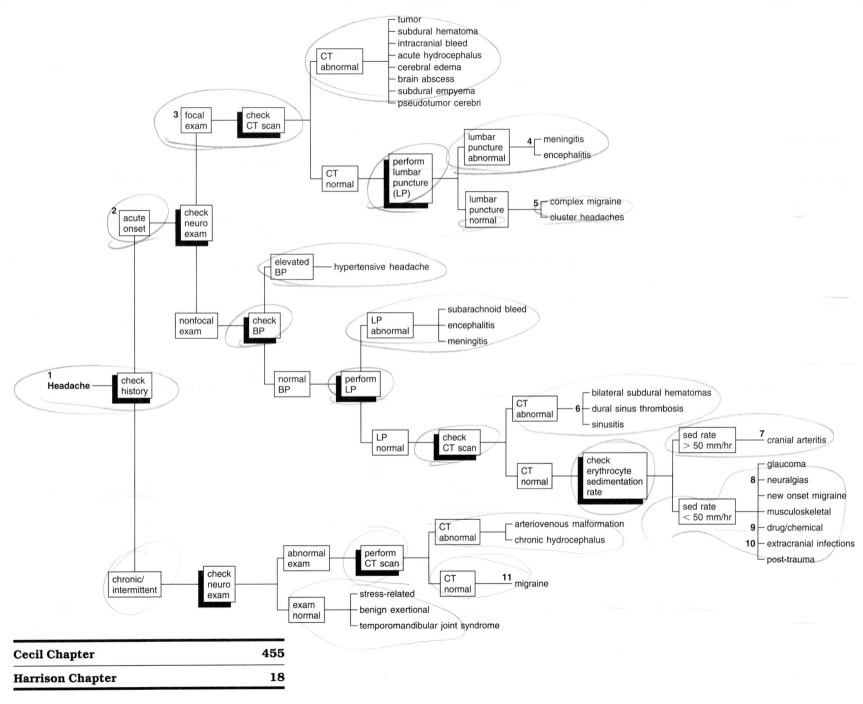

tumor
subdural hematoma
intracranial bleed
CT abnormal — acute hydrocephalus
cerebral edema
brain abscess
subdural empyema
pseudotumor cerebri

3 focal exam — check CT scan

lumbar puncture abnormal — **4** meningitis / encephalitis

CT normal — perform lumbar puncture (LP)

lumbar puncture normal — **5** complex migraine / cluster headaches

2 acute onset — check neuro exam

elevated BP — hypertensive headache

nonfocal exam — check BP

1 Headache — check history

normal BP — perform LP

LP abnormal — subarachnoid bleed / encephalitis / meningitis

LP normal — check CT scan

CT abnormal — **6** bilateral subdural hematomas / dural sinus thrombosis / sinusitis

CT normal — check erythrocyte sedimentation rate

sed rate > 50 mm/hr — **7** cranial arteritis

sed rate < 50 mm/hr — glaucoma / **8** neuralgias / new onset migraine / musculoskeletal / **9** drug/chemical / **10** extracranial infections / post-trauma

chronic/ intermittent — check neuro exam

abnormal exam — perform CT scan

CT abnormal — arteriovenous malformation / chronic hydrocephalus

CT normal — **11** migraine

exam normal — stress-related / benign exertional / temporomandibular joint syndrome

Cecil Chapter	455
Harrison Chapter	18

Vertigo

1 Vertigo is the sensation of rotary movement. The patient may feel either that he is turning or that the environment around him is turning. Vertigo is usually accompanied by nausea and visual disturbances. Vertigo implies a disorder in the vestibular apparatus. This disturbance may be in the vestibular labyrinth itself or in the central nervous system. Injury or disease in any of these areas will cause an imbalance in the symmetry of the impulses from the right and left vestibules and result in vertigo. The vertigo may be continuous or intermittent, and this finding may be useful in the differential diagnosis. Dizziness is any nonrotary sense of disequilibrium. Dizziness is not a labyrinthine phenomenon.

2 Although much can be learned from a skilled neurologic examination, electronystagmography (ENG) is a useful test in the diagnosis of disorders of balance. ENG is a battery of tests that consist first of a recording of tracking gaze, as well as vertical, spontaneous, and optokinetic nystagmus. Abnormalities in this portion of the test are consistent with a central nervous system origin for the vertigo. A second part of the test evaluates positional nystagmus, and the third part tests caloric response of the inner ear. Abnormalities in these last two portions of the ENG are associated with labyrinthine disorders, or positional vertigo. A normal ENG eliminates true vertigo. The patient is more likely unable to differentiate vertigo from dizziness.

3 A formal audiogram should be performed on any patient with vertigo and evidence of hearing loss. Audiometry tests the ability to sense pure tones via both air and bone conduction. The loss of the ability to hear only selected tones is most consistent with certain forms of ototoxicity. A more complete hearing loss in one ear in association with vertigo may indicate nerve damage through entrapment or replacement by tumor. Further evaluation including CT scanning is necessary in this setting. The brain stem evoked response may also be useful in further evaluating the magnitude of the hearing loss and differentiating between disorders of the cochlea, eighth nerve, and brain stem lesions.

4 The most common tumor affecting the cerebropontine angle is an acoustic neuroma. A high index of suspicion is necessary to make the diagnosis while the tumor is small. An acoustic neuroma must be suspected in any patient with total or severe one-sided hearing loss, a depressed caloric response on ENG, or an abnormal brain stem evoked response. Early diagnosis is extremely important, as the prognosis for large or advanced tumors is poor.

5 Ménière's disease is a common disorder affecting mainly middle-aged persons. The disease is manifested as periods of episodic vertigo, many times accompanied by severe nausea, blurred vision, and at times shortness of breath. The vertigo is usually accompanied by fluctuating hearing loss and tinnitus. Ménière's disease may be progressive, with attacks becoming more frequent. Occasionally progressive disease will result in permanent damage to the inner ear.

6 Ototoxic agents can be associated with hearing loss and occasionally with vertigo. The agents most frequently implicated include alcohol, heavy metals, carbon monoxide, the aminoglycoside antibiotics, furosemide, quinine, cisplatin, and aspirin. Among these groups, the aminoglycosides are potentially the most damaging to the vestibular and cochlear sensory cells. The ototoxicity of the aminoglycosides appears to be related to elevated peak serum levels. Furosemide has been associated with severe vertigo. The rapidity of the intravenous administration of furosemide is thought to be associated with its ototoxicity.

7 Temporomandibular joint neuralgia, or TMJ syndrome, is frequently associated with dizziness and tinnitus. The joint itself is tender to palpation. Joint radiographs are usually diagnostic.

8 Benign positional vertigo is a disorder consisting of sudden attacks of vertigo related to changes in position. There is no associated tinnitus or hearing loss. The vertigo is brought on by placing the diseased ear in a dependent position. Nystagmus toward the affected ear is invariably present. The disorder is self-limited, usually resolving in several months, but may last up to a year.

9 True vertigo occurs in up to one third of patients with multiple sclerosis. Nystagmus is almost always present and creates an abnormal ENG. The onset of the disease is usually between 20 and 50 years of age and should be suspected when central-type vertigo or visual disturbances are noted in this age group. The magnetic resonance imaging (MRI) may demonstrate findings consistent with this diagnosis, but there is no single diagnostic test available.

10 Herpes zoster may affect the geniculate ganglion (the Ramsay Hunt syndrome) in the petrous portion of the temporal bone. Severe otalgia and seventh nerve paralysis may occur. Tinnitus, vertigo, and hearing loss may also be noted. Herpetic lesions may be seen in the distribution of the seventh cranial nerve, the external ear, or the tympanic membrane.

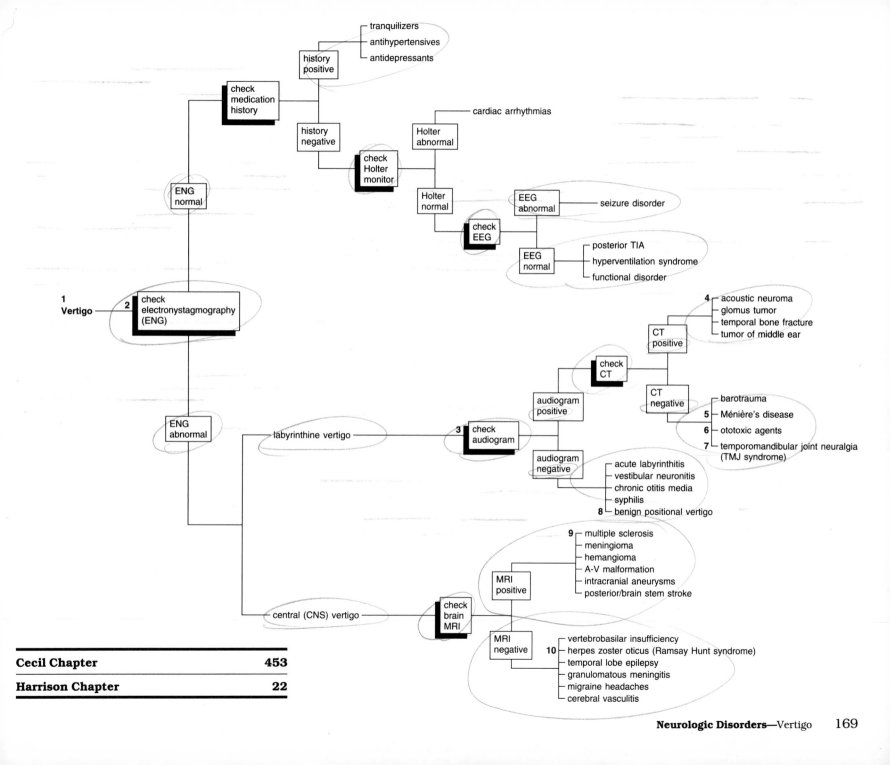

tranquilizers

antihypertensives

antidepressants

history positive

check medication history

history negative

cardiac arrhythmias

Holter abnormal

check Holter monitor

Holter normal

EEG abnormal

seizure disorder

check EEG

EEG normal

posterior TIA

hyperventilation syndrome

functional disorder

ENG normal

1
Vertigo

2 check electronystagmography (ENG)

ENG abnormal

labyrinthine vertigo

3 check audiogram

audiogram positive

check CT

CT positive

4 acoustic neuroma

glomus tumor

temporal bone fracture

tumor of middle ear

CT negative

barotrauma

5 Ménière's disease

6 ototoxic agents

7 temporomandibular joint neuralgia (TMJ syndrome)

audiogram negative

acute labyrinthitis

vestibular neuronitis

chronic otitis media

syphilis

8 benign positional vertigo

9 multiple sclerosis

meningioma

hemangioma

A-V malformation

intracranial aneurysms

posterior/brain stem stroke

MRI positive

central (CNS) vertigo

check brain MRI

MRI negative

vertebrobasilar insufficiency

10 herpes zoster oticus (Ramsay Hunt syndrome)

temporal lobe epilepsy

granulomatous meningitis

migraine headaches

cerebral vasculitis

Cecil Chapter 453

Harrison Chapter 22

Dementia

1 Dementia is an acquired condition in which mental capacity is diminished. Dementia is not a diagnosis, but a symptom of an underlying disorder. Dementia may affect memory, language, cognition, spatial orientation, or personality. Usually several of these functions are impaired. Dementia is a global phenomenon and should be distinguished from focal defects such as aphasia or amnesia. Dementia should also be distinguished from acute confusional states that last only hours or days. Dementia may affect as many as 15 per cent of persons over the age of 65 as well as a smaller percentage of younger persons. As many as 50 per cent of these patients may have treatable metabolic or structural causes for the dementia.

2 Focal neurologic findings are signs or symptoms referable to one area of the central nervous system with relative sparing of other functions. The abnormality most commonly involves motor or sensory functions, but more subtle changes in balance, memory, and other cognitive functions must also be sought.

3 Brain imaging can now be performed utilizing several modalities. The suspected underlying condition should govern the choice of available techniques. CT scanning has become the standard for the evaluation of structural lesions within the brain and ventricles. MRI may be more reliable for certain subtle changes in white or gray matter, as seen in lacunar syndromes and multiple sclerosis. New techniques like positron emission tomography (PET) may help to delineate many metabolic disorders.

4 Multiple sclerosis may be one of the causes of early age dementia. The dementia is usually accompanied by other clinical signs involving scattered areas of the brain as well as the optic nerve and spinal cord. The age of onset is between 15 and 50 years. MRI has been shown to be a sensitive tool for diagnosis by revealing typical areas of demyelination, but may not be diagnostic.

5 Pick's disease is often confused with the more common Alzheimer's disease (see No. 12) because of the similar form of dementia with prominent motor symptoms. The dementia of Pick's disease is caused by a degeneration of the temporal and frontal lobes. Aphasia may be a prominent symptom. The CT scan will reveal enlarged temporal horns and frontal atrophy. There is no known treatment and the progression is rapid.

6 Normal pressure hydrocephalus is a chronic condition in which there is a slow accumulation of cerebrospinal fluid (CSF) and enlargement of the ventricles. The pressure in the CSF is normal. The etiology of normal pressure hydrocephalus is unclear, as is its clinical significance. Many patients with this nonobstructive or communicating form of hydrocephalus have a syndrome of dementia, psychomotor retardation, unsteady gait, and urinary incontinence. As many as 5 per cent of persons over the age of 60 may have demonstrable hydrocephalus on CT scan, and many of these patients are asymptomatic. The reversibility of this disorder with ventricular shunting procedures is unclear.

7 Progressive supranuclear palsy can resemble Parkinson's disease, but it has a less prominent tremor, and ophthalmoplegia is present. Dementia occurs late in the course of the disease, but there is a more rapid decline in mental capacity than in patients with Parkinson's disease. No effective treatment is known.

8 AIDS dementia is composed of a combination of changes in cognition, motor skills, and behavior. It is thought to be the result of direct infection of the brain with the AIDS virus. The dementia has a slow onset and may progress for months to years. As the disease progresses, leg and arm weakness may develop, along with urinary and fecal incontinence. Tremor and myoclonus may also develop. The disease may progress to complete mutism and render the patient completely helpless. This form of dementia must be distinguished from the more treatable causes of dementia associated with AIDS such as infection, medication effects, and depression.

9 Systemic lupus erythematosus, as well as other forms of vasculitis, may cause an acute cerebritis leading to dementia. The exact mechanism of the dementia is not known. The development of dementia in patients with vasculitis should be treated emergently.

10 The chronic forms of meningitis are usually caused by indolent infections. Fungal infections, especially those caused by *Cryptococcus* and *Coccidioides,* are associated with various forms of dementia. Tuberculosis, sarcoidosis, and carcinomatous forms of meningitis are also commonly associated with dementia.

11 Drugs may be the most frequent cause of dementia. Both therapeutic and toxic chemicals may cause dementia. The drugs most commonly associated with dementia include the major tranquilizers, antidepressants, minor tranquilizers, narcotics, anticonvulsants, antihypertensives, digoxin, and anticholinergic drugs, as well as certain antibiotics and antineoplastic drugs. The dementia-producing effect of any of these drugs is more profound in the elderly. Toxic chemicals known to produce dementia include the heavy metals, organic solvents, and insecticides.

12 Alzheimer's disease is the most common illness producing dementia. It is thought to affect as many as 3 million people in the United States alone. Alzheimer's disease begins insidiously, with failure of recent memory a prominent early symptom. Emotional lability and nominal aphasia may be severe. Primary motor and sensory functions are spared early in the disease, but apraxia and incontinence may appear. The etiology is unknown, but viral diseases, genetic predisposition, and neurochemical disorders have all been implicated. The pathologic changes seen in brain tissue consist of senile plaques, granulovacuolar degeneration, and neurofibrillary tangles. The disease is progressive with eventual loss of most cognitive function.

13 Depression may cause a syndrome virtually indistinguishable from dementia. Depression is most difficult to diagnose in the elderly, in whom the common complaints of sadness, helplessness, insomnia, and weight loss may not be obvious. A thorough psychiatric evaluation is necessary when no other cause of the "dementia" can be found. Many patients with even profound depression can be successfully treated and returned to a functional status.

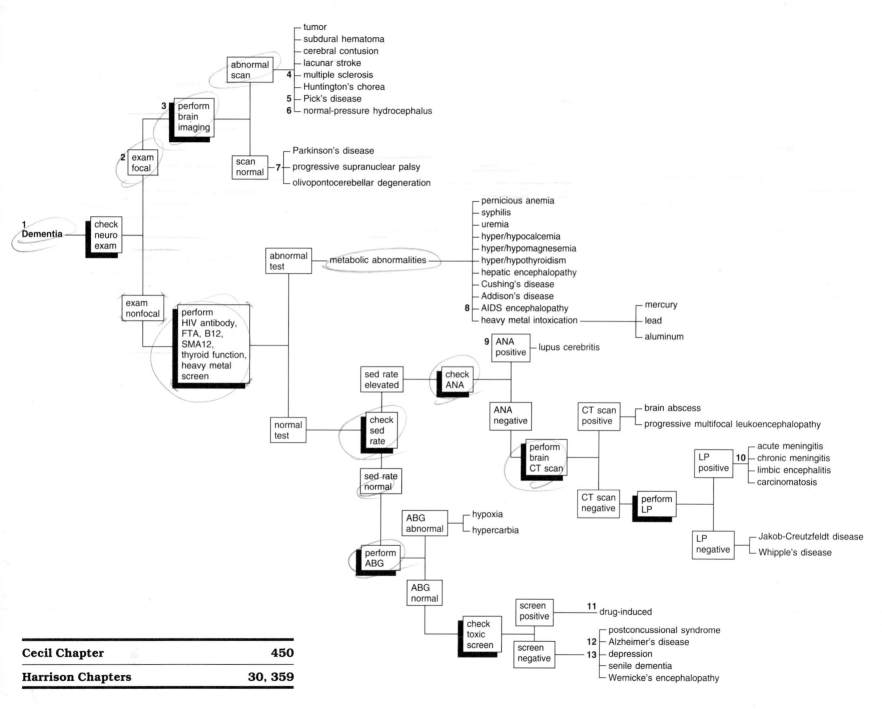

tumor
subdural hematoma
cerebral contusion
lacunar stroke
4 — multiple sclerosis
Huntington's chorea
5 — Pick's disease
6 — normal-pressure hydrocephalus

abnormal scan

3 perform brain imaging

2 exam focal

scan normal **7** — Parkinson's disease
progressive supranuclear palsy
olivopontocerebellar degeneration

1 Dementia — check neuro exam

abnormal test — metabolic abnormalities — pernicious anemia
syphilis
uremia
hyper/hypocalcemia
hyper/hypomagnesemia
hyper/hypothyroidism
hepatic encephalopathy
Cushing's disease
Addison's disease
8 — AIDS encephalopathy
heavy metal intoxication — mercury
lead
aluminum

exam nonfocal

perform HIV antibody, FTA, B12, SMA12, thyroid function, heavy metal screen

9 ANA positive — lupus cerebritis

sed rate elevated — check ANA

ANA negative

CT scan positive — brain abscess
progressive multifocal leukoencephalopathy

normal test — check sed rate

perform brain CT scan

LP positive **10** — acute meningitis
chronic meningitis
limbic encephalitis
carcinomatosis

sed rate normal

CT scan negative — perform LP

ABG abnormal — hypoxia
hypercarbia

LP negative — Jakob-Creutzfeldt disease
Whipple's disease

perform ABG

ABG normal

screen positive **11** — drug-induced

check toxic screen

screen negative — postconcussional syndrome
12 — Alzheimer's disease
13 — depression
senile dementia
Wernicke's encephalopathy

Cecil Chapter	**450**
Harrison Chapters	**30, 359**

Altered Mental Status

1 Altered mental status is defined as a decrease in the level of consciousness. The change in mental status is acute, appearing over minutes to days. The changes may be brief, lasting for minutes to hours, or sustained. A decrease in the level of consciousness is usually classified into three levels of severity—delirium, stupor, and coma. Delirium is confusion and a reduction of awareness. The level of wakefulness is not usually abnormal. Delirium is most often caused by a metabolic brain disorder rather than by trauma or intracranial lesions. Stupor is an unarousability that can be overcome only by vigorous or direct noxious stimuli. The most severe form of altered mental status is coma. In coma, the patient is unarousable to even the strongest external stimuli. Consciousness is controlled mainly in the ascending reticular activating system, a group of neurons extending from the pons to the thalamus. Conditions affecting consciousness must involve the entire brain (metabolic) or the brain stem either directly or indirectly. The more depressed the level of consciousness, and the longer the condition continues, the worse the prognosis. Several severe psychiatric conditions may mimic any of these states (see No. 9).

2 Carbon monoxide poisoning can be acute and is easily detected by history, if obtainable, or the cherry red flush of the skin and mucous membranes. Chronic carbon monoxide poisoning is less easily detected but is seen in a substantial percentage of patients presenting with altered mental status. This form of chronic carbon monoxide exposure usually is the result of faulty indoor heating systems or indoor cooking using charcoal fuel. A carboxyhemoglobin measurement should be included in any arterial blood gas determination when evaluating altered mental status.

3 Extreme changes in body temperature can cause decreased levels of consciousness. Core temperatures greater than 40.5°C or less than 32°C are associated with altered mental status. Hyperthermia may be caused by extremely high fever or heatstroke. Heatstroke is caused by exposure to extremely high ambient temperatures, usually accompanied by some form of impaired bodily heat reduction mechanisms. Drugs that impair sweating, such as anticholinergics, phenothiazines, beta-blockers, and antihistamines, may contribute to the development of heatstroke. Hypothermia is usually associated with metabolic causes such as sepsis, hypoglycemia, uremia, hepatic failure, adrenal insufficiency, and hypothyroidism. Severe brain injury or spinal cord transection can also cause profound hypothermia. Certain drugs such as ethanol and phenothiazines as well as thiamine deficiency (see No. 8) have also been associated with hypothermia.

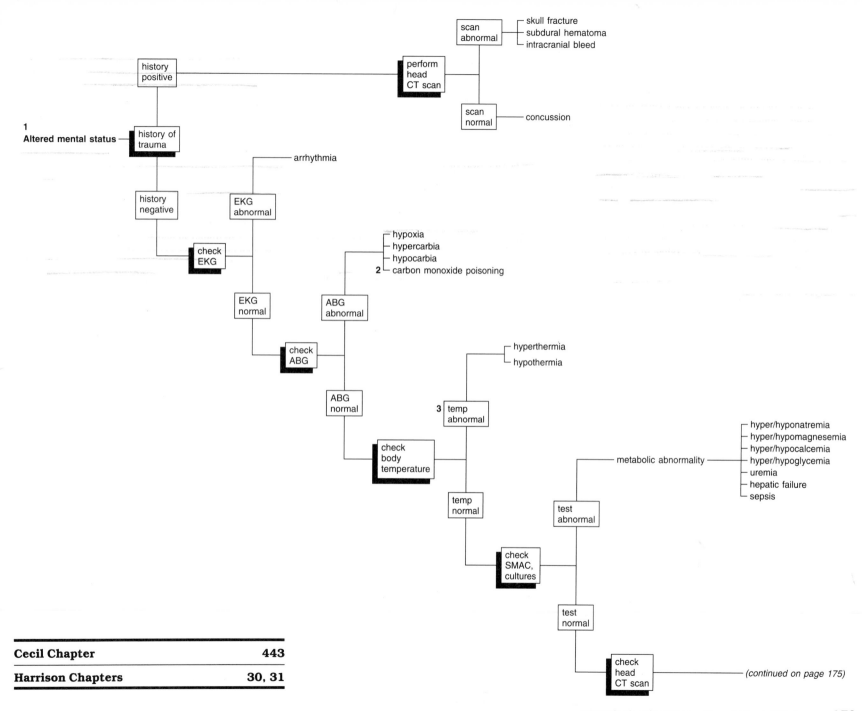

1
Altered mental status

history of trauma

history positive

perform head CT scan

scan abnormal
— skull fracture
— subdural hematoma
— intracranial bleed

scan normal
— concussion

history negative

check EKG

EKG abnormal
— arrhythmia

EKG normal

check ABG

ABG abnormal
— hypoxia
— hypercarbia
— hypocarbia
2 — carbon monoxide poisoning

ABG normal

check body temperature

3 temp abnormal
— hyperthermia
— hypothermia

temp normal

check SMAC, cultures

test abnormal
— metabolic abnormality
— hyper/hyponatremia
— hyper/hypomagnesemia
— hyper/hypocalcemia
— hyper/hypoglycemia
— uremia
— hepatic failure
— sepsis

test normal

check head CT scan
(continued on page 175)

Cecil Chapter	443
Harrison Chapters	30, 31

Altered Mental Status
(Continued)

4 Brain stem herniation is the most ominous cause of altered mental status. Increased intracranial pressure resulting from space-occupying mass lesions or generalized cerebral edema may cause downward displacement of the diencephalon. This displacement causes compression of the midbrain into the tentorial notch (central herniation) or compression of the uncus against the midbrain in the tentorial notch (uncal herniation). Herniation can also be caused by removal of cerebrospinal fluid when intracranial pressure is increased. Therefore, except in extreme circumstances such as the suspicion of bacterial meningitis, lumbar puncture should be performed after the CT scan in patients with altered mental status. Clinical signs of herniation include a rapidly decreasing level of consciousness, sighing, yawning, and periodic respirations. Pupils may shrink to pinpoint size at first. Later one or both of the pupils may dilate. Unless rapid treatment is undertaken, permanent brain damage or brain death is inevitable.

5 Any lesion that directly affects the midbrain region may cause decreased levels of consciousness. These lesions may include rare tumors of the brain stem, ischemia, and degenerative diseases of the central nervous system. Patients who are awake but unable to respond may have a form of "locked-in" syndrome. In this condition, all descending motor pathways are blocked, usually by an infarction or hemorrhage at the base of the pons. The patient may be completely aware of all external stimuli but may be able to communicate only by eye movements.

6 Drugs may be the most common cause of altered mental status. Sedatives, ethanol, tranquilizers, and all of the narcotics are frequent causes of altered mental status. Many other drugs, including tricyclic antidepressants, lithium, steroids, anticonvulsants, heavy metals, cardiac glycosides, cimetidine, salicylates, and amphetamines, have been implicated in decreased levels of consciousness. The random drug screens performed on blood and urine detect only a small percentage of those drugs that may cause an alteration in mental status. It is therefore important to obtain a complete drug history when possible in order to obtain specific drug levels not included in the routine screen. Numerous toxins, including certain pesticides, methanol, ethylene glycol, and cyanide, are also causes of altered mental status.

7 Many forms of vasculitides can affect the cerebral circulation. The most common occurs with systemic lupus erythematosus. Periarteritis nodosa, temporal arteritis, granulomatous vasculitis, drug-induced vasculitis, and isolated vasculitis of the central nervous system are among other forms of vasculitis that affect the central nervous system. The mechanism by which the altered mental status occurs is probably due to ischemia and inflammation with subsequent cerebral edema.

8 Deficiencies of thiamine (causing Wernicke's encephalopathy), niacin, pyridoxine, vitamin B_{12}, and folate are associated with altered mental status.

9 Certain severe psychiatric diseases can be virtually indistinguishable from stupor and coma. Catatonic states and severe hysterical conversion reactions may also mimic stupor and coma. Catatonia may be a manifestation of severe vegetative depression. Many patients with severe depression would now be diagnosed with paranoid schizophrenia.

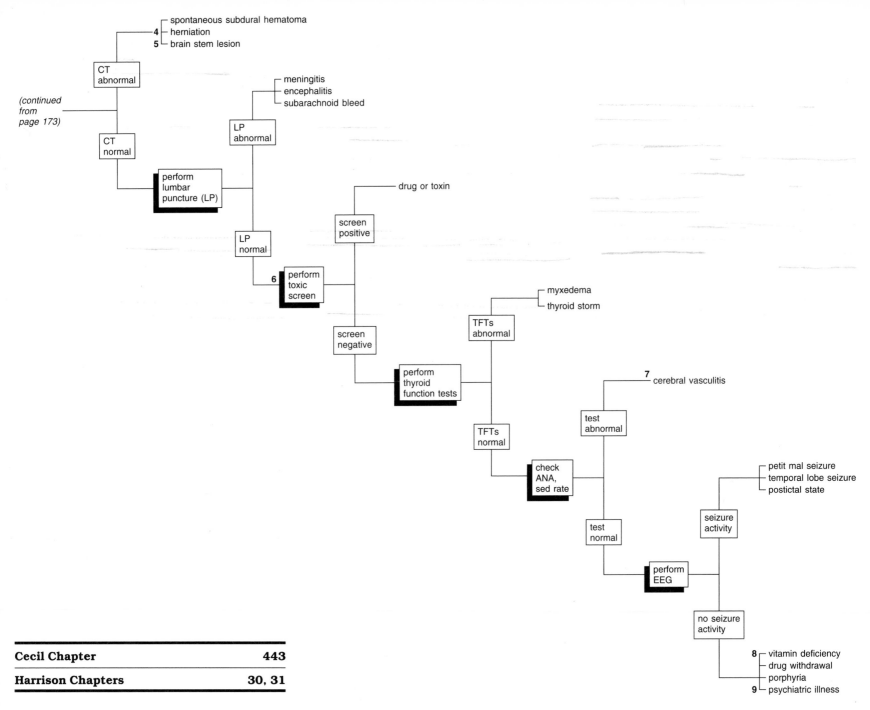

spontaneous subdural hematoma

4 herniation

5 brain stem lesion

CT abnormal

(continued from page 173)

CT normal

meningitis
encephalitis
subarachnoid bleed

LP abnormal

perform lumbar puncture (LP)

LP normal

drug or toxin

screen positive

6 perform toxic screen

screen negative

perform thyroid function tests

myxedema
thyroid storm

TFTs abnormal

TFTs normal

7 cerebral vasculitis

test abnormal

check ANA, sed rate

test normal

petit mal seizure
temporal lobe seizure
postictal state

seizure activity

perform EEG

no seizure activity

8 vitamin deficiency
drug withdrawal
porphyria
9 psychiatric illness

Cecil Chapter	443
Harrison Chapters	30, 31

Seizure

1 Seizures are more frequent than is commonly thought. Approximately 1 per cent of the population has an active seizure disorder, and as many as 10 per cent of the population will suffer at least one seizure in their lifetimes. Seizures may be classified by the area of the brain that is involved. Generalized seizures have no specific focus, whereas partial complex seizures may emanate from a local area of the brain. The specific area of brain involved, i.e., the temporal lobe, may determine the actual manifestation of the seizure. The etiology of any seizure is related to a lowered threshold for seizure, as seen in trauma, toxic reactions, sleep deprivation, stress, or anatomic abnormalities; to genetic traits leading to primary epilepsy; or to some combination of the two.

2 Seizures associated with hypertensive crisis are an extremely ominous sign. This complication is associated with markedly elevated diastolic pressures (usually greater than 140 mm Hg), as well as other manifestations of malignant hypertension. These manifestations may include papilledema, retinal hemorrhages, renal failure, and congestive heart failure. The onset of seizures may reflect a hypertensive stroke or an intracranial hemorrhage.

3 Hypocalcemic seizures are rare and occur when ionized calcium is less than 2.5 mg/100 ml. Causes of hypocalcemia of this severity include renal failure, acute panceatitis, hypoparathyroidism, severe hypomagnesemia, and vitamin D deficiency (see page 92).

4 Hypoglycemia is the most common cause of metabolically induced seizures. Up to 7 per cent of patients with symptomatic hypoglycemia will have at least one seizure episode. The seizures tend to be generalized rather than focal, and they usually occur when the blood glucose is less than 30 mg/dl. Hypoglycemic seizures occur more frequently with the use of insulin than with oral hypoglycemic agents. Generalized seizures may also occur in as many as 25 per cent of patients with nonketotic hyperglycemia. Seizures rarely occur in diabetic ketoacidosis.

5 Both hypo- and hypernatremia have been reported to cause seizures. Seizures appear to be more common with serum sodium below 115 mEq/L than with sodium levels above 160 mEq/L. The rapidity (less than 24 hours) with which either condition develops or the rapidity with which it is corrected may be more important in the causation of seizures than the actual sodium concentration is.

6 Seizures associated with cardiac events are related to cerebral hypoperfusion associated with low output states or arrhythmias. Although the resting electrocardiogram (EKG) may not reveal transient arrhythmias, certain findings associated with some of these arrhythmias may be evident. These include Wolff-Parkinson-White syndrome, abnormal QT intervals, and high-degree atrial ventricular blocks. A 24-hour Holter monitor study may be used when indicated to gain further information.

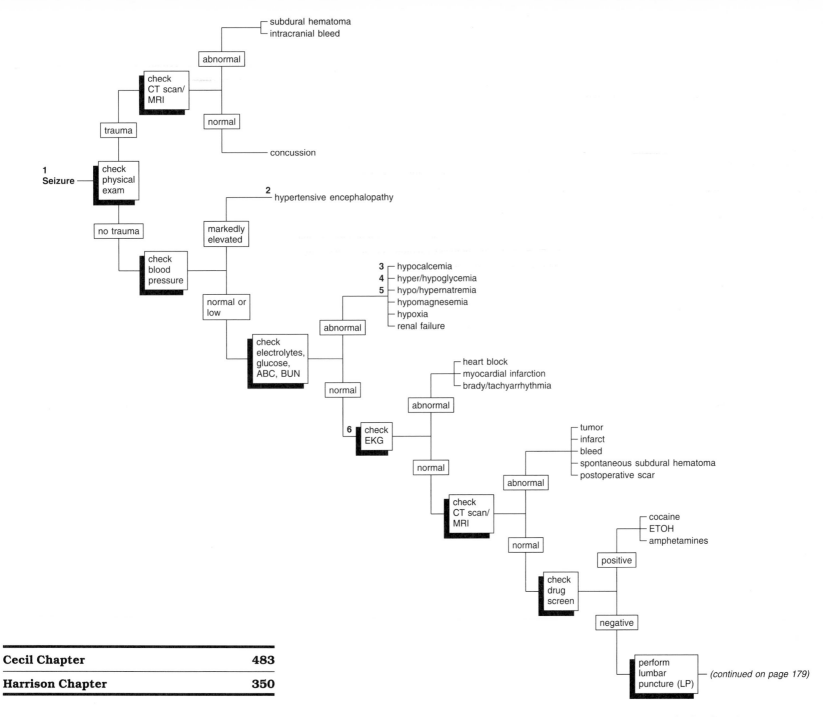

subdural hematoma
intracranial bleed

abnormal

check
CT scan/
MRI

normal

concussion

trauma

1
Seizure — check
physical
exam

2 hypertensive encephalopathy

markedly
elevated

no trauma

check
blood
pressure

3 hypocalcemia
4 hyper/hypoglycemia
5 hypo/hypernatremia
hypomagnesemia
hypoxia
renal failure

normal or
low

abnormal

check
electrolytes,
glucose,
ABC, BUN

heart block
myocardial infarction
brady/tachyarrhythmia

normal

abnormal

6 check
EKG

tumor
infarct
bleed
spontaneous subdural hematoma
postoperative scar

normal

abnormal

check
CT scan/
MRI

cocaine
ETOH
amphetamines

normal

positive

check
drug
screen

negative

perform
lumbar
puncture (LP) — *(continued on page 179)*

Seizure (Continued)

7 Epilepsy is a genetic seizure disorder without associated structural or metabolic abnormalities. Most of the epilepsies have their onset during childhood, but first seizures may occur at any time. Most of the epilepsies have a distinctive pattern on electroencephalogram (EEG) examination, including brief high-amplitude electrical discharges followed by a slower wave, referred to as a spike and wave pattern. Either focal or generalized seizures may be seen, and they involve not only motor abnormalities, but verbal, auditory, sensory, and autonomic phenomena as well.

8 Psychogenic seizures may be manifested in ways that have psychological significance to the patient. They should be suspected in any reported seizure that does not result in even minor injury to the patient, or when the seizure pattern does not fit any known anatomic pathways. Any bizarre behavior may be an epileptic event, so the diagnosis of psychogenic seizures may only be made when the symptoms fit those described above and no abnormalities are found on the EEG.

9 Idiopathic disorders may include seizure-like episodes and at times are distinguishable from true seizure disorders only by sophisticated testing. These disorders may include systemic disorders such as hyperventilation, intermittent porphyria, pheochromocytoma, or dystonic drug reactions. Other neurologic disorders such as dyskinesia and some forms of migraines may be difficult to distinguish from true seizure disorders.

BIBLIOGRAPHY

Cohen NL: The Dizzy Patient. Update in Otolaryngology I. Med Clin North Am 75(6), 1991.

Mahler ME, Cummings JL, Benson DF: Treatable dementias. West J Med 146:705–712, 1987.

Mondell BB: Evaluation of the Patient Presenting with Headache. Med Clin North Am 75(3), 1991.

Plum F, Posner JB: The Diagnosis of Stupor and Coma. 2nd ed. Philadelphia, F. A. Davis Company, 1972.

Taylor RB: Difficult Diagnosis. Philadelphia, W. B. Saunders Company, 1985.

Wyngaarden JB, Smith LH Jr (eds): Cecil Textbook of Medicine. 19th ed. Philadelphia, W. B. Saunders Company, 1991.

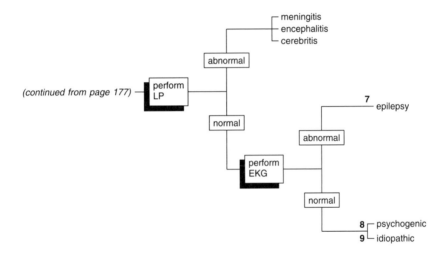

(continued from page 177)

perform
LP

abnormal

— meningitis
— encephalitis
— cerebritis

normal

perform
EKG

abnormal

7 epilepsy

normal

8 — psychogenic
9 — idiopathic

Cecil Chapter	**483**
Harrison Chapter	**350**

9 ▪ Endocrine Disorders

Signs and symptoms:	Labs:
Amenorrhea	Abnormal thyroid
Hirsutism	function tests
Thyroid nodule	Hyperlipidemia
Thyroid enlargement	Hypoglycemia

Amenorrhea

1 Amenorrhea is the absence of menses. Primary amenorrhea is the absence of menses in a phenotypic female by the age of 17. Secondary amenorrhea is the absence of menses for 4 months or more in a previously menstruating female. Oligomenorrhea refers to menstruation that is infrequent and irregular.

2 Pregnancy is the most common physiologic cause of amenorrhea. Despite the most forceful assertions of virginity, a pregnancy test should always be the first test performed in an investigation of secondary amenorrhea.

3 Trophoblastic growths include hydatidiform mole, invasive mole (chorioadenoma destruens), and chorio-carcinoma. These growths are accompanied by unusually high titers of human chorionic gonadotropin (HCG).

4 Once pregnancy has been excluded as a cause of amenorrhea, the serum prolactin level should be measured, particularly if amenorrhea is accompanied by galactorrhea. Hyperprolactinemia is a common cause of secondary amenorrhea, occurring in 15 to 40 per cent of women without galactorrhea and in 80 to 97 per cent of women with galactorrhea. Prolactin secretion can be induced by a variety of factors, including drugs, physical or psychological stress, and pituitary adenomas. The higher the serum prolactin levels, the more likely the presence of a pituitary adenoma. The presence of a pituitary adenoma is almost certain if the serum prolactin level is greater than 300 ng/ml.

5 Secondary amenorrhea can be the earliest manifestation of thyroid dysfunction. Thyroid functions tests (TFTs) should include measurement of free T_4

index and thyroid-stimulating hormone (TSH) to determine whether hypothyroidism is due to pituitary or thyroid dysfunction (see the Abnormal Thyroid Function Tests algorithm). With hypothyroidism owing to thyroid dysfunction, thyrotropin-releasing hormone (TRH) will be elevated and is responsible for a mild prolactinemia. Thyroid hormone replacement should return menstrual function and prolactin levels to normal. Serum prolactin level should be reassayed after thyroid replacement has been achieved. If the prolactin level remains elevated despite adequate thyroid hormone replacement, further investigation is in order (see No. 13).

6 Adequacy of endogenous estrogen production and ovulation can be evaluated by measuring estrogen levels or administering progesterone. The progesterone challenge is performed by administering 100 mg of progesterone in oil intramuscularly, or 10 mg of medroxyprogesterone acetate orally daily for 10 days. Withdrawal bleeding will occur 3 to 5 days after progesterone has been discontinued if endogenous estrogen levels are adequate to stimulate endometrial growth, and the amenorrhea is due to anovulation. If estrogen levels are low or withdrawal bleeding does not occur, the underlying problem is low endogenous estrogen production. Normal estrogen levels vary with the normal cycle phase but will be less than 10 μg/24 hr if endogenous estrogen production is low.

7 High estrogen levels in the setting of secondary amenorrhea may indicate the presence of ovarian or adrenal tumors autonomously secreting androgens or estrogens or both. Secretion of androgens such as androstenedione provides a substrate for peripheral conversion to estrogen. The high levels of androgen or estrogen result in amenorrhea because of the sustained negative feedback effect on the hypothalamic-pituitary control of the ovaries. Androgen produced by ovarian or adrenal tumors may be sufficient to allow peripheral production of estrogen but may not result in signs of virilization.

8 Polycystic ovary disease (PCO), also known as Stein-Leventhal syndrome, is a disorder in which the ovaries are enlarged, with numerous follicular cysts and thecal hyperplasia. High levels of androstenedione are produced by these ovaries. Levels of luteinizing hormone (LH) are increased, but follicle-stimulating hormone

(FSH) is normal or decreased. In addition to secondary amenorrhea, women with this disorder may also be hirsute (90 per cent), overweight (50 per cent), have acne (50 per cent), and show signs of virilization (<25 per cent). Prolactin levels may be mildly elevated in up to 30 per cent of patients with polycystic ovary disease.

9 If estrogen levels are normal but no withdrawal bleeding is observed with progesterone administration, the history becomes important to determine the presence of uterine anomalies responsible for outflow tract abnormalities. Asherman's syndrome is secondary amenorrhea owing to the destruction of the endometrium and the development of intrauterine synechiae. The most common cause of Asherman's syndrome is uterine curettage, which may occur during the course of a therapeutic abortion. Infection is another cause of intrauterine scarring and synechiae formation.

10 Ovarian failure results in low estrogen levels. The etiology of the ovarian failure can be determined by measuring the hypothalamic hormones FSH and LH. Normal levels of FSH and LH vary with the menstrual cycle, but postmenopausal values provide the basis for comparison in amenorrhea. Postmenopausal serum FSH values are 20 to 110 mIU/ml per 24 hr, and serum LH values are 20 to 80 mIU/ml per 24 hr (where mIU/ml = milli-International Units per milliliter). Elevated levels of FSH and LH indicate that ovarian failure is primary. A karyotype should be performed on any woman with primary ovarian failure to rule out a sex chromosome abnormality, especially if ovarian failure occurs before the age of 35. Accelerated follicular atresia with subsequent ovarian failure can occur in patients with Turner's syndrome (XO chromosome abnormality). Thirty per cent of women with the presence of a Y chromosome may be phenotypically female without any signs of virilization. The possibility of malignancy is high in patients with the Y chromosome, so that all gonadal tissue must be removed. Buccal smears are an inadequate means of evaluating karyotype owing to the presence of mosaicism in this tissue.

11 Premature ovarian failure may be due to premature menopause, Savage syndrome (insensitive ovaries), or follicular atresia owing to toxic exposure such as radiation, chemotherapy, or infection. Surgery and au-

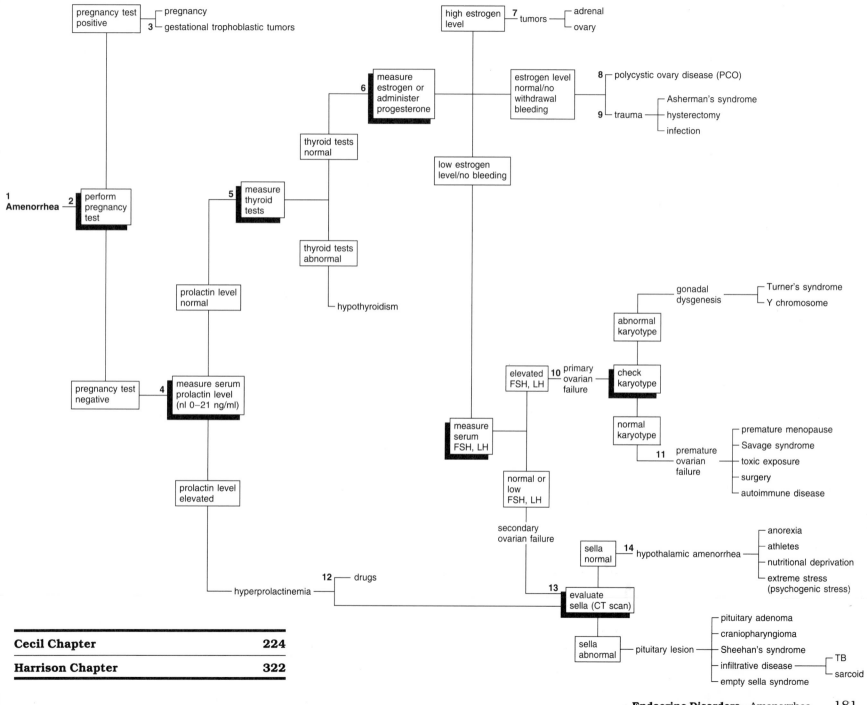

1 Amenorrhea

2 perform pregnancy test

pregnancy test positive — **3** ┌ pregnancy
└ gestational trophoblastic tumors

pregnancy test negative — **4** measure serum prolactin level (nl 0–21 ng/ml)

prolactin level normal — **5** measure thyroid tests

prolactin level elevated — hyperprolactinemia — **12** drugs

thyroid tests normal — **6** measure estrogen or administer progesterone

thyroid tests abnormal — hypothyroidism

high estrogen level — **7** tumors ┌ adrenal
└ ovary

estrogen level normal/no withdrawal bleeding — ┌ **8** polycystic ovary disease (PCO)
└ **9** trauma ┌ Asherman's syndrome
├ hysterectomy
└ infection

low estrogen level/no bleeding — measure serum FSH, LH

elevated FSH, LH — **10** primary ovarian failure — check karyotype

abnormal karyotype — gonadal dysgenesis ┌ Turner's syndrome
└ Y chromosome

normal karyotype — **11** premature ovarian failure ┌ premature menopause
├ Savage syndrome
├ toxic exposure
├ surgery
└ autoimmune disease

normal or low FSH, LH — secondary ovarian failure — **13** evaluate sella (CT scan)

sella normal — **14** hypothalamic amenorrhea ┌ anorexia
├ athletes
├ nutritional deprivation
└ extreme stress (psychogenic stress)

sella abnormal — pituitary lesion ┌ pituitary adenoma
├ craniopharyngioma
├ Sheehan's syndrome
├ infiltrative disease ┌ TB
│   └ sarcoid
└ empty sella syndrome

Cecil Chapter	**224**
Harrison Chapter	**322**

Endocrine Disorders—Amenorrhea   181

Amenorrhea *(Continued)*

toimmune disease may also cause follicular depletion and ovarian failure.

12 Oral contraceptives, progestogens, synthetic estrogens, and TRH may directly stimulate pituitary lactotrophs and cause hyperprolactinemia. Other drugs induce hyperprolactinemia by decreasing dopamine synthesis, which in turn decreases prolactin inhibition. Examples include tricyclic antidepressants, opiates, anorexiants, monoamine oxidase inhibitors, phenothiazines, and thioxanthenes. Prolactin levels usually are no greater than 100 ng/ml when hyperprolactinemia is drug-induced.

13 Pituitary adenomas are a common cause of hyperprolactinemia (see No. 4), and the sella must always be evaluated when prolactin levels are increased. In addition, in women with secondary ovarian failure (i.e., hypothalamic-pituitary dysfunction), the sella must also be evaluated to rule out a pituitary lesion. Evaluation of the sella is most easily accomplished by computed tomography (CT) or magnetic resonance imaging (MRI).

14 Hypothalamic amenorrhea can result from a variety of stresses. Amenorrhea has been well documented in runners and ballet dancers, as well as in patients with anorexia nervosa and nutritional deprivation. Any stress, including surgical or physical trauma, as well as emotional and psychological stress, can result in amenorrhea. Serum prolactin levels are usually elevated with stress as well.

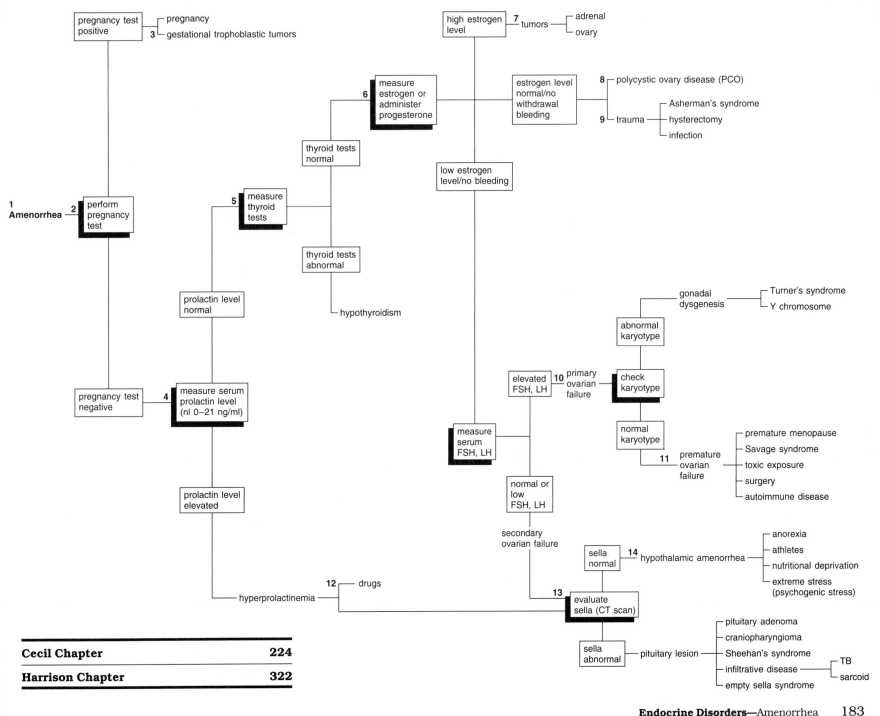

pregnancy test positive
— pregnancy
3 — gestational trophoblastic tumors

high estrogen level
7 tumors
— adrenal
— ovary

6 measure estrogen or administer progesterone

estrogen level normal/no withdrawal bleeding
8 — polycystic ovary disease (PCO)
9 — trauma
— Asherman's syndrome
— hysterectomy
— infection

thyroid tests normal

1 Amenorrhea — **2** perform pregnancy test

5 measure thyroid tests

low estrogen level/no bleeding

thyroid tests abnormal

— hypothyroidism

prolactin level normal

gonadal dysgenesis
— Turner's syndrome
— Y chromosome

abnormal karyotype

pregnancy test negative
4 measure serum prolactin level (nl 0–21 ng/ml)

elevated FSH, LH
10 primary ovarian failure

check karyotype

measure serum FSH, LH

normal karyotype
11 premature ovarian failure
— premature menopause
— Savage syndrome
— toxic exposure
— surgery
— autoimmune disease

prolactin level elevated

normal or low FSH, LH

secondary ovarian failure

sella normal
14 hypothalamic amenorrhea
— anorexia
— athletes
— nutritional deprivation
— extreme stress (psychogenic stress)

12 — drugs

13 evaluate sella (CT scan)

— hyperprolactinemia

sella abnormal — pituitary lesion
— pituitary adenoma
— craniopharyngioma
— Sheehan's syndrome
— infiltrative disease
— empty sella syndrome
— TB
— sarcoid

Cecil Chapter	224
Harrison Chapter	322

Hirsutism

1 Hirsutism is defined as terminal hair growth occurring on the body and face of a woman in a pattern that is typical of the hair growth in men. It is important to know the normal distribution of terminal hair growth in women, because terminal hair on the upper back, shoulders, upper abdomen, and sternum is distinctly abnormal, whereas terminal hair on the lower abdomen, around the areolae, and even on the face may be normal. In addition, the division between normal and abnormal hair growth in a woman is not exact, because there are major variations in the normal pattern owing to racial variations. Therefore, family history and appearance of family members is very important in the overall evaluation of a patient with hirsutism. A family history of hirsutism does not rule out an endocrine cause of abnormal hair growth, however. An evaluation should be performed even in these patients, because familial or idiopathic hirsutism is a diagnosis of exclusion. Androgens are responsible for terminal hair growth in sex hormone–responsive hair follicles. In women, the adrenal glands and the ovaries are equally responsible for androgen production. The adrenal androgens (dehydroepiandrosterone [DHEA], DHEA-sulfate, and androstenedione) do not produce an androgenic effect on the hair follicles directly but do so by peripheral conversion to testosterone and its metabolites (e.g., dihydrotestosterone, or DHT). Testosterone and androstenedione are secreted by the ovary. Androstenedione from the ovary, as from the adrenals, must be converted to testosterone to exert an androgenic effect.

2 The most important hormonal measurement in the evaluation of hirsutism is the free serum testosterone level. The bound fraction of testosterone is biologically inactive so that, although the total measured level of testosterone may be elevated, no conclusions can be made relative to hirsutism if the unbound portion is not measured. If the measurement of free testosterone is not readily available, the ratio of testosterone to sex hormone–binding globulin can identify an abnormality in hirsute women. A majority of hirsute women can be demonstrated to have an increased level of serum testosterone. Measurement of DHEA-sulfate can be done simultaneously but is a nonspecific test in the evaluation of hirsutism (see No. 5).

3 Exogenously administered androgenic agents are a common cause of hirsutism. Women athletes may be reluctant to reveal the use of anabolic steroids.

4 Cushing's disease results from hypersecretion of adrenocorticotrophic hormone (ACTH). Clinical features include diabetes, amenorrhea, hypertension, centripetal obesity, hirsutism, and acne. Cushing first described the disorder secondary to basophilic adenoma of the pituitary, but any ACTH-secreting tumor can produce this disease. ACTH can be produced ectopically by a number of tumors, including small-cell lung carcinomas, pancreatic islet cell tumors, and carcinoid tumors. In patients with Cushing's disease, only about 50 per cent have elevated plasma cortisol levels. Therefore, the 24-hour urinary free cortisol is the most reliable test to identify adrenal hyperactivity.

5 Although the measurement of DHEA and DHEA-sulfate is often recommended as a screening test for the detection of an adrenal carcinoma, the best test for detection of an adrenal tumor is an abdominal CT scan. Extremely high levels of these hormones may be present with adrenal tumors, but the levels of these hormones may be elevated in a variety of other disorders, including Cushing's disease, polycystic ovary disease, ovarian tumors, and idiopathic hirsutism. Similarly, a pelvic examination and pelvic ultrasound are the most sensitive measures to identify an ovarian neoplasm.

6 Both benign and malignant adrenal neoplasms can produce androgens and cause hirsutism. Adrenal carcinomas, however, are usually inefficient in their production of steroid hormones and can grow to large size before they produce enough androgen to cause hirsutism.

7 Ovarian tumors are uncommon causes of androgen production resulting in hirsutism. Sertoli-Leydig cell tumors account for half of all ovarian virilizing tumors but make up less than 0.2 per cent of all ovarian tumors. Most ovarian tumors resulting in hirsutism are benign and well differentiated. Most granulosa-stromal cell tumors are feminizing and rarely cause hirsutism.

8 Congenital adrenal hyperplasia (CAH) is associated with hirsutism because androgen overproduction is the result of the overactivity of the adrenals necessary to maintain normal cortisol secretion. The virilizing forms of CAH are caused by either 21-hydroxylase deficiency, 11-hydroxylase deficiency, or 3-beta-hydroxysteroid dehydrogenase deficiency. The most common cause of CAH is the 21-hydroxylase deficiency, but its incidence is estimated to be only 1 to 10 per cent among women with hirsutism. 21-Hydroxylase deficiency is inherited as an autosomal recessive trait and may present as PCO. The best way to diagnose any of these enzyme deficiencies is to perform an ACTH stimulation test and measure the steroid precursor just prior to the enzyme defect in the adrenal steroidogenic pathway.

9 Increased prolactin secretion is often associated with increased levels of DHEA and DHEA-sulfate. Prolactin has been found to augment the ACTH-induced secretion of these two hormones by the adrenals and is therefore thought to have a direct effect on the adrenal glands. The increased levels of these preandrogens are responsible for the associated hirsutism.

10 Hyperprolactinemia is the most common manifestation of pituitary hyperfunction. In addition to prolactin-secreting adenomas, causes of nonphysiologic hyperprolactinemia include pharmacologic agents such as Aldomet (alpha-methyldopa), reserpine, phenothiazines, estrogens, and narcotics. Inflammatory or infiltrative diseases, such as sarcoidosis and histiocytosis, hypothyroidism, renal failure, and hepatic cirrhosis, as well as idiopathic hyperprolactinemia, may cause elevated prolactin levels. The sella must always be evaluated when prolactin levels are increased.

11 PCO is a diagnosis of exclusion. PCO accounts for 30 per cent of all the diagnoses of hirsutism and is the leading cause of hirsutism in women. The clinical features of this disorder include hirsutism (>90 per cent), obesity (50 per cent), virilization (<25 per cent), and acne (<50 per cent). The etiology of PCO is poorly understood and has been associated with insulin resistance and hyperinsulinemia. In addition, mild elevations of prolactin levels have been found in up to 30 per cent of patients with PCO, which may explain, in part, the increased androgen levels in these women. PCO is diagnosed on the basis of the constellation of clinical findings, which include the aforementioned symptoms, as well as menstrual irregularity, elevated gonadotropin (LH/FSH) levels, and polycystic ovaries detected by pelvic ultrasound examination.

12 Hirsutism for which no abnormality is found can be diagnosed as idiopathic hirsutism. Idiopathic hirsutism accounts for only 10 per cent of all hirsutism and is a diagnosis of exclusion. These patients have excessive male-pattern hair growth, which can be mild or diffuse and severe; normal menstrual cycles; and normal serum testosterone. Because it is the local conversion of androgens to DHT by 5-alpha-reductase that is responsi-

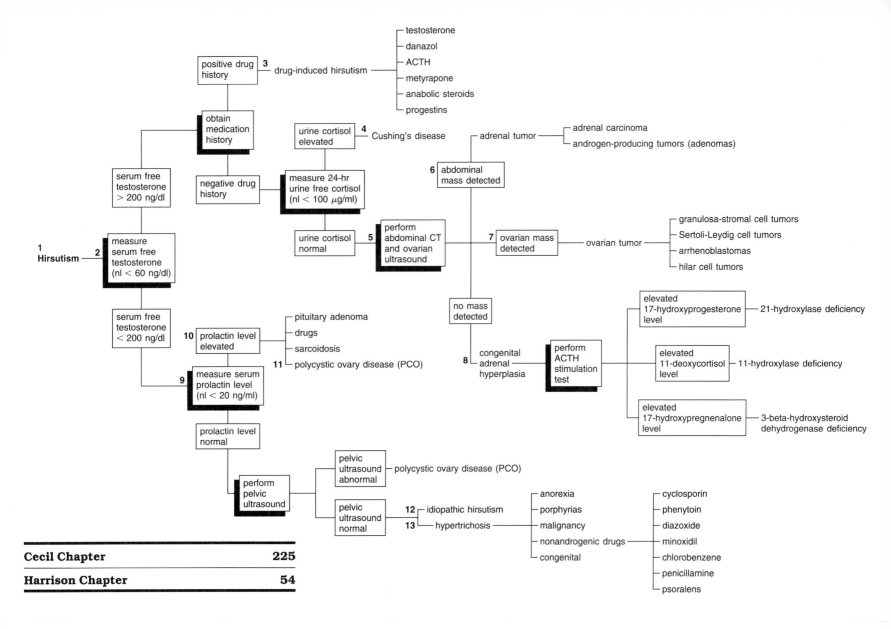

1 Hirsutism

2 measure serum free testosterone (nl < 60 ng/dl)

serum free testosterone > 200 ng/dl → obtain medication history

positive drug history → **3** drug-induced hirsutism
- testosterone
- danazol
- ACTH
- metyrapone
- anabolic steroids
- progestins

negative drug history → measure 24-hr urine free cortisol (nl < 100 μg/ml)

urine cortisol elevated → **4** Cushing's disease

urine cortisol normal → **5** perform abdominal CT and ovarian ultrasound

6 abdominal mass detected → adrenal tumor
- adrenal carcinoma
- androgen-producing tumors (adenomas)

7 ovarian mass detected → ovarian tumor
- granulosa-stromal cell tumors
- Sertoli-Leydig cell tumors
- arrhenoblastomas
- hilar cell tumors

no mass detected → **8** congenital adrenal hyperplasia → perform ACTH stimulation test

elevated 17-hydroxyprogesterone level → 21-hydroxylase deficiency

elevated 11-deoxycortisol level → 11-hydroxylase deficiency

elevated 17-hydroxypregnenalone level → 3-beta-hydroxysteroid dehydrogenase deficiency

serum free testosterone < 200 ng/dl → **9** measure serum prolactin level (nl < 20 ng/ml)

10 prolactin level elevated
- pituitary adenoma
- drugs
- sarcoidosis
- **11** polycystic ovary disease (PCO)

prolactin level normal → perform pelvic ultrasound

pelvic ultrasound abnormal → polycystic ovary disease (PCO)

pelvic ultrasound normal → **12** idiopathic hirsutism

13 hypertrichosis
- anorexia
- porphyrias
- malignancy
- nonandrogenic drugs
  - cyclosporin
  - phenytoin
  - diazoxide
  - minoxidil
  - chlorobenzene
  - penicillamine
  - psoralens
- congenital

ble for the end-organ response (hair growth) to androgens, it has been hypothesized that the hirsutism in these patients may be due to an increase in 5-alpha-reductase activity in the skin.

13 Hirsutism must be differentiated from hypertrichosis, in which there is an increase in the non-androgen-dependent, nonsexual hair of the body. Hypertrichosis can be localized or generalized and typically is more vellus than terminal hair growth. Nonandrogenic drugs, the porphyrias, a variety of congenital syndromes (including the fetal alcohol syndrome), and malignant tumors can be associated with diffuse hair growth.

Thyroid Nodule

1 Although most solitary thyroid nodules are benign, the discovery of a thyroid nodule requires investigation to rule out the possibility of malignancy. In addition, even if a thyroid nodule is identified to be a benign lesion, its function and growth are important to identify and follow. A hyperfunctioning autonomous benign nodule may lead to thyrotoxicosis. Thyroid nodules occur in 1 to 5 per cent of the adult population, and are four times more common in women than in men. The incidence of single thyroid nodules that are malignant is estimated to be between 0.1 and 0.2 per cent.

2 Although many tests have been proposed for the initial evaluation of a thyroid nodule, a needle aspiration biopsy is the most informative and cost-effective initial test if it is performed by an experienced operator. Needle aspiration biopsy is indicated, because open biopsy of the thyroid presents unnecessary risks to important neck structures, especially because most solitary nodules are benign. Many other "first tests" have been suggested to rule out thyroid carcinoma, including thyroid function tests (carcinomas are usually poorly functioning, so thyroid function tests are usually normal), radioiodine thyroid scan (most thyroid nodules are "cold" on scan), and ultrasonography (cystic lesions are less likely cancerous). All of these tests are nonspecific, however, because hyperfunctioning lesions ("hot" nodules) can be cancerous, "cold" nodules are often benign, and cystic lesions may occasionally be cancerous. All of these tests can add information in the evaluation of thyroid nodules but are of limited usefulness because they do not accurately differentiate between benign and malignant lesions.

3 Needle aspiration biopsy is most useful if cytology is interpreted as definitely benign or definitely malignant, which can be done for 60 to 80 per cent of the patients. In the other 20 to 40 per cent, however, cytology is not as clear, and approximately one fourth of patients with thyroid nodule aspirates of unclear cytology will ultimately be found to have thyroid malignancy. A suspicious aspirate should therefore be considered a positive result and be followed by open biopsy of the thyroid. Papillary carcinoma of the thyroid is the most common type of thyroid carcinoma and carries the best prognosis. Approximately 50 to 60 per cent of thyroid carcinomas are papillary or mixed papillary-follicular carcinoma. An-

other 25 per cent of malignant thyroid nodules are follicular carcinoma. Needle aspiration biopsy may not always distinguish between a benign follicular adenoma and follicular carcinoma. Because these lesions can be well differentiated, only the presence of capsular and vascular invasion will indicate that the lesion is malignant and is found on open biopsy. Undifferentiated carcinoma accounts for 15 per cent and medullary carcinoma for 5 per cent of thyroid carcinomas. Metastatic carcinoma to the thyroid is rare, as is lymphoma involving the thyroid, but they can also be identified by needle aspiration biopsy.

4 If the needle aspiration biopsy is inadequate or equivocal, benign disease is a diagnosis of exclusion (see No. 3). Sampling error can occur, especially when the nodule is large. Numerous samples from various areas of a large nodule must be performed before a nodule can be considered benign. Risk factors that would direct the clinician toward surgical intervention with an equivocal needle aspiration cytology, include any history of prior head and neck irradiation (e.g., acne, thymic enlargement, tonsillar enlargement), male sex (malignant nodule is twice as likely in men than in women), age under 20 or over 60, family history (medullary carcinoma), palpable lymph nodes, or a hard, fixed nodule on palpation. Patients with risk factors for thyroid carcinoma should undergo surgical removal and histologic diagnosis of the nodule, rather than simply periodic follow-up examinations.

5 In patients with negative needle aspiration results and no risk factors for thyroid carcinoma, imaging techniques may be helpful in evaluating the thyroid nodule. If a radioiodine scan is performed, a nonfunctioning or cold nodule is more likely carcinoma (thyroid carcinoma is not very efficient at trapping iodine and synthesizing thyroid hormone), whereas a functioning or hot nodule is less likely to be carcinoma. Likewise, with ultrasonography, a cystic nodule is less likely to be carcinoma, although cystic degeneration can occur in any mass, including carcinoma. Because imaging techniques are poor predictors of malignancy, close clinical observation and repeat needle aspiration biopsy are necessary until a definite diagnosis is made.

6 If thyroid scan reveals a cold nodule, needle aspiration biopsy is negative, and risk factors for thyroid carcinoma are absent, a repeat needle aspiration

biopsy is indicated prior to open biopsy. If a second aspiration biopsy is negative, then suppression of the nodule should be undertaken by administering thyroid hormone. If the nodule increases in size despite suppression, open biopsy is indicated.

7 A warm nodule is a nodule that functions the same as the surrounding thyroid tissue. A hot nodule is a hyperfunctioning nodule. Most functioning nodules are benign. Both hot and warm nodules can be followed clinically without treatment if the patient remains asymptomatic. Functional suppression of the nodule can be attempted by administering thyroid hormone. If the nodule increases in size despite suppression, or the patient remains hyperthyroid, treatment is indicated.

8 Most solitary thyroid nodules are benign adenomas. Ninety to 95 per cent of thyroid adenomas are nonfunctioning and exist as asymptomatic neck masses. With growth, these lesions may rarely cause problems secondary to compression of other neck structures. Functioning follicular adenomas usually do not cause hyperthyroidism unless they are greater than 3 cm in diameter.

9 A colloid nodule is a mixed cystic-solid area that results from cycles of hyperplasia followed by involution of a thyroid lobule. The nodule may contain areas of necrosis, fibrosis, and hemorrhage, but it mainly consists of large colloid-filled follicles lined by typical cuboidal epithelium. A colloid nodule can form clusters leading to a multinodular goiter.

10 Owing to its anatomic location, a parathyroid adenoma can present as an apparent "thyroid" mass. Parathyroid adenomas presenting as neck masses are extremely rare.

11 Multinodular goiters may contain hyperfunctioning and hypofunctioning areas, visible as hot and cold nodules on thyroid scan. If risk factors for thyroid carcinoma are present (see No. 4), surgical intervention is necessary. If a single cold nodule continues to enlarge despite absence of risk factors, needle biopsy of that nodule may be adequate to determine the presence or absence of malignancy.

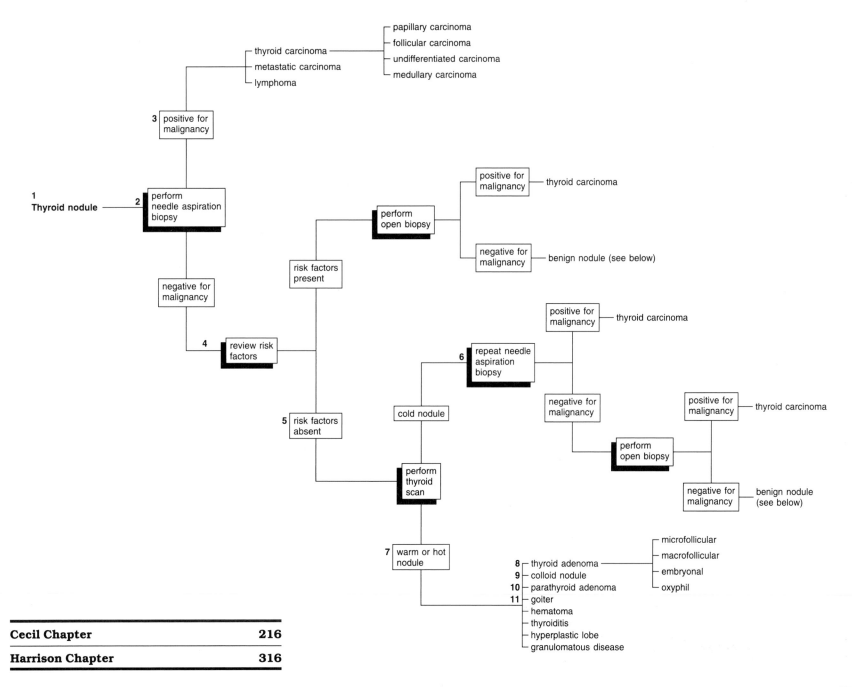

1

Thyroid nodule

2 perform needle aspiration biopsy

3 positive for malignancy

thyroid carcinoma ──┬── papillary carcinoma
├── follicular carcinoma
├── undifferentiated carcinoma
└── medullary carcinoma

metastatic carcinoma

lymphoma

negative for malignancy

4 review risk factors

risk factors present

perform open biopsy ──┬── positive for malignancy ── thyroid carcinoma
└── negative for malignancy ── benign nodule (see below)

5 risk factors absent

perform thyroid scan

cold nodule

repeat needle aspiration biopsy 6 ──┬── positive for malignancy ── thyroid carcinoma
└── negative for malignancy

perform open biopsy ──┬── positive for malignancy ── thyroid carcinoma
└── negative for malignancy ── benign nodule (see below)

7 warm or hot nodule

8 ├ thyroid adenoma ──┬── microfollicular
├── macrofollicular
├── embryonal
└── oxyphil

9 ├ colloid nodule
10 ├ parathyroid adenoma
11 ├ goiter
├ hematoma
├ thyroiditis
├ hyperplastic lobe
└ granulomatous disease

Cecil Chapter	**216**
Harrison Chapter	**316**

Thyroid Enlargement

1 An enlarged thyroid can be diffusely enlarged (goiter), multinodular (multinodular goiter), or partially enlarged (single thyroid nodule). Enlargement of the thyroid suggests nothing about the thyroid's function, because an enlarged thyroid can be hyperfunctioning (hyperthyroid), normal functioning (euthyroid), or hypofunctioning (hypothyroid). The evaluation of an enlarged thyroid is undertaken principally to determine the thyroid function and metabolic status and to evaluate for the presence or absence of malignancy.

2 Lithium ingestion may cause thyroid enlargement but is most often associated with hypothyroidism. Thyroid hormone replacement can cause iatrogenic hyperthyroidism if the replacement dose is too high. Thyroid hormone is often ingested by patients (usually women) as a method of weight control. Many times, thyroid hormone is ingested surreptitiously, and any history of exogenous thyroid ingestion is denied.

3 Thyroid function tests, along with the history and physical examination, are very useful clues to the diagnosis of an enlarged thyroid. Despite thyroid gland enlargement, however, most of these thyroid diseases may be accompanied by varying degrees of hyper-, hypo-, and euthyroid states at various times during the course of the disease. Hashimoto's thyroiditis, for example, often presents as hyperthyroidism but ultimately results in hypothyroidism. Hashimoto's autoimmune thyroiditis is the most common cause of hypothyroidism. Thyroid function can be determined by measuring TSH and the free T_4 index and free T_3 index (referred to in the algorithm as "indices"). The combination of these measurements can help to determine the source of the thyroid gland dysfunction. (See page 190.)

4 Thyroid carcinoma is a rare cause of hyperthyroidism. Most thyroid carcinomas are nonfunctioning so that the patient is euthyroid despite thyroid enlargement. Thyroid enlargement, therefore, is more often due to tumor infiltration and growth than to hyperfunctioning thyroid tissue.

5 Acute thyroiditis is rare. The condition is due to bacterial infection of the thyroid gland, and thyroid function tests are usually normal. Clinical symptoms include an enlarged, tender thyroid and fever.

6 Graves' disease (diffuse toxic goiter) is the most common cause of goiter and hyperthyroidism. It is an autoimmune disease in which a serum immunoglobulin (antibody) acts to stimulate thyroid function. Clinical features of Graves' disease (also known as Basedow's disease in Europe) include symptoms of hyperthyroidism, a diffusely enlarged thyroid gland (goiter), exophthalmos with symptoms of burning, itching, and tearing, and pretibeal dermopathy.

7 Rarely, trophoblastic tumors can stimulate thyroid gland hypertrophy and hyperfunction via secretion of large amounts of HCG. HCG has some biologic cross-reactivity with TSH and can stimulate the thyroid gland directly.

8 The jodbasedow phenomenon refers to hyperthyroidism induced by iodine supplementation. Most cases of this phenomenon are patients with underlying Graves' disease who are given iodine in sufficient amounts to provide substrate for the diseased gland's overproduction of thyroid hormone.

9 Subacute granulomatous thyroiditis (de Quervain's thyroiditis) presents as a painful thyroid enlargement, often with systemic symptoms of fever, malaise, and chills. It occurs more commonly in women (3:1), usually in their third to fifth decades of life. Although the etiology is unknown, the condition usually follows a viral infection by several weeks. Histologically, the thyroid gland is infiltrated with lymphocytes, neutrophils, and multinucleate giant cells characteristic of granulomata.

10 Subacute lymphocytic thyroiditis, in contrast to de Quervain's disease, is a painless thyroiditis with hyperthyroidism, thyroid gland enlargement, and histologic lymphocytic infiltration of the thyroid gland. The etiology of the disorder is unknown but is thought to be an autoimmune mechanism. The features of subacute lymphocytic thyroiditis are similar to early Hashimoto's disease and to Graves' disease. Subacute lymphocytic thyroiditis can be differentiated from Graves' disease on the basis of the low radioactive iodine uptake, and from Hashimoto's disease by a low antimicrosomal antibody titer (see No. 11).

11 Hashimoto's thyroiditis, also known as chronic lymphocytic thyroiditis, is an autoimmune disease of the thyroid gland. Hashimoto's disease is the most common thyroid disorder in the United States. It most often presents with a painless palpable goiter, usually initially euthyroid but ultimately almost always hypothyroid. In 5 to 10 per cent of patients, Hashimoto's disease presents with hyperthyroidism, which must be distinguished from Graves' disease. Most often the serum free T_4 index is low and the TSH is elevated, but the diagnosis is based on the demonstration of circulating antimicrosomal antibodies, which are present in approximately 95 per cent of the patients with the disease. Approximately 50 to 60 per cent of patients also have circulating antithyroglobulin antibodies in their serum as well. Radioactive iodine uptake may be normal, low, or increased in Hashimoto's thyroiditis.

12 Riedel's thyroiditis is a rare disorder of unknown etiology in which the thyroid gland is gradually infiltrated by a sclerosing fibrous infiltration, ultimately resulting in hypothyroidism and a firm, enlarged gland.

13 Endemic goiter refers to thyroid enlargement found in a large fraction of the population, usually caused by environmental influences. Most commonly a result of iodine deficiency, the disorder is now very rare in the United States owing to the iodinization of salt. The thyroid enlargement is due to hypersecretion of TSH, which occurs in response to a decreased production of thyroid hormone, especially T_4.

14 Sporadic goiter is presumed to be due to an enzymatic defect in one of the steps of thyroid hormone production, leading to low thyroid hormone levels and elevated levels of serum TSH.

15 Pituitary adenoma may secrete TSH autonomously without sensitivity to negative feedback regulation.

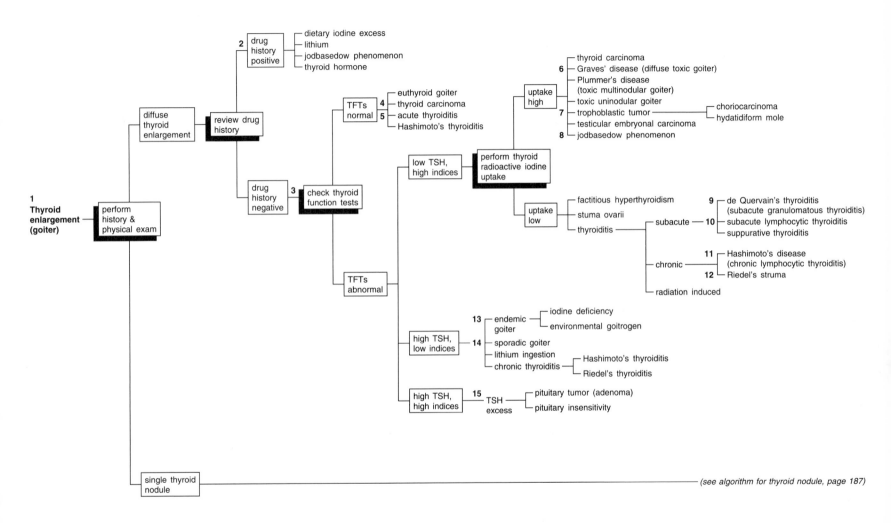

1
Thyroid enlargement (goiter) — perform history & physical exam

- diffuse thyroid enlargement — review drug history
  - **2** drug history positive
    - dietary iodine excess
    - lithium
    - jodbasedow phenomenon
    - thyroid hormone
  - drug history negative — **3** check thyroid function tests
    - TFTs normal
      - euthyroid goiter
      - **4** thyroid carcinoma
      - **5** acute thyroiditis
      - Hashimoto's thyroiditis
    - TFTs abnormal
      - low TSH, high indices — perform thyroid radioactive iodine uptake
        - uptake high
          - thyroid carcinoma
          - **6** Graves' disease (diffuse toxic goiter)
          - Plummer's disease (toxic multinodular goiter)
          - toxic uninodular goiter
          - **7** trophoblastic tumor
            - choriocarcinoma
            - hydatidiform mole
          - testicular embryonal carcinoma
          - **8** jodbasedow phenomenon
        - uptake low
          - factitious hyperthyroidism
          - stuma ovarii
          - thyroiditis
            - subacute — **10**
              - **9** de Quervain's thyroiditis (subacute granulomatous thyroiditis)
              - subacute lymphocytic thyroiditis
              - suppurative thyroiditis
            - chronic
              - **11** Hashimoto's disease (chronic lymphocytic thyroiditis)
              - **12** Riedel's struma
            - radiation induced
      - high TSH, low indices
        - **13** endemic goiter
          - iodine deficiency
          - environmental goitrogen
        - **14** sporadic goiter
        - lithium ingestion
        - chronic thyroiditis
          - Hashimoto's thyroiditis
          - Riedel's thyroiditis
      - high TSH, high indices — **15** TSH excess
        - pituitary tumor (adenoma)
        - pituitary insensitivity
- single thyroid nodule ——— *(see algorithm for thyroid nodule, page 187)*

Cecil Chapter	**216**
Harrison Chapter	**316**

Abnormal Thyroid Function Tests

1 Thyroid function may be assessed as part of a routine chemistry panel even in the absence of any clinical signs of thyroid abnormality. Thyroid dysfunction can be difficult to recognize clinically when the disorder is early or mild or when the patient is elderly. The prevalence of clinically inapparent thyroid disorders in elderly women makes this subgroup a population in which thyroid testing is an important adjunct to the history and physical examination. A free T_4 index (FT_4I) is the most commonly used means for screening for thyroid abnormalities. The index is a measurement that takes into account the amount of thyroxine-binding globulin (TBG) and the number of binding sites on TBG available to bind thyroxine. The index corrects for falsely elevated levels of measured T_4 seen in conditions with increased TBG, such as pregnancy or estrogen administration, and falsely low levels of T_4 with decreased levels of TBG as occurs in cirrhosis of the liver. In 5 per cent of cases with hyperthyroidism, the T_4 level is within the reference range and only the T_3 level is elevated. This condition is known as T_3-toxicosis and can be confirmed by measuring the total T_3 level. T_3-toxicosis can represent mild or early hyperthyroidism and can occur with any cause of hyperthyroidism.

2 An elevated FT_4I indicates possible hyperthyroidism, but hyperthyroidism must then be confirmed by measuring the free T_3 index (FT_3I). Hyperthyroidism is confirmed if both the FT_4I and the FT_3I are elevated.

3 Measuring the TSH level helps to establish the source of hyperthyroidism. If hyperthyroidism is primary (owing to primary thyroid gland dysfunction), the TSH level will be low. An ultrasensitive TSH assay is now available in some laboratories. The accuracy of this test is so great that it may preclude the use of a TRH stimulation test (see Nos. 11 and 12). In fact, if available, a third-generation TSH immunoradiometric assay is the best test of thyroid function (to detect both hyper- and hypothyroidism) in any patient suspected of having thyroid disease.

4 Thyroid carcinoma is a rare cause of hyperthyroidism, because thyroid carcinoma makes thyroid hormone inefficiently. Occasionally a large, well-differentiated thyroid carcinoma can make sufficient thyroid hormone to result in clinically apparent hyperthyroidism.

5 The most common cause of hyperthyroidism is Graves' disease. The disease is apparently due to the presence in the circulation of abnormal thyroid-stimulating globulins.

6 Toxic multinodular goiter is a cause of hyperthyroidism, usually occurring in an elderly patient with a long history of goiter. The onset of hyperthyroidism is gradual and is due to growth of nodules within the goiter. Some of these nodules may eventually become autonomous in their secretion of thyroid hormone.

7 HCG has a slight biologic cross-reactivity with TSH. Rarely, trophoblastic tumors such as hydatidiform mole and choriocarcinoma, as well as embryonal carcinoma of the testis, can secrete HCG in large enough quantities to result in hyperthyroidism.

8 Thyroiditis may result in the release of excessive amounts of thyroid hormone and cause hyperthyroidism. Examples include inflammation following treatment with irradiation or ^{131}I therapy, and chronic lymphocytic thyroiditis.

9 Thyroid hormone replacement therapy of hypothyroidism can result in iatrogenic hyperthyroidism if the replacement dose is too high. When hyperthyroidism is due to surreptitious ingestion of thyroid hormone, serum thyroglobulin levels and radioactive iodine uptake will be low.

10 Struma ovarii refers to the presence of thyroid tissue in an ovarian teratoma or dermoid tumor that may produce excess amounts of thyroid hormones.

11 If the FT_4I is elevated but the FT_3I is within the reference range, hyperthyroidism is not excluded, but the possibility of a nonthyroidal illness as the source of thyroid function abnormalities must be investigated. At times, a hyperthyroid patient with a nonthyroidal illness will have this constellation of laboratory findings despite the presence of hyperthyroidism. The clinical settings will determine the need for further investigation. In general, further testing can be deferred until the patient has sufficiently recovered from a nonthyroidal illness. In some instances, however, a TRH (thyrotropin-releasing hormone) stimulation test can be used to clarify borderline thyroid function tests. The TRH test is most useful when the FT_4I and the FT_3I levels are equivocal and hyperthyroidism is suspected, or when the FT_4I level is low and TSH is not clearly elevated. A rise in TSH after TRH stimulation excludes the presence of hyperthyroidism and effectively explains the constellation of laboratory abnormalities to be due to the nonthyroidal illness (see No. 19). Some drugs, such as high-dose propranolol, amiodarone, and radioiodinated contrast agents, can inhibit the conversion of T_4 to T_3 so that the FT_4I will be elevated and the FT_3I will be low.

12 The TRH stimulation test is performed by injecting 400 to 500 μg of synthetic TRH and measuring the TSH level just prior to injection and at 30 minutes after the injection. Normally the TSH rises to 5 to 25 μIU/ml at 30 minutes after TRH injection. If hypothyroidism is present and is due to thyroid gland dysfunction, the TSH response is markedly increased. In secondary hypothyroidism, TSH will not rise, or a delayed rise will be seen. Even mild hyperthyroidism eliminates TSH response to TRH. In addition, glucocorticoids, somatostatin, and dopamine inhibit TSH secretion and blunt the TSH response to exogenously administered TRH.

13 If the FT_4I is decreased or in the low normal range, hypothyroidism is suspected but must be confirmed by measuring the serum TSH level. An FT_3I is not helpful in this setting, because the value will be within the reference range in up to 20 per cent of patients with hypothyroidism. The combination of a low FT_4I and an elevated TSH (>20mIU/L) is diagnostic of primary hypothyroidism.

14 The most common cause of hypothyroidism is Hashimoto's thyroiditis, also known as chronic lymphocytic thyroiditis or autoimmune thyroiditis. The exact nature of the autoimmune disorder is not known. Transition from the hypothyroidism of autoimmune thyroiditis to hyperthyroid Graves' disease has been described.

15 Antithyroid drugs used for the treatment of hyperthyroidism can result in hypothyroidism. Drugs such as lithium can block the release of thyroid hormones and result in hypothyroidism. Iodine can inhibit release of thyroid hormone as well and can occasionally cause hypothyroidism. Other agents that may rarely cause hypothyroidism include resorcinol, para-aminosalicylic acid, phenylbutazone, and cobalt.

16 The second most common cause of hypothyroidism is iatrogenic hypothyroidism resulting from the destruction of the thyroid by surgical procedures, radioactive iodine, or radiation treatment of hyperthyroidism.

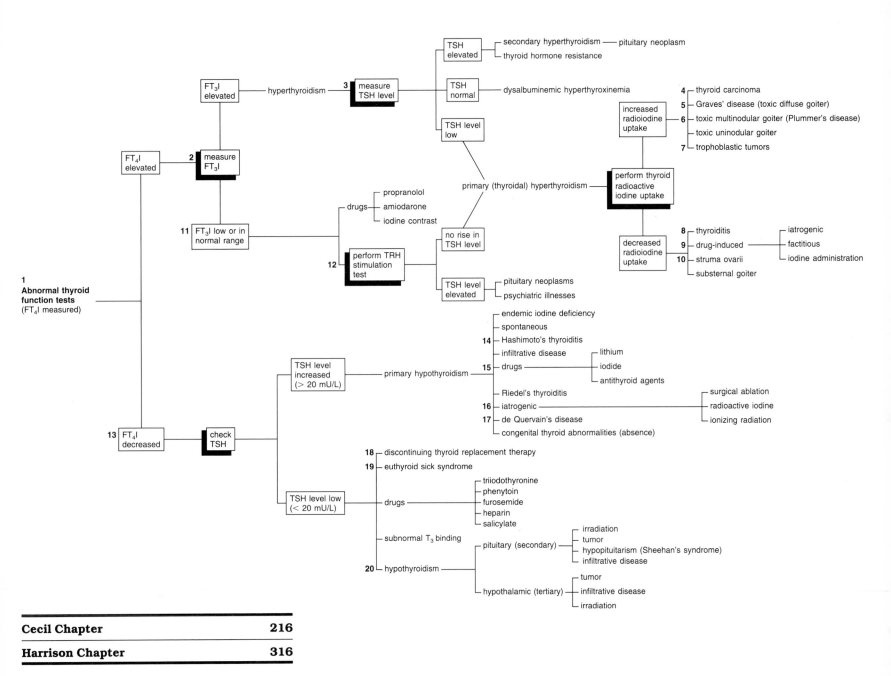

1
Abnormal thyroid function tests
(FT₄I measured)

2 measure FT₃I

3 measure TSH level

FT₄I elevated

FT₃I elevated — hyperthyroidism

TSH elevated — secondary hyperthyroidism — pituitary neoplasm
— thyroid hormone resistance

TSH normal — dysalbuminemic hyperthyroxinemia

TSH level low

primary (thyroidal) hyperthyroidism — **perform thyroid radioactive iodine uptake**

increased radioiodine uptake
— **4** thyroid carcinoma
— **5** Graves' disease (toxic diffuse goiter)
— **6** toxic multinodular goiter (Plummer's disease)
— toxic uninodular goiter
— **7** trophoblastic tumors

decreased radioiodine uptake
— **8** thyroiditis
— **9** drug-induced — iatrogenic
— **10** struma ovarii — factitious
— substernal goiter — iodine administration

11 FT₃I low or in normal range

drugs — propranolol
— amiodarone
— iodine contrast

12 perform TRH stimulation test

no rise in TSH level

TSH level elevated — pituitary neoplasms
— psychiatric illnesses

13 FT₄I decreased — check TSH

TSH level increased (> 20 mU/L) — primary hypothyroidism
— endemic iodine deficiency
— spontaneous
— **14** Hashimoto's thyroiditis
— infiltrative disease
— **15** drugs — lithium
— iodide
— antithyroid agents
— Riedel's thyroiditis
— **16** iatrogenic — surgical ablation
— radioactive iodine
— ionizing radiation
— **17** de Quervain's disease
— congenital thyroid abnormalities (absence)

TSH level low (< 20 mU/L)
— **18** discontinuing thyroid replacement therapy
— **19** euthyroid sick syndrome
— drugs — triiodothyronine
— phenytoin
— furosemide
— heparin
— salicylate
— subnormal T₃ binding
— **20** hypothyroidism — pituitary (secondary) — irradiation
— tumor
— hypopituitarism (Sheehan's syndrome)
— infiltrative disease
— hypothalamic (tertiary) — tumor
— infiltrative disease
— irradiation

Cecil Chapter	**216**
Harrison Chapter	**316**

Abnormal Thyroid Function Tests (Continued)

17 Subacute thyroiditis (de Quervain's thyroiditis) is a disease of unclear etiology in which transient hypothyroidism may be present for periods of 1 month to 1 year. Also known as subacute granulomatous thyroiditis, it often follows an acute viral infection by several weeks. Although adenovirus, coxsackievirus, and influenza virus have all been implicated, the precise etiology remains unknown. Permanent hypothyroidism is rare with this disorder.

18 The half-life of T_4 is 6 days. When thyroid replacement is discontinued in a hypothyroid patient, the FT_4I falls rapidly but the TSH level may remain within the reference range for 4 to 6 weeks.

19 Euthyroid sick syndrome refers to abnormalities of thyroid function tests associated with nonthyroidal illness. In the setting of an acute illness, a low T_4 with a normal or slightly elevated TSH may be due to the acute illness rather than to true thyroid disease. The tests should be repeated once the illness has resolved. If the diagnosis of hypothyroidism is strongly suspected in the setting of equivocal laboratory values and nonthyroidal illness, a TRH stimulation test can be helpful in establishing a diagnosis (see Nos. 11 and 12).

20 Pituitary and hypothalamic (secondary and tertiary) causes of hypothyroidism are rare. Lesions that would produce secondary or tertiary hypothyroidism would interfere with other endocrine functions as well, so the clinical setting and the presence of other signs and symptoms of endocrine dysfunction should be present before further laboratory evaluation is performed. A TRH stimulation test will add valuable information to determine the presence of secondary hypothyroidism (see No. 12). In primary hypothyroidism, the TSH rise is exaggerated (>25 μIU/ml) with TRH stimulation. In secondary or tertiary hypothyroidism, the rise in TSH may be delayed, blunted, prolonged, or absent after TRH stimulation.

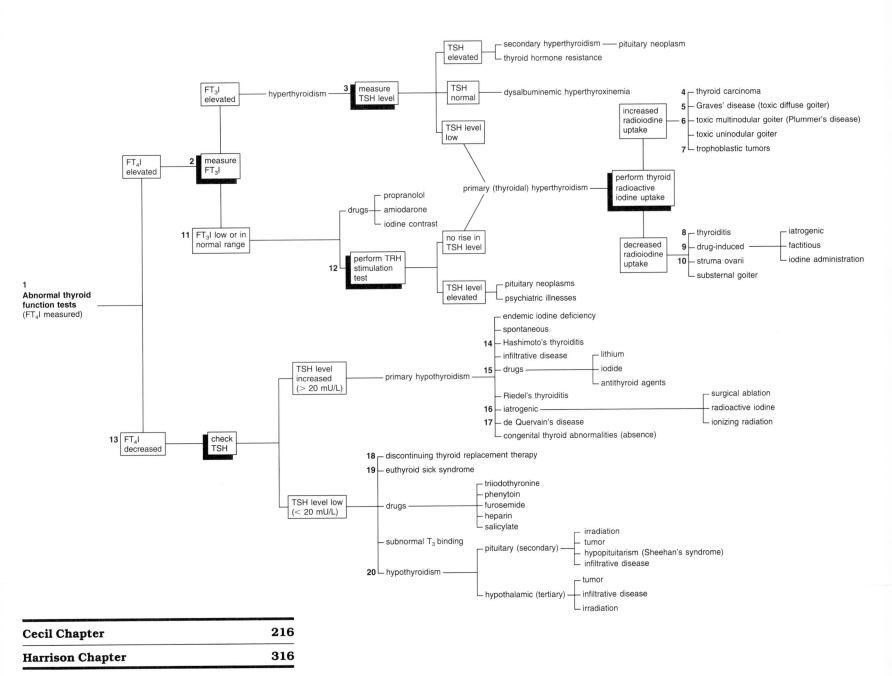

TSH elevated
— secondary hyperthyroidism —— pituitary neoplasm
— thyroid hormone resistance

3 measure TSH level

FT₃I elevated —— hyperthyroidism

TSH normal —— dysalbuminemic hyperthyroxinemia

increased radioiodine uptake
4 — thyroid carcinoma
5 — Graves' disease (toxic diffuse goiter)
6 — toxic multinodular goiter (Plummer's disease)
— toxic uninodular goiter
7 — trophoblastic tumors

TSH level low

FT₄I elevated

2 measure FT₃I

perform thyroid radioactive iodine uptake

primary (thyroidal) hyperthyroidism

11 FT₃I low or in normal range

drugs
— propranolol
— amiodarone
— iodine contrast

no rise in TSH level

decreased radioiodine uptake
8 — thyroiditis —— iatrogenic
9 — drug-induced —— factitious
10 — struma ovarii —— iodine administration
— substernal goiter

12 perform TRH stimulation test

TSH level elevated
— pituitary neoplasms
— psychiatric illnesses

1
Abnormal thyroid function tests
(FT₄I measured)

TSH level increased (> 20 mU/L) —— primary hypothyroidism

— endemic iodine deficiency
— spontaneous
14 — Hashimoto's thyroiditis
— infiltrative disease
15 — drugs
— lithium
— iodide
— antithyroid agents
— Riedel's thyroiditis
16 — iatrogenic
— surgical ablation
— radioactive iodine
— ionizing radiation
17 — de Quervain's disease
— congenital thyroid abnormalities (absence)

13 FT₄I decreased

check TSH

TSH level low (< 20 mU/L)

18 — discontinuing thyroid replacement therapy
19 — euthyroid sick syndrome

drugs
— triiodothyronine
— phenytoin
— furosemide
— heparin
— salicylate

— subnormal T₃ binding

20 — hypothyroidism

pituitary (secondary)
— irradiation
— tumor
— hypopituitarism (Sheehan's syndrome)
— infiltrative disease

hypothalamic (tertiary)
— tumor
— infiltrative disease
— irradiation

Hyperlipidemia

1 Hyperlipidemia is defined as an increase in the concentration of plasma triglycerides, cholesterol, or both. Hyperlipidemia can be discovered inadvertently, because measurements of triglycerides and cholesterol are included in many routine blood panels. Blood must be obtained from patients after a 12- to 14-hour fast, however, because postprandial chylomicronemia can increase triglyceride levels substantially. The cut-off points for diagnosing hyperlipidemia are largely arbitrary, because the distribution of lipoprotein concentrations in the population is continuous. The importance of the diagnosis of hyperlipidemia lies in the fact that there is a positive correlation between plasma cholesterol levels and the prevalence of coronary artery disease (CAD). Hypercholesterolemia is defined as the ninetieth percentile of the population distribution, separated by age and sex. Hypertriglyceridemia is defined by values in the upper 5 per cent of the distribution. The prevalence of genetic disorders increases at higher cut-off points. The hyperlipidemias have been classified most commonly on the basis of lipid phenotype. This classification has been outlined and described as types I through V based upon laboratory findings independent of genetic or pathophysiologic mechanisms. The primary hyperlipidemias can also be classified on the basis of genetic mechanisms. Management of hyperlipidemia depends primarily upon which of the blood lipids are elevated (either triglycerides or cholesterol), regardless of the genetic or phenotypic subtype. Therefore, these classification schemes are not of practical significance in the diagnosis and treatment of the hyperlipidemias. The lipoprotein profile for an individual can change with time and will change as other diseases are superimposed.

2 If hyperlipidemia is discovered inadvertently, testing should be repeated on a fasting blood sample. The basic testing that should be performed includes total cholesterol level, triglyceride (TG) level, and high density lipoprotein (HDL) level. Low density lipoprotein (LDL) levels can be estimated from the formula: $LDL = $ total serum cholesterol $- HDL - TG/5$, although the triglyceride level must be less than 400 mg/dl for this estimation to be accurate. The level of LDL cholesterol is important to know, because increased levels of LDL are associated with increased incidence of atherosclerosis. High levels of HDL cholesterol are correlated with a decreased prevalence of atherosclerosis. The combination of these tests should provide enough information to determine the abnormal lipoprotein type. Electrophoresis will also identify very low density lipoprotein (VLDL), chylomicrons, LDL, and HDL levels. However, even with electrophoresis it may not always be possible to distinguish between the primary and secondary causes of hyperlipidemia. Primary hyperlipidemias have a genetic basis, and the molecular defect is known in at least five of these disorders. Secondary hyperlipidemias are due to systemic diseases in otherwise normolipemic persons. Secondary causes of hyperlipidemia must be sought and treated on an individual basis before the diagnosis of a primary disorder can be diagnosed. In addition, it is possible for an individual to have a primary disorder upon which a secondary disorder is superimposed. In such cases, the abnormal lipid profile owing to the systemic disorder can alter the lipid profile of the primary disorder.

3 Elevated triglyceride levels are due to increased chylomicrons or increased VLDL levels. In general, patients with triglyceride levels of less than 1000 mg/dl rarely have chylomicronemia, and the presence of chylomicronemia suggests that the patient did not fast. Patients who have eaten a large dinner accompanied by a large amount of alcohol will manifest a transiently high fasting triglyceride level. If chylomicronemia is absent, serum triglyceride levels are correlated with elevated VLDL triglycerides.

4 Familial lipoprotein lipase (LPL) deficiency is classified as type I hyperlipidemia. It is characterized by grossly lipemic fasting plasma with elevated chylomicrons. The disease is rare and manifests its symptoms in childhood. Symptoms include eruptive xanthomas of the skin, recurrent episodes of pancreatitis and abdominal pain, hepatosplenomegaly, and lipemia retinalis. A deficiency of the activator of LPL, apoC-II, results in a similar syndrome.

5 The most common but most poorly defined pattern of hyperlipidemia is the so-called polygenic hypercholesterolemia. The term refers to a group of patients with increased levels of total cholesterol with LDL above the 90th percentile for the population, but without a well-defined mode of inheritance. It is thought that environmental influences (primarily dietary) superimposed on a permissive genetic background are responsible for this disorder. This lipid disorder probably accounts for 80 to 90 per cent of the individuals with a type II lipid profile.

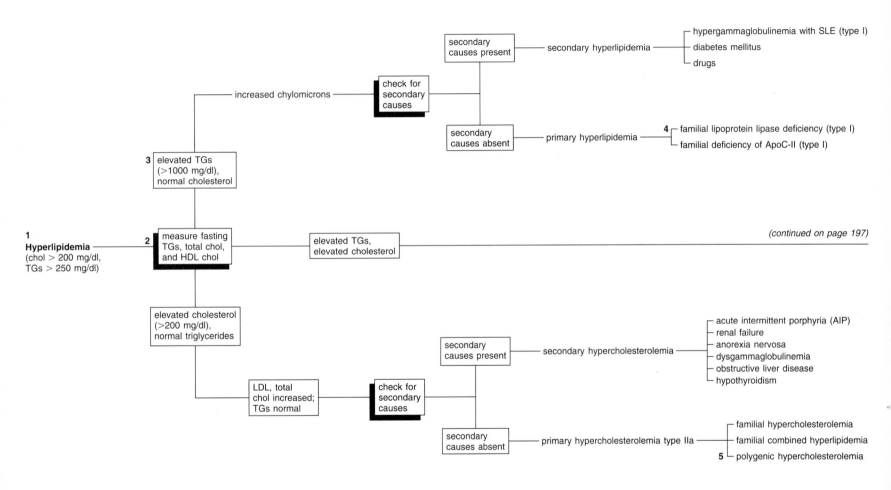

1
Hyperlipidemia —
(chol > 200 mg/dl,
TGs > 250 mg/dl)

2 measure fasting
TGs, total chol,
and HDL chol

3 elevated TGs
(>1000 mg/dl),
normal cholesterol

increased chylomicrons — check for
secondary
causes

secondary
causes present — secondary hyperlipidemia — hypergammaglobulinemia with SLE (type I)
— diabetes mellitus
— drugs

secondary
causes absent — primary hyperlipidemia — **4** — familial lipoprotein lipase deficiency (type I)
— familial deficiency of ApoC-II (type I)

elevated TGs,
elevated cholesterol

(continued on page 197)

elevated cholesterol
(>200 mg/dl),
normal triglycerides

LDL, total
chol increased;
TGs normal — check for
secondary
causes

secondary
causes present — secondary hypercholesterolemia — acute intermittent porphyria (AIP)
— renal failure
— anorexia nervosa
— dysgammaglobulinemia
— obstructive liver disease
— hypothyroidism

secondary
causes absent — primary hypercholesterolemia type IIa — familial hypercholesterolemia
— familial combined hyperlipidemia
5 — polygenic hypercholesterolemia

Cecil Chapter	172
Harrison Chapter	326

Hyperlipidemia (Continued)

6 In the absence of chylomicronemia, hypertriglyceridemia can be attributed to elevated levels of VLDL. However, if an increased level of VLDL is responsible for hypertriglyceridemia, there will be an increase in the cholesterol level as well, because VLDL contains both cholesterol and TGs. This combination of findings defines type IV hyperlipidemia.

7 Drugs such as alcohol, estrogens, diuretics, and beta-blocking agents may elevate levels of triglycerides, but the effect is usually mild unless these drugs are superimposed on a genetically hyperlipidemic patient. Oral contraceptives can cause hypertriglyceridemia. Estrogen replacement in postmenopausal women raises the total cholesterol level, but the LDL level is actually decreased and the HDL level is increased, thereby possibly decreasing overall cardiovascular risk.

8 Familial hypertriglyceridemia (FHT) can be manifested with a type IV lipid profile. The diagnosis of type IV FHT is suspected when the triglyceride level is elevated and the total cholesterol level is mildly elevated. Eruptive xanthomas are uncommon in type IV FHT. Superimposed disorders, such as diabetes mellitus, obesity, alcoholism, hypothyroidism, or estrogen use, can markedly worsen the lipid profiles in type IV FHT.

9 Familial combined hyperlipidemia (FCH) can manifest itself by a variety of different lipid profiles, most commonly as types IIa, IIb, and IV. Profiles may be different among members of the same family. In addition, lipid profiles may change in any individual with time. The disorder is thought to be inherited as an autosomal dominant condition. The diagnosis of type IV FCH is suspected when the triglyceride level is elevated and the total cholesterol level is mildly elevated.

10 Diabetes mellitus is often associated with hypertriglyceridemia. The increase in TGs in these patients may be due to insulin deficiency or associated with obesity and hyperinsulinemia. Marked elevations of TGs, however, should lead to the suspicion of an underlying familial form of hypertriglyceridemia upon which diabetic hypertriglyceridemia has been superimposed.

11 Type V FHT is usually more severe than type IV FHT (see No. 8). Type V FHT causes elevated levels of chylomicrons, VLDL, and cholesterol, whereas type IV FHT causes elevated VLDL and mildly elevated levels of cholesterol, without associated chylomicronemia. It may be difficult to distinguish the familial form of a type V pattern from secondary causes of this lipid pattern, such as estrogen use, alcohol use, and diabetes mellitus, but family screening may be useful. Clinically, patients with type V FHT demonstrate eruptive xanthomas and recurrent bouts of abdominal pain or pancreatitis. Superimposed estrogen use, alcohol excess, and diabetes may decrease the age of onset of symptomatic disease, which is usually between 20 and 50 years of age. These modifying influences may also markedly increase the triglyceride levels.

12 Familial dysbetaproteinemia is a lipoprotein disorder in which levels of total cholesterol and triglycerides are elevated to an equal degree. Serum cholesterol between 300 and 1000 mg/dl may be seen. Clinically, patients manifest coronary artery disease, peripheral vascular disease, and xanthomas, including tendon xanthomas of the Achilles and extensor tendons of the hands. Tuberous xanthomas are common. Lipid electrophoresis will help to identify this abnormal lipoprotein profile in which the pre-beta band (VLDL) is increased. Although the total cholesterol level is elevated, levels of HDL and LDL are low (type III pattern). The increase in total cholesterol can therefore be explained on the basis of the VLDL fraction, which differs from normal VLDL in that it has an increase in the ratio of cholesterol to the triglyceride content. Concurrent disease such as obesity, hypothyroidism, diabetes mellitus, and excessive alcohol consumption will exaggerate the expression of this disorder.

13 Hypothyroidism can cause familial lipoprotein disorders to become clinically manifest or to worsen. By itself, hypothyroidism can be associated with a type II hyperlipedemic pattern. Cholesterol level may increase as hypothyroidism becomes more profound.

14 Nephrotic syndrome usually results in increased levels of TGs and total cholesterol owing to increased VLDL and LDL with a type IIb lipid profile. These abnormalities are directly related to an increase in hepatic lipid synthesis. The severity of the lipid abnormality is directly related to the degree of hypoalbuminemia and proteinuria.

15 Familial hypercholesterolemia (FHC) can exist in two forms with two different lipid profiles, type IIa and type IIb. In type IIa, LDL cholesterol is increased and TGs are normal. In type IIb, LDL cholesterol and TGs (primarily VLDL) are increased. Both of these disorders are associated with tendon xanthomas, xanthalasma, premature coronary artery disease, and peripheral vascular disease. Approximately two thirds of the heterozygote patients will demonstrate tuberous or tendon xanthomas during their lifetimes. Total cholesterol levels are usually in the 300 to 500 mg/dl range for these patients. In contrast, in the homozygous form, cholesterol levels range from 600 to 1200 mg/dl. Clinically, the homozygous form demonstrates xanthomas over the extremities, buttocks, knees, and palms, in addition to premature atherosclerosis.

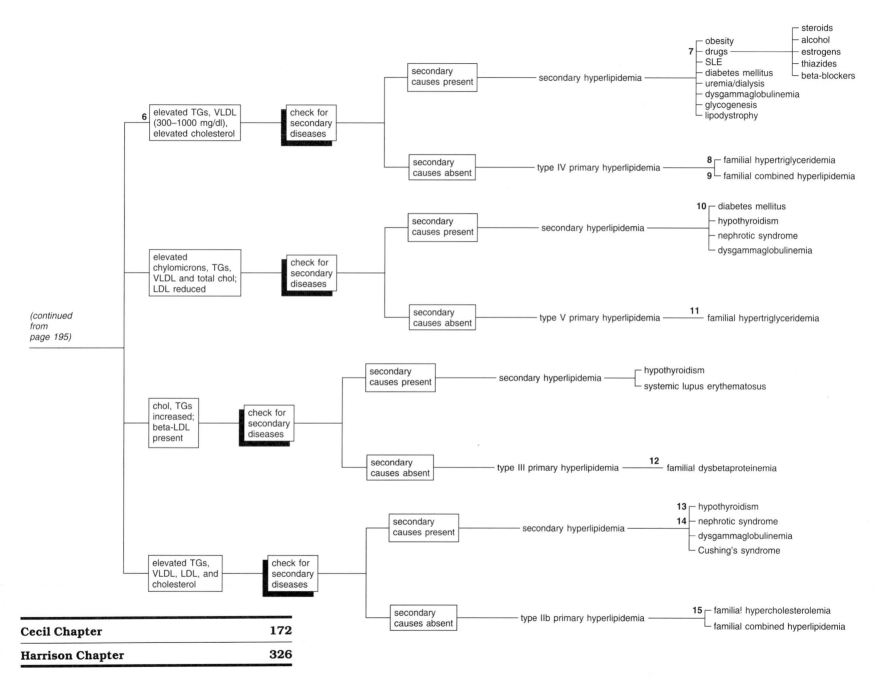

(continued from page 195)

6 elevated TGs, VLDL (300–1000 mg/dl), elevated cholesterol → check for secondary diseases

secondary causes present → secondary hyperlipidemia →
- obesity
- **7** drugs
  - steroids
  - alcohol
  - estrogens
  - thiazides
  - beta-blockers
- SLE
- diabetes mellitus
- uremia/dialysis
- dysgammaglobulinemia
- glycogenesis
- lipodystrophy

secondary causes absent → type IV primary hyperlipidemia →
- **8** familial hypertriglyceridemia
- **9** familial combined hyperlipidemia

elevated chylomicrons, TGs, VLDL and total chol; LDL reduced → check for secondary diseases

secondary causes present → secondary hyperlipidemia →
- **10** diabetes mellitus
- hypothyroidism
- nephrotic syndrome
- dysgammaglobulinemia

secondary causes absent → type V primary hyperlipidemia → **11** familial hypertriglyceridemia

chol, TGs increased; beta-LDL present → check for secondary diseases

secondary causes present → secondary hyperlipidemia →
- hypothyroidism
- systemic lupus erythematosus

secondary causes absent → type III primary hyperlipidemia → **12** familial dysbetaproteinemia

elevated TGs, VLDL, LDL, and cholesterol → check for secondary diseases

secondary causes present → secondary hyperlipidemia →
- **13** hypothyroidism
- **14** nephrotic syndrome
- dysgammaglobulinemia
- Cushing's syndrome

secondary causes absent → type IIb primary hyperlipidemia →
- **15** familia! hypercholesterolemia
- familial combined hyperlipidemia

Cecil Chapter	172
Harrison Chapter	326

Hypoglycemia

1 Hypoglycemia may be a symptom or "diagnosis" reported by the patient, may be discovered by routine blood glucose measurement, or may be suspected on the basis of the group of signs and symptoms reported by the patient. Hypoglycemia is a measured glucose level lower than the lower limit of normal. In general, it can be defined as a plasma glucose level of less than 50 mg/dl, but it is considered in a patient with any low glucose level in whom symptoms occur. All patients with a blood glucose level less than 50 mg/dl should be evaluated whether or not symptoms occur.

2 If low blood glucose is discovered by random glucose measurement but symptoms are absent, the hypoglycemia may be artifactual. Excessive numbers of leukocytes or red cells may result in spuriously low whole blood values for glucose. A plasma glucose level should be normal, however.

3 Some patients can have an asymptomatic hypoglycemia that is not artifactual (see No. 2). These patients may have mild symptoms that are difficult to recognize or may have a long-standing hypoglycemia to which they have adapted.

4 Because the signs and symptoms of hypoglycemia are nonspecific, symptomatic hypoglycemia must be confirmed by measuring glucose levels at the time the patient complains of symptoms. Symptoms include anxiety, palpitations, headache, blurred vision, irritability, weakness, diaphoresis, nervousness, drowsiness, fatigue, hunger, and paresthesias. Some of the symptoms are due to an adrenergic response caused by the release of epinephrine (e.g., palpitations, nervousness), and some of the symptoms are due to a neuroglycopenia (e.g., headache, confusion, slurred speech). There is a triad of conditions known as Whipple's triad, that must be demonstrated prior to further evaluation of hypoglycemia: the patient must be shown to have symptoms concomitantly with documented hypoglycemia and resolution of symptoms when glucose or food is administered.

5 The majority of patients who present with a symptomatic hypoglycemia are diabetics who take oral hypoglycemic agents or insulin injections. The most common cause of hypoglycemia in these patients is the use of the hypoglycemic agent without an associated sufficient carbohydrate intake. Other causes of hypoglycemia in these patients include incorrect dosing (overdos-

ing), strenuous exercise, alcohol intake, and the simultaneous use of potentiating drugs. Commonly used drugs that can potentiate the effect of sulfonylureas, for example, include barbiturates, salicylates, sulfonamides, and thiazides. Of note, beta-adrenergic blocking agents (e.g., propranolol) can block the adrenergic symptoms of hypoglycemia and can be dangerous when prescribed to diabetics because the early symptoms of hypoglycemia may then go unrecognized. At times, pharmacy error leads to the ingestion of sulfonylureas when another medication has been prescribed.

6 A food tolerance test can be performed with a standard solid or liquid meal rather than the oral glucose tolerance test. If hypoglycemia cannot be documented, it is important to consider other causes for the patient's symptoms. Because similar adrenergic responses can occur in many emotional and psychiatric states, it is important to document true hypoglycemia prior to proceeding with further evaluation. A food-stimulated hypoglycemia, also known as a reactive hypoglycemia, usually results in adrenergic symptoms. A fasting (food-deprived) hypoglycemia usually results in symptoms of neuroglycopenia (see No. 4).

7 Postprandial hypoglycemia (after a food tolerance test), with spontaneous recovery from the symptoms, is considered to be a reactive (or food-stimulated) hypoglycemia. Reactive hypoglycemia may be due to dumping syndrome or may represent a precursor form of diabetes mellitus. Dumping syndrome can occur postgastrectomy. The hypoglycemia is due to the rapid dumping of carbohydrates into the intestine from the stomach, causing an oversecretion of insulin and resultant hypoglycemia. Very few patients demonstrate idiopathic reactive hypoglycemia. Symptoms occur several hours postprandially and usually resolve spontaneously. These patients may have an early precursor of non–insulin-dependent diabetes.

8 Serum glucose that does not return to normal spontaneously after a glucose load is usually indicative of a serious underlying disorder. A 72-hour fast (food-deprived hypoglycemia) is performed in order to detect a possible insulin-secreting tumor. The fast is monitored in a controlled environment (i.e., a hospital) and is usually begun after an evening meal that contains high glucose levels. The patient is allowed to drink only water during the subsequent fast. Blood glucose levels, C-peptide levels (see No. 10), and insulin are measured for a baseline and then every 6 hours. When symptoms are

reported, a quick finger-stick glucose test is done to confirm the low blood glucose; then, insulin, glucose, and C-peptide levels are immediately drawn and the test terminated. Almost 100 per cent of patients with insulinoma will develop hypoglycemia within a 72-hour fasting period.

9 Insulin-producing tumors are not subject to the usual regulatory feedback mechanism in which a low blood sugar causes insulin secretion to decrease. The best measurement of the relationship between glucose and insulin is the glucose-to-insulin ratio, calculated as follows:

$$\frac{\text{Glucose (mg/dl)}}{\text{Insulin } (\mu\text{IU/ml})}$$

This ratio is usually greater than 2:1. If endogenous insulin is increased, the ratio is less than 2:1, as usually occurs with insulinoma. Perhaps more useful to demonstrate relative hyperinsulinemia is a plasma insulin level that will remain inappropriately high in the presence of hypoglycemia. A plasma insulin level greater than 6 μIU/ml is considered the value above which hyperinsulinemic states are defined.

10 If factitial hypoglycemia is suspected, a C-peptide level will be helpful. C-peptide is the fragment of endogenously produced proinsulin that is cleaved off the proinsulin to form insulin. If endogenous insulin production increases, the level of C-peptide increases in equal amounts. Therefore, when exogenous insulin is surreptitiously injected, endogenous insulin production will be suppressed and blood levels of insulin will be high, whereas blood levels of C-peptide will be disproportionately low. Becasue insulin is cleared by the liver and C-peptide is cleared by the kidneys, C-peptide levels will be elevated in renal failure. C-peptide levels may be elevated when renal failure and insulinoma coexist. Provocative tests are performed to strengthen evidence for an insulin-secreting tumor. Tests include the C-peptide suppression test, the intravenous tolbutamide test, and the intravenous glucagon suppression test. The C-peptide suppression test documents excess production of endogenous insulin by demonstrating the lack of suppression of C-peptide when intravenous (IV) insulin is exogenously administered. An IV tolbutamide test is performed over a 3-hour period. Patients with insulinoma respond to IV tolbutamide with exaggerated suppression of plasma glucose levels. Plasma insulin levels are of less use diagnostically with this test. The administration of IV glucagon increases blood glucose with simultaneous release of insulin. If the peak

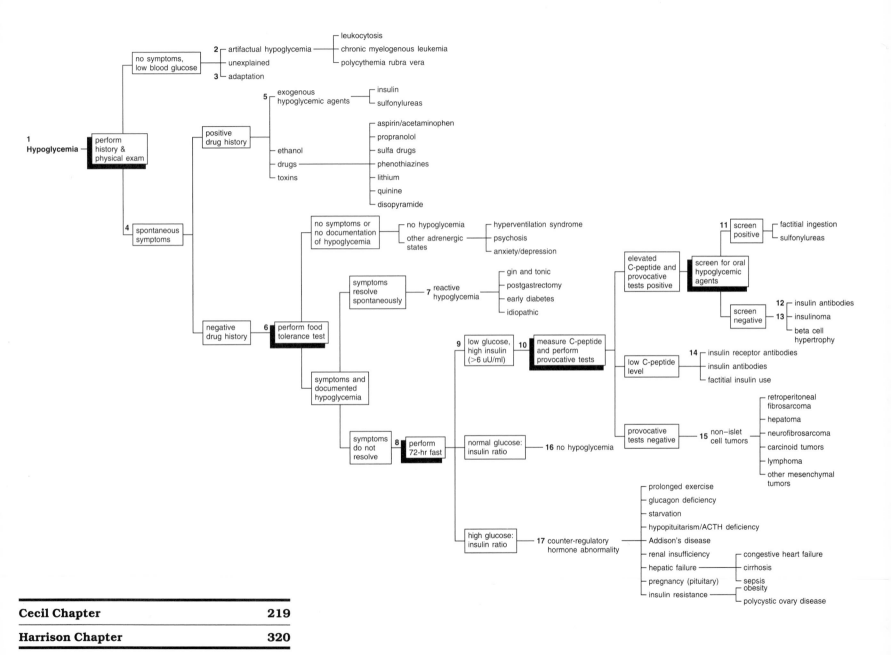

1
Hypoglycemia

perform history & physical exam

no symptoms, low blood glucose

2 artifactual hypoglycemia
- leukocytosis
- chronic myelogenous leukemia
- polycythemia rubra vera

unexplained

3 adaptation

4 spontaneous symptoms

positive drug history

5 exogenous hypoglycemic agents
- insulin
- sulfonylureas

ethanol

drugs
- aspirin/acetaminophen
- propranolol
- sulfa drugs
- phenothiazines
- lithium
- quinine
- disopyramide

toxins

negative drug history

6 perform food tolerance test

no symptoms or no documentation of hypoglycemia
- no hypoglycemia
- other adrenergic states
  - hyperventilation syndrome
  - psychosis
  - anxiety/depression

symptoms resolve spontaneously

7 reactive hypoglycemia
- gin and tonic
- postgastrectomy
- early diabetes
- idiopathic

symptoms and documented hypoglycemia

symptoms do not resolve

8 perform 72-hr fast

9 low glucose, high insulin (>6 uU/ml)

10 measure C-peptide and perform provocative tests

elevated C-peptide and provocative tests positive

screen for oral hypoglycemic agents

11 screen positive
- factitial ingestion
- sulfonylureas

screen negative
- **12** insulin antibodies
- **13** insulinoma
- beta cell hypertrophy

low C-peptide level
- **14** insulin receptor antibodies
- insulin antibodies
- factitial insulin use

provocative tests negative

15 non-islet cell tumors
- retroperitoneal fibrosarcoma
- hepatoma
- neurofibrosarcoma
- carcinoid tumors
- lymphoma
- other mesenchymal tumors

normal glucose: insulin ratio — **16** no hypoglycemia

high glucose: insulin ratio

17 counter-regulatory hormone abnormality
- prolonged exercise
- glucagon deficiency
- starvation
- hypopituitarism/ACTH deficiency
- Addison's disease
- renal insufficiency
- hepatic failure
  - congestive heart failure
  - cirrhosis
  - sepsis
- pregnancy (pituitary)
- insulin resistance
  - obesity
  - polycystic ovary disease

Cecil Chapter	219
Harrison Chapter	320

Hypoglycemia (Continued)

insulin response exceeds 130 µIU/ml, the diagnostic accuracy for insulinoma is 50 to 80 per cent.

11 Oral hypoglycemic agents (sulfonylureas) can stimulate proinsulin secretion with C-peptide production. Test results for insulinoma will not identify the patient who secretly ingested a sulfonylurea prior to the test. Therefore, a screen for these agents must also be performed prior to pursuing further localization studies for insulinoma. Sulfonylurea concentration can be measured if surreptitious ingestion is suspected.

12 Insulin antibodies are almost always formed after repeated injection of insulin, so that insulin antibodies can also be measured to support the suspicion of exogenously administered insulin. Some patients, however, have developed insulin antibodies without ever having had an insulin injection.

13 Insulinoma is rare, occurring in fewer than 1 in 4000 people. The median age at diagnosis is 50, and the majority of patients with insulinoma are women (60 per cent). Insulinoma occurs as part of the multiple endocrine neoplasia syndrome type 1 (MEN 1), and these patients are usually diagnosed in their twenties. The majority of insulinomas are solitary benign tumors (80 per cent), but some can be multiple or malignant. The hypoglycemia associated with insulinoma usually occurs more than 5 hours after a meal. The diagnosis lies with the demonstration of inappropriately high insulin levels while the glucose level is low, but a number of endocrine provocative tests (see No. 10) can also be performed to strengthen the diagnosis. Ultimately, the tumor must be localized anatomically, which can be achieved with various techniques including ultrasound and pancreatic angiography. Insulinomas are usually highly vascular tumors. If provocative tests are negative but radiographic evaluation reveals tumor, a non–islet cell tumor may be present.

14 Rarely, some patients produce insulin receptor antibodies that act like insulin agonists and cause hypoglycemia. Most of these patients have insulin-resistant diabetes, and the insulin receptor antibodies are thought to be due to autoimmune disease.

15 Hypoglycemia has been associated with many different mesenchymal tumors. About 65 per cent of these tumors are localized to the abdomen, the most common of which is retroperitoneal fibrosarcoma. Approximately 35 per cent of mesenchymal tumors are found in the chest. The etiology of the associated hypoglycemia is multifactorial and may be due to high glucose utilization by the tumor, interference with glucose regulation, or metastatic destruction of glands such as the adrenals, to name a few possible mechanisms. In general, measured insulin levels remain relatively low in relation to the low glucose levels in these non–insulin-producing tumors, unlike the high insulin levels seen with insulin-producing tumors. Nonpancreatic tumors may produce an insulin-like growth factor (IGF-like) that is responsible for the associated hypoglycemia. Tumors that have been found to produce IGF-like material include fibrosarcoma, neurilemmoma, leiomyosarcoma, mesothelioma, and hemangiopericytoma.

16 If hypoglycemia cannot be documented during a 72-hour fast, the patient is unlikely to have hypoglycemia. Less than 2 per cent of patients with insulinoma remain undetected (i.e., do not demonstrate hypoglycemia) within 72 hours of a prolonged, supervised fast. In addition to a rare undetected patient with an insulinoma, this group of patients may include nondiabetics who secretly take sulfonylureas or insulin, but are unable to use them during the supervised fasting period. Surreptitious use of oral hypoglycemic agents and insulin is most likely to occur in 30- to 40-year-old women in health-related occupations (e.g., nurses).

17 Hepatic disease and dysfunction is a common cause of hypoglycemia because of the liver's role in glucose homeostasis. The liver is able to maintain normal glucose homeostasis with as little as 20 per cent of the parenchymal cells functioning, but biochemical hypoglycemia can occur in a wide variety of diseases in which the liver is primarily or secondarily involved. The hypoglycemia reported with congestive heart failure and sepsis, for example, is likely due to hepatic dysfunction.

BIBLIOGRAPHY

Burnett RG: Diagnostic strategies for amenorrhea. Postgrad Med 87(5):241–250, 1990.

Cox MR, Marshall SG, Spence RAJ: Solitary thyroid nodule: a prospective evaluation of nuclear scanning and ultrasonography. Br J Surg 78:90–93, 1991.

Erkkola R, Ruutiainen K: Hirsutism: definitions and etiology. Ann Med 22:99–103, 1990.

Fitzpatrick TB (ed): Dermatology in General Medicine. 3rd ed. New York, McGraw-Hill Book Company, 1987.

Fredrickson DS, Levy RI, et al.: Dietary Management of Hyperlipoproteinemia: A Handbook for Physicians and Dieticians. Bethesda, MD, National Heart and Lung Institute, 1974.

Fritz MA, Speroff L: Current concepts of the endocrine characteristics of normal menstrual funtion: The key to diagnosis and management of menstrual disorders. Clin Obstet Gynecol 26(3):647–679, 1983.

Gold JJ, Josimovich JB (eds): Gynecologic Endocrinology. 3rd ed. Hagerstown, MD, Harper & Row, 1980.

Gotto AM, Jones PH, Scott LW: The diagnosis and management of hyperlipidemia. DM 32(5):245–311, 1986.

Hare JW: Signs and Symptoms in Endocrine and Metabolic Disorders. Philadelphia, J. B. Lippincott Company, 1986.

Harvey HK: Diagnosis and management of the thyroid nodule. Otolaryngol Clin North Am 23(2):303–330, 1990.

Havel RJ (ed): Lipid Disorders. Med Clin North Am 66(2): 1982.

Helfand M, Crapo LM: Screening for thyroid disease. Ann Intern Med 112:840–849, 1990.

Herschman JM: Endocrine Pathophysiology: A Patient Oriented Approach. Philadelphia, Lea & Febiger, 1977.

Howanitz PJ, Howanitz JH (eds): Issues in Laboratory Endocrinology. Clin Lab Med 4(4), 1984.

Judd HL: Endocrinology of polycystic ovarian disease. Clin Obstet Gynecol 21(1):99–114, 1978.

Kaplan MM, Larsen PR (eds): Thyroid Disease. Med Clin North Am 69, 1985.

Keller PJ: Hormonal Disorders in Gynecology. New York, Springer-Verlag, 1981.

Kohler PO (ed): Clinical Endocrinology. New York, John Wiley & Sons, 1986.

Malo JW, Bezdicek BJ: Secondary amenorrhea. Postgrad Med 79(3):86–95, 1986.

Margolis S: Diagnosis and management of abnormal plasma lipids. J Clin Endocrinol Metab 70(4):821–825, 1990.

McFarland KF: A clinical approach to amenorrhea. J SC Med Assoc 81(9):481–483, 1985.

Mitchell AJ, Krull EA (eds): Hair Disorders. Dermatol Clin 5(3):1987.

Nanji AA: Disorders of gonadal function. Clin Lab Med 4(4):717–728, 1984.

Rifkind BM, Levy RI (eds): Hyperlipidemia: Diagnosis and Therapy. New York, Grune & Stratton, 1977.

Rittmaster RS, Loriaux DL: Hirsutism. Ann Intern Med 106:95–107, 1987.

Toft AD (ed): Hyperthyroidism. Clin Endocrinol Metab 14(2):1985.

White PC, New MI, Dupont B: Congenital adrenal hyperplasia. N Engl J Med 316:1519–1524, 1987.

Williams ED (ed): Pathology and Management of Thyroid Disease. Clin Endocrinol Metab 10:1981.

Wong, ET, Steffes MW: A fundamental approach to the diagnosis of diseases of the thyroid gland. Clin Lab Med 4(4):655–670, 1984.

Wyngaarden JB, Smith LH Jr (eds): Cecil Textbook of Medicine. 18th ed. Philadelphia, W. B. Saunders Company, 1988.

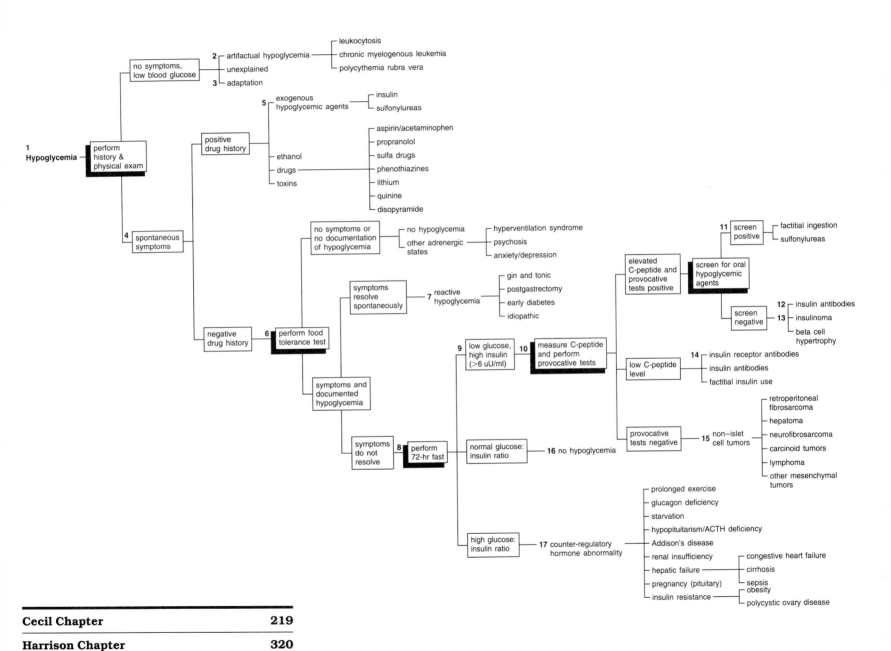

1 **Hypoglycemia**

perform history & physical exam

no symptoms, low blood glucose

2 artifactual hypoglycemia
— leukocytosis
— chronic myelogenous leukemia
— polycythemia rubra vera

unexplained

3 adaptation

positive drug history

5 exogenous hypoglycemic agents
— insulin
— sulfonylureas

ethanol
drugs
toxins
— aspirin/acetaminophen
— propranolol
— sulfa drugs
— phenothiazines
— lithium
— quinine
— disopyramide

4 spontaneous symptoms

negative drug history

6 perform food tolerance test

no symptoms or no documentation of hypoglycemia

no hypoglycemia

other adrenergic states
— hyperventilation syndrome
— psychosis
— anxiety/depression

symptoms resolve spontaneously

7 reactive hypoglycemia
— gin and tonic
— postgastrectomy
— early diabetes
— idiopathic

symptoms and documented hypoglycemia

symptoms do not resolve

8 perform 72-hr fast

9 low glucose, high insulin (>6 uU/ml)

10 measure C-peptide and perform provocative tests

elevated C-peptide and provocative tests positive

screen for oral hypoglycemic agents

11 screen positive
— factitial ingestion
— sulfonylureas

screen negative

12 insulin antibodies
13 insulinoma
— beta cell hypertrophy

low C-peptide level

14 insulin receptor antibodies
— insulin antibodies
— factitial insulin use

provocative tests negative

15 non–islet cell tumors
— retroperitoneal fibrosarcoma
— hepatoma
— neurofibrosarcoma
— carcinoid tumors
— lymphoma
— other mesenchymal tumors

normal glucose: insulin ratio

16 no hypoglycemia

high glucose: insulin ratio

17 counter-regulatory hormone abnormality
— prolonged exercise
— glucagon deficiency
— starvation
— hypopituitarism/ACTH deficiency
— Addison's disease
— renal insufficiency
— hepatic failure
— pregnancy (pituitary)
— insulin resistance

— congestive heart failure
— cirrhosis
— sepsis
— obesity
— polycystic ovary disease

Cecil Chapter	219
Harrison Chapter	320

10 ▪ Skin Disorders

Signs and symptoms:	Purpura
Pruritus	Alopecia
Urticaria	

Pruritus

1 Pruritus is the sensation in the skin that induces the desire to scratch. Itching is the most common symptom in dermatology; it may be generalized without evidence of skin disease. In the absence of primary skin lesions, generalized pruritus can be indicative of an underlying systemic disorder. Some systemic disorders, such as diabetes mellitus and cholestasis, can present with localized itching as well. Most patients with pruritus do not have a systemic disorder, however, and generalized itching is usually due to a widespread cutaneous disorder.

2 Examination of the skin may be abnormal even in the absence of any primary skin lesions. The skin may have secondary lesions such as excoriations owing to the scratching induced by pruritus. A number of skin disorders will not have primary skin lesions. Atopic dermatitis, for example, will demonstrate only secondary skin lesions, because the sensation of itching results in the disease. A complete history and physical examination may elucidate the source of pruritus, but in addition, a series of screening laboratory tests can be performed that will be useful in diagnosis of pruritus. These tests include a complete blood count (CBC), an electrolyte and liver function test (LFT) panel (Sequential Multiple Analyzer, SMA 12/60), thyroid function tests (TFTs), a urinalysis (UA), and a chest radiograph (CXR).

3 Pruritus is a rare, nonspecific symptom of underlying malignancy, most commonly pancreatic or stomach carcinoma. A variety of neurologic diseases can also be associated with itching on rare occasions. The diagnosis is made by examination, which may reveal focal neurologic findings. Paroxysmal itching has been reported with multiple sclerosis. Severe pruritus of the nostrils has been associated with frontal brain tumors.

4 Notalgia paresthetica is a form of pruritus in which itching is localized to an area of the back, medial to the left scapula. Notalgia paresthetica is thought to be a variant form of peripheral neuropathy.

5 Chronic renal failure is the most common systemic disorder responsible for pruritus. Pruritus has been estimated to affect as many as 90 per cent of patients with chronic renal failure on hemodialysis. Almost 50 per cent of the patients are most bothered by pruritus during or shortly after dialysis. The etiology of the pruritus accompanying renal failure is unclear. The pruritus of renal failure has been attributed to secondary hyperparathyroidism or to elevated phosphorus and magnesium levels. Itching tends to resolve when serum phosphorus levels are decreased.

6 Cholestatic liver disease is frequently associated with generalized pruritus. The itching may precede other signs and symptoms of cholestatic disease. Initially the itching may be localized, limited to the hands and feet and to areas of pressure, becoming worse at night. Although the accumulation of bile acids in the skin has been implicated in the pathogenesis of cholestatic pruritus, bile levels do not always correlate with the presence or absence of pruritus, or with its severity. The pruritus that accompanies benign cholestatic jaundice of pregnancy is most severe in the third trimester and resolves after delivery. Women who develop cholestatic jaundice during pregnancy are at greater risk of developing jaundice and pruritus with use of oral contraceptives at a later date. Primary biliary cirrhosis is a disease of unknown etiology, with the progressive destruction of the small intrahepatic bile ducts. The destruction is thought to be due to an immunologic process. The disease occurs primarily in women. The initial manifestation of the disease is usually pruritus, and the diagnosis is made at this stage when hepatomegaly is found upon physical examination and abnormal LFTs are found on an automated screening panel (SMA 12/60). Like cholestasis of pregnancy, the pruritus may develop during pregnancy, but in contrast to the cholestasis of pregnancy, the pruritus in primary biliary cirrhosis continues after delivery.

7 Rarely, pruritus may be associated with iron deficiency anemia and resolves with effective therapy. Pruritus has been reported in 15 to 50 per cent of patients with polycythemia vera. The itching is usually more severe with temperature changes, the patients often complaining of severe itching after showering. Pruritus is also one of the most common cutaneous manifestations of leukemia.

8 Approximately 6 per cent of patients with Hodgkin's lymphoma present with generalized severe pruritus without any other symptoms to suggest the diagnosis. It is unclear whether the presence of pruritus is a bad prognostic symptom, but pruritus has been dropped as a criterion for the B category in classifying Hodgkin's lymphoma. Itching usually starts on the legs, is continuous, and is associated with a burning sensation.

9 As many as 8 per cent of patients with thyrotoxicosis are bothered by generalized itching. Itching resolves when the euthyroid state is achieved after treatment. Itching associated with hypothyroidism is thought to be due primarily to dry skin.

10 Generalized pruritus is rare in diabetes mellitus (DM), estimated to affect about 3 per cent of patients with this disease. The severity of the itching does not generally correlate with the severity of the underlying disease. Localized itching is common in DM and may be associated with secondary fungal infections of the skin or mucous membranes, e.g., crural candidiasis.

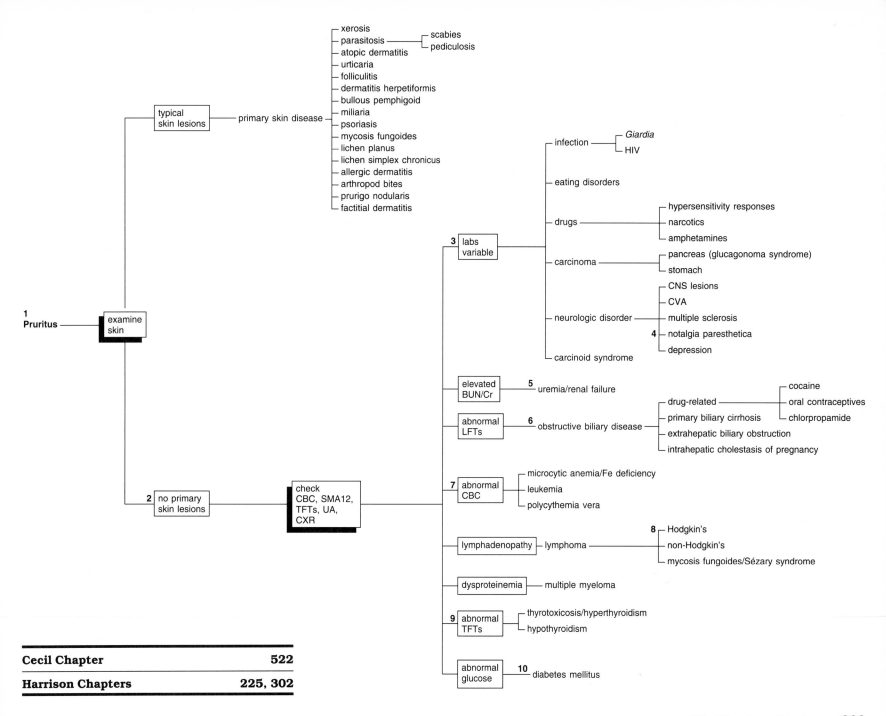

1
Pruritus

examine skin

typical skin lesions — primary skin disease
- xerosis
- parasitosis — scabies / pediculosis
- atopic dermatitis
- urticaria
- folliculitis
- dermatitis herpetiformis
- bullous pemphigoid
- miliaria
- psoriasis
- mycosis fungoides
- lichen planus
- lichen simplex chronicus
- allergic dermatitis
- arthropod bites
- prurigo nodularis
- factitial dermatitis

2 no primary skin lesions — check CBC, SMA12, TFTs, UA, CXR

3 labs variable
- infection — *Giardia* / HIV
- eating disorders
- drugs — hypersensitivity responses / narcotics / amphetamines
- carcinoma — pancreas (glucagonoma syndrome) / stomach
- neurologic disorder — CNS lesions / CVA / multiple sclerosis / **4** notalgia paresthetica / depression
- carcinoid syndrome

elevated BUN/Cr — **5** uremia/renal failure

abnormal LFTs — **6** obstructive biliary disease
- drug-related — cocaine / oral contraceptives / chlorpropamide
- primary biliary cirrhosis
- extrahepatic biliary obstruction
- intrahepatic cholestasis of pregnancy

7 abnormal CBC
- microcytic anemia/Fe deficiency
- leukemia
- polycythemia vera

lymphadenopathy — lymphoma — **8** Hodgkin's / non-Hodgkin's / mycosis fungoides/Sézary syndrome

dysproteinemia — multiple myeloma

9 abnormal TFTs — thyrotoxicosis/hyperthyroidism / hypothyroidism

10 abnormal glucose — diabetes mellitus

Cecil Chapter	**522**
Harrison Chapters	**225, 302**

Urticaria

1 Urticaria is the term used to describe evanescent skin lesions that are edematous (raised), circumscribed, erythematous, and usually intensely pruritic. Individual lesions of true urticaria typically last less than 6 hours and almost always less than 24 hours. Lesions persisting longer than 24 hours suggest the presence of angioedema or urticaria-like dermatoses such as drug eruptions or vasculitis. Angioedema, related to urticaria and initiated by similar mechanisms, is due to the extension of edema into the deep dermis or subcutaneous and submucosal layers. Urticaria and angioedema differ mainly in the depth of edema and may coexist in the same patient. Mediators of urticaria include IgE, complement, mast cells, and basophils, which release histamine and chemotactic factors.

2 Urticaria can be differentiated into acute and chronic forms on the basis of clinical duration. Even if the etiology of the urticaria is not apparent by initial history and physical examination, extensive evaluation is unwise because most urticaria clears spontaneously within a few months. Associated symptoms, such as fever or arthralgias, may warrant immediate further evaluation, however. In the majority of cases, further evaluation is warranted only if the lesions are recurrent for longer than 6 to 8 weeks. The condition is then known as chronic urticaria. The cause of both acute and chronic urticaria is rarely uncovered. In fact, up to 70 per cent of chronic urticaria is idiopathic. Although idiopathic urticaria is the most common form, it is a diagnosis of exclusion.

3 Urticaria results from the administration of radiocontrast media in as many as 5 per cent of patients. Opiates and antibiotics are other drugs commonly causing urticaria. The mechanism of drug-induced urticaria is thought to be histamine release from mast cells and basophils. Aspirin, nonsteroidal anti-inflammatory agents, azo dyes, benzoates, and thiazides are also well-known causes of urticaria, although the pathogenesis is unclear. Aspirin may exacerbate existing urticaria without being the etiologic agent of the underlying chronic urticaria.

4 Urticaria that occurs after direct contact with a variety of agents is known as contact urticaria. Chemicals, arthropod hairs, and stinging nettles may cause contact urticaria.

5 Serum sickness is manifested by fever, urticaria, lymphadenopathy, arthralgia, and myalgia. The reaction occurs 1 to 3 weeks following the administration of the offending agent, usually heterologous serum. As many as 70 per cent of patients with serum sickness manifest urticaria. The symptoms are thought to be due to an immune complex–induced vasculitis in which activation of complement may contribute the anaphylatoxins that induce mast cell degranulation.

6 Urticaria may occur during the prodrome of acute hepatitis B infection. The urticaria is thought to represent a necrotizing venulitis owing to complement activation.

7 Urticaria-like dermatoses are primary skin disorders that mimic urticaria but are distinctive and diagnostic histologically. Strictly speaking, a skin biopsy of a true urticarial lesion shows normal skin.

8 Angioedema is edema of the deep dermis and subcutaneous layers of skin, more often involving mucous membranes such as the lips. Lesions of angioedema, in contrast to those of urticaria, can last up to 72 hours. Measurement of the serum complement levels is helpful in detecting patients with angioedema. Serum C4 levels can be measured as a screening test. If serum C4 levels are low, further evaluation should include measurement of C1, C2, and C3 levels, as well as the levels and function of C1-esterase inhibitor protein. Low levels of or dysfunctional C1-esterase inhibitor is diagnostic of hereditary angioedema, which can be life-threatening. A low C1q level can be due to a paraneoplastic syndrome that consumes C1q, causing an acquired angioedema, such as occurs in rare cases with B-cell lymphoma.

9 Chronic urticaria may be a manifestation of a cutaneous vasculitis, which is an urticaria-like dermatosis. The urticaria may be associated with arthralgia, arthritis, glomerulonephritis, and abdominal pain. The disorder has been called the hypocomplementemic-urticaria-vasculitis syndrome.

10 Urticaria pigmentosa (cutaneous mastocytosis) is a condition in which increased numbers of mast cells are present in the skin. Urticaria is the result of mast cell degranulation that occurs with stroking of the skin lesions. Individual lesions of urticaria pigmentosa are hyperpigmented and papular when not urticated. Biopsy is diagnostic by demonstrating collections of mast cells in the dermis.

11 Pressure urticaria may arise immediately or be delayed 4 to 6 hours after constant pressure has been applied to the skin. The diagnosis is suggested by the location of the urticaria: under shoulder straps and belts, on the hands after manual labor, or on the feet after running.

12 Cold urticaria is induced by cold foods or liquids and may be associated with headache, syncope, and wheezing. Cold urticaria may be acquired or inherited as a dominant trait. Cryoproteins (including cold agglutinins) can be demonstrated in less than one third of these patients.

13 Pruritus and urticaria may accompany exposure to the sun or an artificial light source emitting certain wavelengths of light. The diagnosis is suggested by the distribution of lesions in light-exposed areas. Solar urticaria may be a manifestation of systemic lupus erythematosus (SLE), erythropoietic protoporphyria (EPP), or drug photosensitivity.

14 Heat urticaria is rare. The condition is manifested as urticaria at the site of locally applied heat.

15 The role of food as a cause of urticaria is difficult to assess. Foods frequently implicated as a source of urticaria include strawberries, shellfish, nuts, fish, and eggs. It is difficult to establish most foods as a source of urticaria with any objective certainty, but a dietary log can be used if foods are suspected. Elimination diets can also be helpful.

16 Chronic urticaria is considered idiopathic if no underlying cause can be found. The role of food and occult infection as causes of urticaria are difficult to assess because the urticaria can be coincident. Urticaria rarely precedes neoplasia but may be a presenting sign of lymphoma. The course of urticaria is unpredictable, although most patients experience gradual waning of lesions by 3 to 6 months.

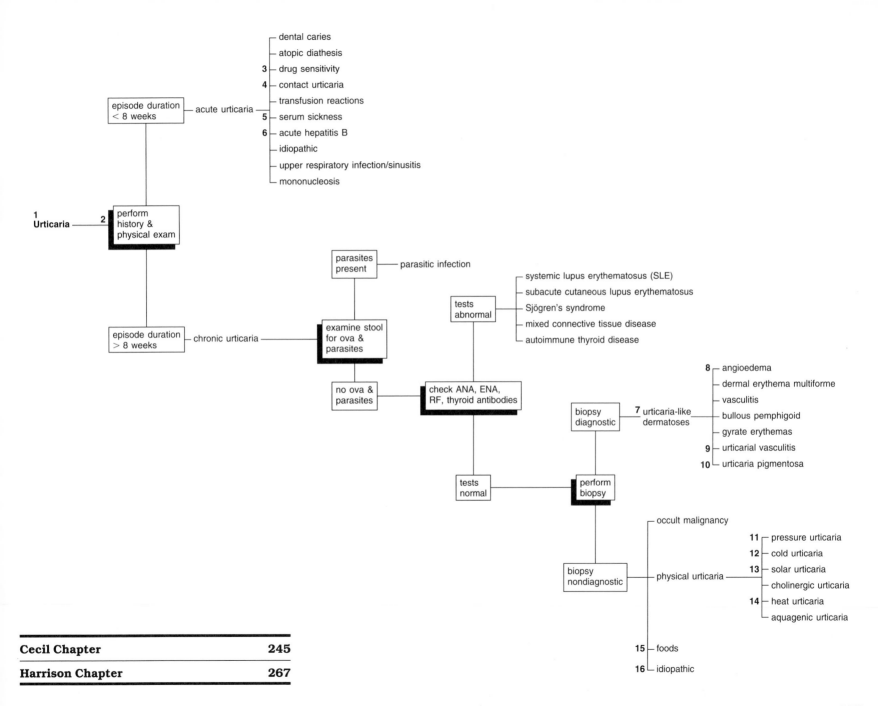

dental caries

atopic diathesis

3 drug sensitivity

4 contact urticaria

transfusion reactions

5 serum sickness

6 acute hepatitis B

idiopathic

upper respiratory infection/sinusitis

mononucleosis

episode duration < 8 weeks — acute urticaria

1
Urticaria — **2** perform history & physical exam

episode duration > 8 weeks — chronic urticaria

parasites present — parasitic infection

examine stool for ova & parasites

tests abnormal — systemic lupus erythematosus (SLE)

subacute cutaneous lupus erythematosus

Sjögren's syndrome

mixed connective tissue disease

autoimmune thyroid disease

no ova & parasites

check ANA, ENA, RF, thyroid antibodies

biopsy diagnostic — **7** urticaria-like dermatoses

8 angioedema

dermal erythema multiforme

vasculitis

bullous pemphigoid

gyrate erythemas

9 urticarial vasculitis

10 urticaria pigmentosa

tests normal

perform biopsy

biopsy nondiagnostic

occult malignancy

physical urticaria

11 pressure urticaria

12 cold urticaria

13 solar urticaria

cholinergic urticaria

14 heat urticaria

aquagenic urticaria

15 foods

16 idiopathic

Purpura

1 Purpura is a result of hemorrhage into the skin. Purpura includes petechiae, which are purpuric lesions less than 3 mm in diameter. Ecchymoses are larger purpuric lesions. Purpura is due to a qualitative or quantitative platelet disorder, a coagulation abnormality, or abnormal or inflamed blood vessels. If the platelet count is decreased, purpura is likely due to thrombocytopenia (see page 158).

2 If the platelet count and coagulation tests are normal, a bleeding time should be determined to ascertain platelet function. Platelet dysfunction is common with uremia and can also be responsible for the purpura accompanying dysproteinemias such as Waldenström's macroglobulinemia or multiple myeloma (see page 162).

3 If tests of platelet number and function are normal, purpura is due to abnormalities of the blood vessels. Blood vessels may lose their integrity owing to inflammation, which occurs with vasculitis, or to loss of adequate tissue support for the vessel, as seen in senile purpura.

4 Except for the presence of extravasated red blood cells, a biopsy of a purpuric lesion will be otherwise normal in steroid purpura, senile purpura, and purpura owing to trauma. Autoerythrocyte sensitization syndrome (Gardner-Diamond syndrome) is thought to be factitial, secondary to self-induced skin trauma.

5 Hereditary hemorrhage telangiectasia, or Osler-Weber-Rendu disease, is an autosomal dominant disorder in which purpura can occur secondary to vascular fragility. A developmental abnormality of the vasculature results in thin vessel walls with poor support and contractility. Mucous membrane bleeding, including gastrointestinal bleeding, is the most common clinical manifestation. The disorder is easily recognized by the presence of numerous telangiectasias, especially on the mucous membranes.

6 Amyloid deposition in the walls of cutaneous blood vessels is responsible for their fragility and subsequent bleeding. Common dermatologic manifestations of amyloidosis include petechiae and ecchymoses, most commonly on the eyelids and periorbital region. Minor trauma can cause these lesions, leading to the designation "pinch purpura."

7 Inflammatory change in the walls of blood vessels is known as vasculitis. Leukocytoclastic vasculitis is the term used pathologically to describe a constellation of changes that occur in and around the blood vessel wall owing to inflammation. A variety of conditions appear as a leukocytoclastic vasculitis histologically, the prototype being Henoch-Schönlein purpura. Palpable purpura is the clinical lesion that corresponds to a leukocytoclastic vasculitis histologically.

8 Purpuric drug eruptions represent a leukocytoclastic vasculitis believed to be due to immune complex deposition in the blood vessels. Drugs that have been associated with vasculitis include allopurinol, thiazides, sulfonamides, quinidine, phenytoin, nonsteroidal anti-inflammatory agents, tetracycline, penicillin, cimetidine, and ketoconazole.

9 Petechiae and purpura in the setting of acute infection are manifestations of vasculitis. Although vasculitis may accompany a variety of bacteremic infections, these skin findings are most diagnostically significant in acute and chronic meningococcemia and rickettsial infections. The presence of thrombi in the blood vessels is characteristic of the vasculitis that accompanies infection.

10 Henoch-Schönlein purpura is the prototype of leukocytoclastic vasculitis. In this condition, petechiae and palpable purpura are accompanied by arthralgias, abdominal pain with melena, hematuria resulting from glomerulonephritis, and occasionally dyspnea with pulmonary infiltrates. Both the skin and systemic manifestations are thought to be due to an IgA immune complex-induced vasculitis.

11 The cryoglobulins that occur in mixed cryoglobulinemia consist of circulating immune complexes, of which the most common combination is IgG-IgM. Mixed cryoglobulinemia may occur in association with autoimmune diseases such as Sjögren's syndrome, rheumatoid arthritis, and SLE. A leukocytoclastic vasculitis is usually not a feature of monoclonal cryoglobulinemia.

12 Wegener's granulomatosis is defined by the triad of necrotizing granulomata of the upper and lower respiratory tract, necrotizing vasculitis, and necrotizing glomerulitis. Skin lesions may consist of papulonecrotic lesions with ulceration in addition to purpura. These skin lesions are present in about 25 per cent of patients in the early stage of the disease, and in about half of the patients when the disease is more advanced.

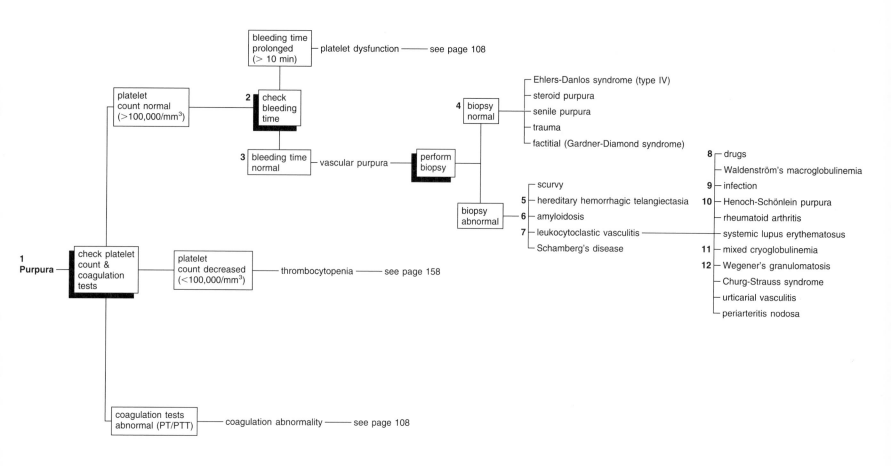

1 Purpura → check platelet count & coagulation tests

- platelet count normal (>100,000/mm³)
  - **2** check bleeding time
    - bleeding time prolonged (> 10 min) — platelet dysfunction ——— see page 108
    - **3** bleeding time normal — vascular purpura — perform biopsy
      - **4** biopsy normal
        - Ehlers-Danlos syndrome (type IV)
        - steroid purpura
        - senile purpura
        - trauma
        - factitial (Gardner-Diamond syndrome)
      - biopsy abnormal
        - scurvy
        - **5** hereditary hemorrhagic telangiectasia
        - **6** amyloidosis
        - **7** leukocytoclastic vasculitis
        - Schamberg's disease
- platelet count decreased (<100,000/mm³) — thrombocytopenia ——— see page 158
- coagulation tests abnormal (PT/PTT) — coagulation abnormality ——— see page 108

leukocytoclastic vasculitis:
- **8** drugs
- Waldenström's macroglobulinemia
- **9** infection
- **10** Henoch-Schönlein purpura
- rheumatoid arthritis
- systemic lupus erythematosus
- **11** mixed cryoglobulinemia
- **12** Wegener's granulomatosis
- Churg-Strauss syndrome
- urticarial vasculitis
- periarteritis nodosa

Cecil Chapters	154, 525
Harrison Chapter	59

Alopecia

1 Alopecia is the term used to describe hair loss. Most commonly the term refers to scalp hair loss, but it can be used to describe hair loss in other body regions. Hair loss secondary to structural abnormalities resulting in hair breakage are excluded from this classification of alopecia. The most common cause of alopecia is male pattern baldness (androgenetic alopecia).

2 The etiology of hair loss cannot always be determined, and the cause of certain alopecias is not fully understood. The most useful observation to help establish the diagnosis of alopecia, however, is the presence or absence of scarring. Scarring is a useful diagnostic as well as prognostic finding. The presence of scarring precludes hair regrowth because the hair follicle has been damaged or destroyed and it can no longer produce hair.

3 Both malignant and benign neoplasms can be responsible for follicular destruction and hair loss. Neoplasm is usually apparent on examination, and a biopsy will establish the diagnosis. At times, the biopsy will reveal an unsuspected tumor. Metastatic carcinoma to the skin, although rare, affects the scalp 3 to 8 per cent of the time. Almost half of metastatic tumors to the scalp, however, are unsuspected at the time of biopsy.

4 Infection is also apparent on examination, although at times the inflammation is so severe that the causative organism is difficult to culture and identify. Severe fungal infections, including kerions (severe, diffuse scalp inflammation complicating fungal infection of the hair), can lead to extensive scarring and hair loss. Viral infections, including herpes, can result in scarring and hair loss, usually because of the complication of secondary infection.

5 Discoid lupus erythematosus (DLE) may involve the scalp with a scarring alopecia. Although scarring alopecia may be seen in SLE, a noncicatricial alopecia is more commonly seen in this disorder. The lesions in DLE are usually atrophic and telangiectatic. Immunofluorescent staining of a biopsy specimen can be useful when an LE diagnosis is suspected.

6 Follicular mucinosis, also known as alopecia mucinosa, can lead to a scarring alopecia when mucin deposition in the outer root sheath causes follicular destruction. The alopecia is usually reversible and non-scarring. Fifteen per cent of patients over 40 years of age with follicular mucinosis have been reported to have concomitant mycosis fungoides, a T-cell lymphoma of the skin.

7 The presence of scar will be confirmed on biopsy but will be nondiagnostic when the scarring alopecia is due to traumatic destruction of the hair follicles by mechanical or physical means. History will provide the important clues to diagnosis as seen after radiation exposure or repeated trauma.

8 Nonscarring alopecia can accompany both hyper- and hypothyroidism, as well as hyper- and hypopituitarism, and may be either patchy or diffuse. Most commonly, hypothyroidism is accompanied by a diffuse alopecia that may also affect the lateral third of the eyebrows. Hair regrowth can usually be expected once the euthyroid state is reached.

9 Secondary or tertiary syphilis can be accompanied by a "moth-eaten" scalp alopecia. The lateral eyebrows may also manifest hair loss.

10 Rarely, alopecia can be due to iron deficiency.

11 Alopecia accompanying SLE is usually nonscarring. In addition to the patches of alopecia that can occur with SLE, a diffuse nonscarring alopecia can accompany acute disease exacerbations.

12 When scarring is absent, diagnosis of hair loss can be established on the basis of patient history and the pattern of the hair loss. Nutritional deficiencies in general can result in a diffuse alopecia, as has been observed in patients on prolonged inadequate parenteral hyperalimentation. Hair loss in this setting may have been due to zinc deficiency, as is observed in acrodermatitis enteropathica.

13 Telogen effluvium is a diffuse hair loss that occurs when the majority of hair follicles have synchronously entered the telogen (resting) stage of the hair cycle. Normally, approximately 20 per cent of follicles are in the telogen stage, resulting in a loss of less than 50 hairs a day. The anagen (growing) stage of the hair cycle accounts for the other 80 per cent of the hair follicles on a normal scalp. Hair loss is diffuse and may not be clinically apparent. The patient usually presents with the complaint of increased hair loss with shampooing, or greater numbers of hair noted in the comb or brush. The hair loss usually follows a physical or emotional stress by 3 to 6 months. Causes include severe illness, high fever, rapid weight loss, or severe psychiatric or emotional stress. The most common presentation is that of postpartum telogen effluvium, in which marked hair loss is noted several months post partum. A similar presentation has been observed in patients who have discontinued long-term use of birth control pills or high-dose systemic steroids.

14 Subconscious frequent hair manipulation may lead to the alopecia found in trichotillomania. A biopsy may be confirmatory, as distinct changes can be identified histologically. Histologic features include distorted hair follicles and perifollicular extravasated blood. Alopecia as a result of traction is apparent by the pattern of hair loss and the observed hair style.

15 Alopecia has been associated with a variety of hereditary syndromes as either a primary or a secondary feature. Many hereditary alopecias are considered to be congenital, although the alopecia may not be apparent at birth. Progeria is an example of a hereditary nonscarring alopecia in which there is a progressive loss of scalp, eyebrow, and eyelash hair in association with scleroderma-like changes in the skin.

16 Drugs are common causes of nonscarring alopecia. The most striking example is the anagen effluvium that accompanies treatment with chemotherapeutic agents. Anti-mitotic drugs such as cyclophosphamide, methotrexate, and actinomycin affect the rapidly dividing cells in anagen hair follicles. Because anagen hairs are primarily found on the scalp, the hair loss is usually confined to the scalp. Hair loss is rapid and diffuse, but regrowth can be expected when the drug is discontinued. Other drugs that result in hair loss include heparin, coumadin, vitamin A, propranolol, levodopa, and lithium.

17 Alopecia areata is also a common cause of non-cicatricial alopecia. The presence of exclamation-point hairs is a clue to diagnosis. The exclamation-point hair is due to a gradual taper of the proximal portion of the hair shaft as a result of a follicular insult. The alopecia may be mild or severe, ranging from coin-sized patches of hair loss in the scalp to a generalized loss of all body hair, which is known as alopecia universalis. Alopecia areata is not limited to the scalp and may occur in patches on the forearm, beard, or axillae, even if the scalp is not involved. Prognosis varies with the extent of hair loss and

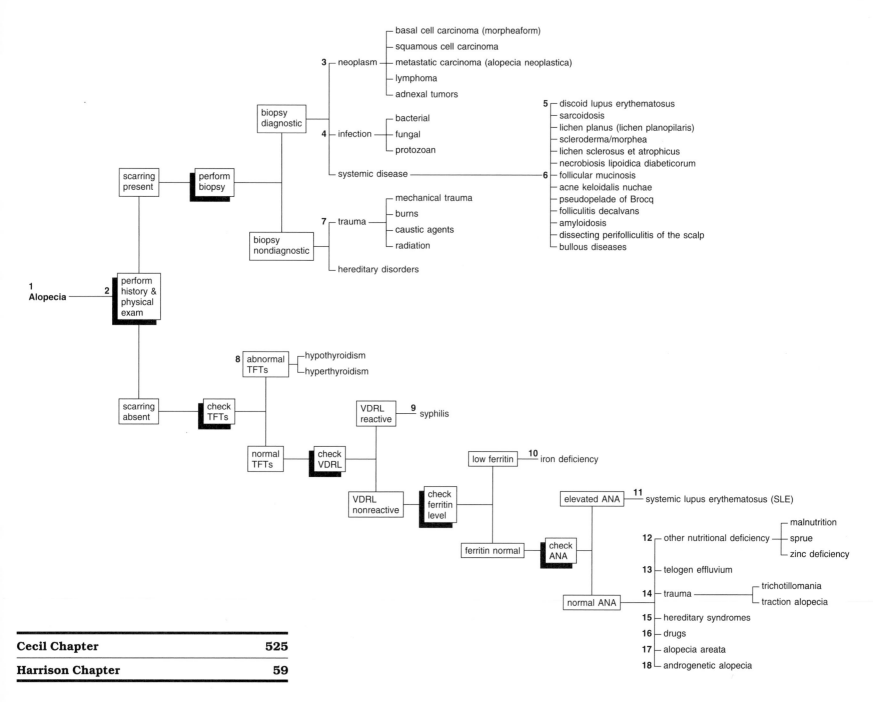

1
Alopecia

2 perform history & physical exam

scarring present

perform biopsy

biopsy diagnostic

3 neoplasm
- basal cell carcinoma (morpheaform)
- squamous cell carcinoma
- metastatic carcinoma (alopecia neoplastica)
- lymphoma
- adnexal tumors

4 infection
- bacterial
- fungal
- protozoan

systemic disease

5
- discoid lupus erythematosus
- sarcoidosis
- lichen planus (lichen planopilaris)
- scleroderma/morphea
- lichen sclerosus et atrophicus
- necrobiosis lipoidica diabeticorum
6 - follicular mucinosis
- acne keloidalis nuchae
- pseudopelade of Brocq
- folliculitis decalvans
- amyloidosis
- dissecting perifolliculitis of the scalp
- bullous diseases

biopsy nondiagnostic

7 trauma
- mechanical trauma
- burns
- caustic agents
- radiation

hereditary disorders

scarring absent

check TFTs

8 abnormal TFTs
- hypothyroidism
- hyperthyroidism

normal TFTs

check VDRL

VDRL reactive — **9** syphilis

VDRL nonreactive

check ferritin level

low ferritin — **10** iron deficiency

ferritin normal

check ANA

elevated ANA — **11** systemic lupus erythematosus (SLE)

normal ANA

12 other nutritional deficiency
- malnutrition
- sprue
- zinc deficiency

13 telogen effluvium

14 trauma
- trichotillomania
- traction alopecia

15 hereditary syndromes

16 drugs

17 alopecia areata

18 androgenetic alopecia

Cecil Chapter	525
Harrison Chapter	59

Alopecia (Continued)

the age of onset. Poor prognosis accompanies the loss of extensive amounts of hair or onset prior to puberty. When a small, stable number of patches is present, spontaneous regrowth can be anticipated within 6 to 12 months.

18 Androgenetic alopecia is the common "male-pattern" baldness that results from the combination of androgen level and an appropriate genetic make-up. The pattern of this type of hair loss in males is typical and presents as hair loss in the frontotemporal and vertex areas of the scalp, eventuating in a rim of hair on the posterior and lateral aspects of the scalp. Androgenetic alopecia occurs in women as well, although the pattern is one of diffuse hair loss that begins on the vertex of the scalp. In contrast to men, women with androgenetic alopecia tend to retain a thin rim of frontal hair while hair loss progresses on the top of the head. The presentation of a young woman with androgenetic alopecia should instigate a search for the source of excessive androgens, especially if other signs of virilization are also present. Women with hair loss beginning at age 50 or older should be considered to have senile or involutional alopecia.

BIBLIOGRAPHY

Cooper KD: Urticaria and angioedema: diagnosis and evaluation. J Am Acad Dermatol 25:166–176, 1991.

Denman ST: A review of pruritus. J Am Acad Dermatol 14(3):375–388, 1986.

Fitzpatrick TB, Eisen AZ, Wolff K, et al.: Dermatology in General Medicine. 3rd ed. New York, McGraw-Hill Book Company, 1987.

Kitchens CS: The purpuric disorders. Semin Thromb Hemost 10(3):36; 1984.

Lever WF, Schaumburg-Lever G: Histopathology of the Skin. 6th ed. Philadelphia, J. B. Lippincott Company, 1983.

Moschella SL, Hurley HJ: Dermatology. 2nd ed. Philadelphia, W. B. Saunders Company, 1985.

Olsen EA: Alopecia: evaluation and management. Prim Care 16(3):765–785, 1989.

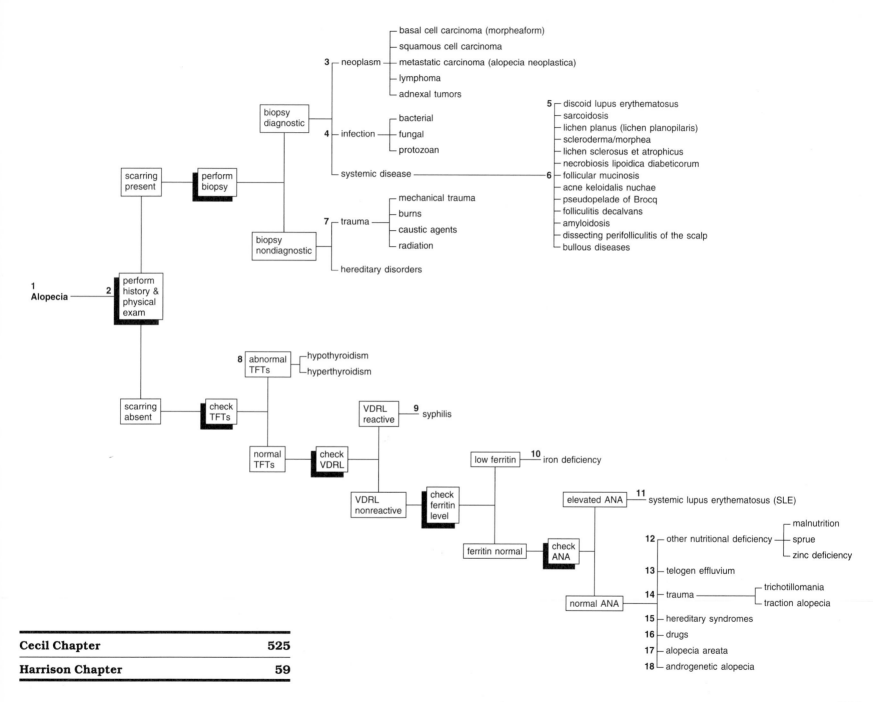

1
Alopecia

2 perform history & physical exam

scarring present

perform biopsy

biopsy diagnostic

3 neoplasm
- basal cell carcinoma (morpheaform)
- squamous cell carcinoma
- metastatic carcinoma (alopecia neoplastica)
- lymphoma
- adnexal tumors

4 infection
- bacterial
- fungal
- protozoan

systemic disease

6
- discoid lupus erythematosus
- sarcoidosis
- lichen planus (lichen planopilaris)
- scleroderma/morphea
- lichen sclerosus et atrophicus
- necrobiosis lipoidica diabeticorum
- follicular mucinosis
- acne keloidalis nuchae
- pseudopelade of Brocq
- folliculitis decalvans
- amyloidosis
- dissecting perifolliculitis of the scalp
- bullous diseases

biopsy nondiagnostic

7 trauma
- mechanical trauma
- burns
- caustic agents
- radiation

hereditary disorders

scarring absent

check TFTs

8 abnormal TFTs
- hypothyroidism
- hyperthyroidism

normal TFTs

check VDRL

VDRL reactive — **9** syphilis

VDRL nonreactive

check ferritin level

low ferritin — **10** iron deficiency

ferritin normal

check ANA

elevated ANA — **11** systemic lupus erythematosus (SLE)

normal ANA

12 other nutritional deficiency
- malnutrition
- sprue
- zinc deficiency

13 telogen effluvium

14 trauma
- trichotillomania
- traction alopecia

15 hereditary syndromes

16 drugs

17 alopecia areata

18 androgenetic alopecia

Cecil Chapter   **525**

Harrison Chapter   **59**

11 · Musculoskeletal Disorders

Signs and symptoms: Muscle weakness
Arthralgias/arthritis   Low back pain

Arthralgias/Arthritis

1 The differential diagnosis of arthralgias and arthritis is broad, encompassing more than 200 separate entities. The history and physical examination are aimed at defining the nature of the pain and identifying associated systemic factors that aid in diagnosis. Factors that must be weighed heavily include the number, pattern of distribution, and size of the joints involved, as well as the presence or absence of other systemic signs or symptoms. Whether pain is monoarticular, oligoarticular, or polyarticular and whether the joint is small or large are important factors to take into account diagnostically.

2 When a patient complains of arthralgia (joint pain), the initial step is to determine whether arthritis is also present. The signs of arthritis (true joint inflammation) include swelling, heat, redness, evidence of synovial thickening, tenderness upon palpation, and evidence of joint effusion. All joints must be assessed despite complaints of pain limited to one joint.

3 If no objective signs of arthritis are present, periarticular pain syndromes must be considered. Nonarticular or periarticular pain encompasses a large group of miscellaneous conditions that can be diagnosed on the basis of history and physical examination.

4 With objective evidence for true joint involvement, other clues obtained from the history and physical examination should be taken into account. It may be difficult to determine whether the arthritis is due to a primary rheumatic disease or secondary to some underlying systemic disease. Although an underlying disorder may already be diagnosed, it must be determined whether the joint symptoms are due to the disease or represent a separate, unrelated problem. Therefore, with any new onset of arthritis, joint fluid should be examined when possible. The clinical setting should always be taken into account prior to invasive diagnostic procedures such as a joint aspiration. Depending upon the clinical picture, sup-portive treatment can be undertaken initially, with joint rest and analgesics. Evaluation with radiographic examination and joint aspiration is undertaken if symptoms persist or progress.

5 Joint fluid examination is the most useful test in diagnosing joint inflammation. Radiologic examination may not be helpful in acute disease because many of the bone and joint space changes characteristic for a particular disease do not occur until late in the course of the disease. Synovial fluid should be analyzed for cell count and differential. Normal fluid contains a small number of mononuclear white cells, whereas infected joints contain primarily polymorphonuclear white cells. The fluid should also be examined for the presence of crystals and stained for bacterial, fungal, and acid-fast organisms. Measurement of joint fluid complement level is rarely diagnostic.

6 Examination of fluid for the presence of crystals must be performed with a polarizing microscope because crystals are difficult to identify with brightfield microscopy. The sodium urate crystals of gout are negatively birefringent and needle-shaped under the polarizing microscope. Clinically, gout presents as acute monoarticular arthritis. The first metatarsophalangeal joint is typically involved, but any joint or multiple joints can also be affected. Pseudogout presents in a similar manner to gout with acute monoarticular arthritis, but the crystals are calcium pyrophosphate. The calcium pyrophosphate crystals show positive birefringence under the polarizing microscope. Pseudogout may occur as a complication of hyperparathyroidism.

7 Stain for bacterial, fungal, and acid-fast organisms as well as the corresponding cultures should always be performed on aspirated joint fluid regardless of suspected diagnosis. Septic arthritis is considered on the basis of cell count and differential, because white cell counts are extremely elevated (50,000 to 200,000 cells/cm³) and neutrophils predominate (>80 per cent). Tuberculous arthritis results in fewer inflammatory cells (<25,000), and the differential is variable. Fungal and acid-fast stains are important because fungal and mycobacterial cultures may take many weeks to grow. Gonococcal arthritis may be missed unless a special medium (modified Thayer-Martin medium) is used to culture the joint fluid.

8 Common causes of pyogenic arthritis include staphylococci (accounting for approximately two thirds of cases), streptococci (15 per cent of cases), pseudomonas (15 per cent of cases), and pneumococci. Gram-negative bacillary joint infections are most often seen in immunocompromised patients. Gonococcal arthritis can be polyarticular early, but later typically affects one large joint. The initial joint symptoms in gonococcal arthritis are due to immune complex deposition and can involve many joints. Aspirated joint fluid at this stage will be culture-negative. As the disease progresses, true gonococcal infection settles, usually into one large joint, and aspirated joint fluid may reveal the gonococci on smear or culture. Because gonococcal arthritis is a complication of untreated primary gonorrhea, women may be affected more frequently, as gonococcal infections may progress undiagnosed because of the paucity of symptoms of primary infection in women. A skin rash consisting of a few periarticular pustules can be a clue to the diagnosis of gonococcal arthritis.

9 The white cell count and differential will help differentiate between inflammatory joint disease and degenerative joint disease. Markedly elevated white cell counts with a predominance of neutrophils are found in inflammatory joint disease such as crystalline arthritis (gout and pseudogout), infection, and inflammatory conditions of unknown etiology, such as rheumatoid arthritis.

10 Viral infections most commonly cause arthralgias without true arthritis but can cause transient polyarthritis, which usually resolves without sequelae. Rubella can cause viral arthritis, and symptoms may occur even following rubella vaccination. Varicella, viral hepatitis, infectious mononucleosis, and mumps are other viral diseases associated with polyarthritis. Arthritis as a result of viral joint involvement will be culture-negative, and the joint fluid can range from noninflammatory to severely inflammatory.

11 Metabolic conditions that result in noninflammatory arthritis include alkaptonuria (ochronosis), Wilson's disease, hemochromatosis, amyloidosis, and ac-

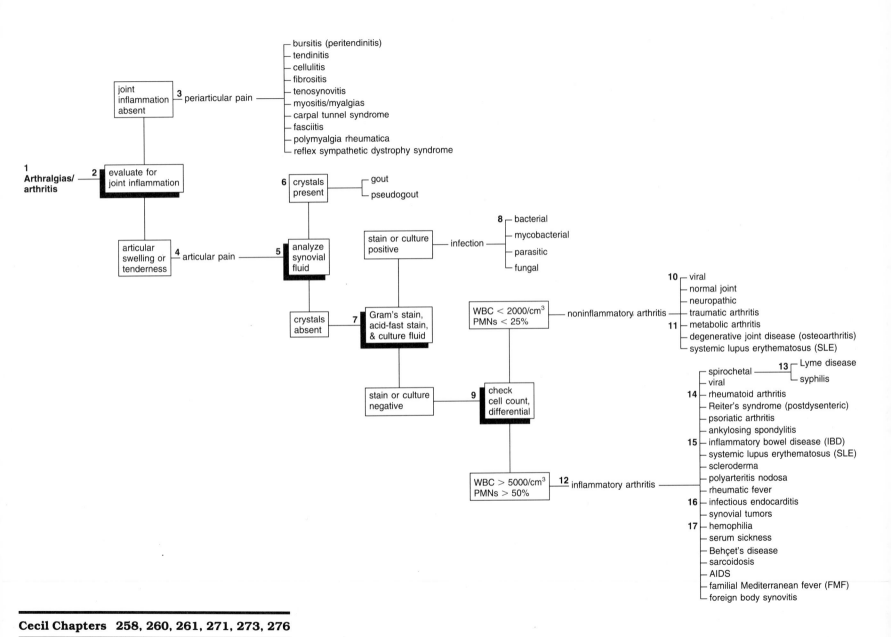

bursitis (peritendinitis)
tendinitis
cellulitis
fibrositis
tenosynovitis
myositis/myalgias
carpal tunnel syndrome
fasciitis
polymyalgia rheumatica
reflex sympathetic dystrophy syndrome

1
Arthralgias/
arthritis

2 evaluate for joint inflammation

joint inflammation absent — **3** periarticular pain

articular swelling or tenderness — **4** articular pain — **5** analyze synovial fluid

6 crystals present — gout / pseudogout

crystals absent — **7** Gram's stain, acid-fast stain, & culture fluid

stain or culture positive — infection — **8** bacterial / mycobacterial / parasitic / fungal

stain or culture negative — **9** check cell count, differential

WBC < 2000/cm³ PMNs < 25% — noninflammatory arthritis — **10** viral / normal joint / neuropathic / traumatic arthritis / **11** metabolic arthritis / degenerative joint disease (osteoarthritis) / systemic lupus erythematosus (SLE)

WBC > 5000/cm³ PMNs > 50% — **12** inflammatory arthritis —
spirochetal — **13** Lyme disease / syphilis
viral
14 rheumatoid arthritis
Reiter's syndrome (postdysenteric)
psoriatic arthritis
ankylosing spondylitis
15 inflammatory bowel disease (IBD)
systemic lupus erythematosus (SLE)
scleroderma
polyarteritis nodosa
rheumatic fever
16 infectious endocarditis
synovial tumors
17 hemophilia
serum sickness
Behçet's disease
sarcoidosis
AIDS
familial Mediterranean fever (FMF)
foreign body synovitis

Cecil Chapters 258, 260, 261, 271, 273, 276

Harrison Chapter   280

Arthralgias/Arthritis (Continued)

romegaly. Storage disease (Gaucher's) can also result in a noninflammatory arthritis.

12 The inflammatory arthritides that have not been identified as crystalline or infectious in nature must be differentiated on the basis of detailed history, physical examination, and serologies. Important factors that must be taken into account include the number, size, and pattern of joint involvement, the presence or absence of systemic symptoms, and the subsequent clinical course. Other helpful diagnostic aids include radiographic examination of both involved and noninvolved joints and needle biopsy of the synovium, which may be supportive or diagnostic. Both computed tomography (CT) and magnetic resonance imaging (MRI) are being used to evaluate joints (such as the sacroiliac joints), that are difficult to evaluate clinically with MRI particularly useful in visualizing the synovium.

13 Lyme disease is caused by the spirochete *Borrelia burgdorferi*. Arthritis follows infection by a tick bite. A characteristic skin rash (erythema chronicum migrans) can precede the arthritis by several weeks and can be the hallmark of the disease. If the rash is identified and the patient treated, subsequent arthritis may be avoided. Serologic Lyme titers can be measured if the patient's history is suggestive of a risk of infection.

14 Rheumatoid arthritis is a chronic systemic disease without known etiology. The disease manifestations are primarily articular, with progressive symmetric inflammatory destruction of the peripheral joints. Systemic manifestations are rare and diverse and include pleural effusions, splenomegaly, and peripheral neuropathy. The onset of the disease is usually insidious, with complaints of fatigue, weakness, myalgia, and morning joint stiffness as the initial manifestations.

15 Arthritis may accompany ulcerative colitis in approximately one fifth of patients and affects approximately 10 per cent of patients with Crohn's disease. Arthritis may also affect as many as 60 per cent of patients with Whipple's disease.

16 Infectious endocarditis can be accompanied by an acute polyarthritis of the large joints. The polyarthritis may be migratory and resembles septic arthritis clinically, but the joint fluid is sterile. The arthritis is thought to be immunologically mediated.

17 Bleeding diatheses such as hemophilia result in recurrent hemarthrosis and gradual joint destruction. The diagnosis can be suspected in the presence of a bloody joint aspiration with a history of minimal trauma.

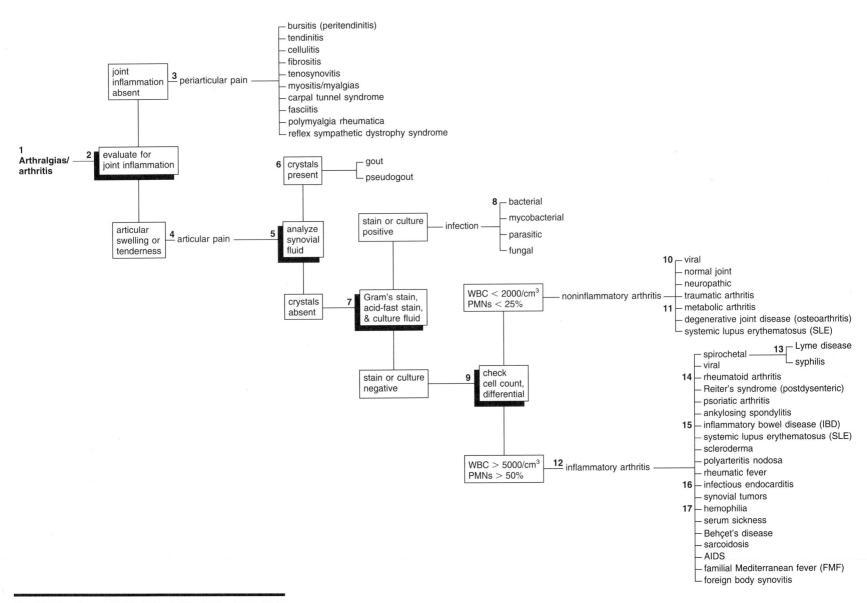

bursitis (peritendinitis)
tendinitis
cellulitis
fibrositis
tenosynovitis
myositis/myalgias
carpal tunnel syndrome
fasciitis
polymyalgia rheumatica
reflex sympathetic dystrophy syndrome

joint
inflammation
absent

3 periarticular pain

1
Arthralgias/
arthritis

2 evaluate for
joint inflammation

6 crystals
present

gout
pseudogout

8 bacterial
mycobacterial
parasitic
fungal

stain or culture
positive

infection

articular
swelling or
tenderness

4 articular pain

5 analyze
synovial
fluid

crystals
absent

7 Gram's stain,
acid-fast stain,
& culture fluid

10 viral
normal joint
neuropathic
traumatic arthritis
11 metabolic arthritis
degenerative joint disease (osteoarthritis)
systemic lupus erythematosus (SLE)

WBC < 2000/cm³
PMNs < 25%

noninflammatory arthritis

stain or culture
negative

9 check
cell count,
differential

spirochetal
13 Lyme disease
syphilis
viral
14 rheumatoid arthritis
Reiter's syndrome (postdysenteric)
psoriatic arthritis
ankylosing spondylitis
15 inflammatory bowel disease (IBD)
systemic lupus erythematosus (SLE)
scleroderma
polyarteritis nodosa
rheumatic fever
16 infectious endocarditis
synovial tumors
17 hemophilia
serum sickness
Behçet's disease
sarcoidosis
AIDS
familial Mediterranean fever (FMF)
foreign body synovitis

WBC > 5000/cm³
PMNs > 50%

12 inflammatory arthritis

Cecil Chapters   258, 260, 261, 271, 273, 276

Harrison Chapter   280

Muscle Weakness

1 The diagnosis of muscle weakness is difficult owing to the diversity of causes and to the fact that there are no tests that, taken alone, are diagnostic for a particular disorder. Muscle weakness is diagnosed by the evaluation of both clinical and laboratory abnormalities. The constellation of abnormalities, including age of onset, pattern of muscle involvement, associated systemic symptoms, and clinical course, is the key to diagnosis. There is considerable overlap among the various clinical manifestations of muscle disease, making accurate diagnosis more difficult. Multiple tests may be necessary to confirm a suspected diagnosis.

2 Muscle weakness can be due to a primary muscle disorder or to neurologic dysfunction. A complete neurologic examination is essential as part of the history and physical examination. Muscle pain, however, may prevent full effort by the patient, resulting in perceived muscle weakness by the examiner. Cerebral and upper motor neuron disease is not difficult to identify, because weakness in these disorders is usually manifested as hemiparesis or other gross abnormalities. A primary myopathy may be difficult to differentiate from a neurogenic myopathy when neurologic dysfunction involves the anterior horn cells, the nerve roots, or the peripheral nerves. A variety of both clinical clues and test abnormalities helps to distinguish a neuropathic myopathy from a primary myopathy. In general, distal limb weakness is likely secondary to a neurogenic disorder, whereas proximal limb weakness is more likely myopathic. Muscle fasciculation never occurs in myopathy and is seen primarily with chronic motor neuron diseases but rarely with peripheral neuropathy. Cutaneous sensory loss suggests peripheral neuropathy. Laboratory data such as muscle enzymes, electromyogram (EMG), or muscle biopsy can confirm the diagnosis.

3 The source of myopathy can be a metabolic derangement or one of the collagen-vascular diseases or muscular dystrophies. Appropriate metabolic tests should be performed based on the history and physical examination. In general, metabolic abnormalities result in an acute or subacute onset of muscle weakness in which the weakness progresses over days to weeks. Transient or intermittent muscle weakness is usually due to a metabolic derangement and can be secondary to hypoka-lemia caused by drug use or due to familial periodic paralysis. The latter is an autosomal dominant disorder in which serum potassium falls precipitously during attacks of muscle weakness.

4 Rhabdomyolysis is the rapid destruction of muscle tissue. With muscle destruction, large amounts of myoglobin and other cellular products are released into the bloodstream and excreted by the kidney. Approximately 50 per cent of patients with rhabdomyolysis develop acute renal failure as a result of the release of these proteins. Myoglobinuria can be seen in approximately 50 per cent of patients with dermatomyositis, polymyositis, and many of the other progressive muscle diseases. Acute alcoholic myopathy is due to muscle necrosis occurring after a heavy bout of drinking. Urine myoglobin and serum muscle enzymes are markedly elevated. Chronic alcoholic myopathy is probably secondary to a progressive peripheral neuropathy rather than being a primary myopathy.

5 Polymyositis (PM) and dermatomyositis (DM) are relatively common diseases that manifest clinically as proximal limb weakness and aching. Dermatomyositis is accompanied by characteristic skin changes. The clinical manifestations of polymyositis can occur in isolation or can be associated with other collagen diseases such as rheumatoid arthritis, scleroderma, or systemic lupus erythematosus. An underlying malignancy is thought to account for the clinical symptoms in approximately 10 per cent of patients with DM and PM. The muscle changes can precede the detection of malignancy by as much as 2 years. The diagnosis of idiopathic PM/DM is based on the clinical picture, elevated muscle enzymes, EMG, and muscle biopsy. No single criterion is diagnostic. Probably less than one fourth of all patients demonstrate the characteristic abnormalities in all four categories.

6 The muscular dystrophies are a group of genetic diseases that cause progressive muscle weakness and wasting. Most of these disorders begin in infancy or childhood, although a few manifest as late as middle age. Serum muscle enzymes are markedly elevated in some of the muscular dystrophies and are normal in others. The diagnosis is based upon the clinical picture, including the mode of inheritance, the localization of involvement, the disease's progression, and its associated features. Serum muscle enzyme abnormalities, EMG abnormalities, and muscle biopsy are not diagnostic but are used as adjunctive information in defining the myopathy and in ruling out other myopathic or neuropathic disorders.

7 Although nonspecific, an elevated erythrocyte sedimentation rate (ESR) may allow for identification of one of the collagen-vascular disease-associated myopathies. If muscle enzymes are not elevated, an elevation of the ESR in the face of clinical weakness would justify the use of the EMG to identify disease.

8 Polymyalgia rheumatica (PMR) presents as shoulder or hip girdle pain in the elderly. Muscles appear weak clinically owing to the poor effort by the patient secondary to pain. The diagnosis is made when the EMG is normal but the erythrocyte sedimentation rate (ESR) is markedly elevated. PMR is associated with an increased incidence of temporal arteritis.

9 A variety of drugs can cause muscle weakness, but more commonly drugs unmask muscle weakness that was not clinically apparent. Even in the face of drug use, other etiologies of muscle weakness should be sought. However, if evaluation of muscle weakness is negative, the drug should be discontinued and the patient observed clinically. If weakness resolves, the muscle weakness can be assumed to be drug-induced. If the weakness persists despite discontinuation of the drug, an EMG and a muscle biopsy should be performed.

10 Steroid myopathy is muscle weakness resulting from the administration of systemic steroids. A similar myopathy may accompany Cushing's syndrome, in which adrenal corticosteroids are elevated. The proximal muscles of the limbs are primarily affected. The severity of muscle weakness is poorly correlated with steroid dose, and the onset of the symptoms is variable, occurring within weeks to months after the initiation of corticosteroids.

11 Congenital myopathies are due to a metabolic or structural abnormality of the muscle fiber. Serum muscle enzyme levels are usually normal, the disease is slowly progressive over many years, and muscle biopsy is usually diagnostic. Muscle biopsy alone is diagnostic of the rare congenital myopathies and of myopathy associated with infection, sarcoidosis, amyloidosis, and vasculitis.

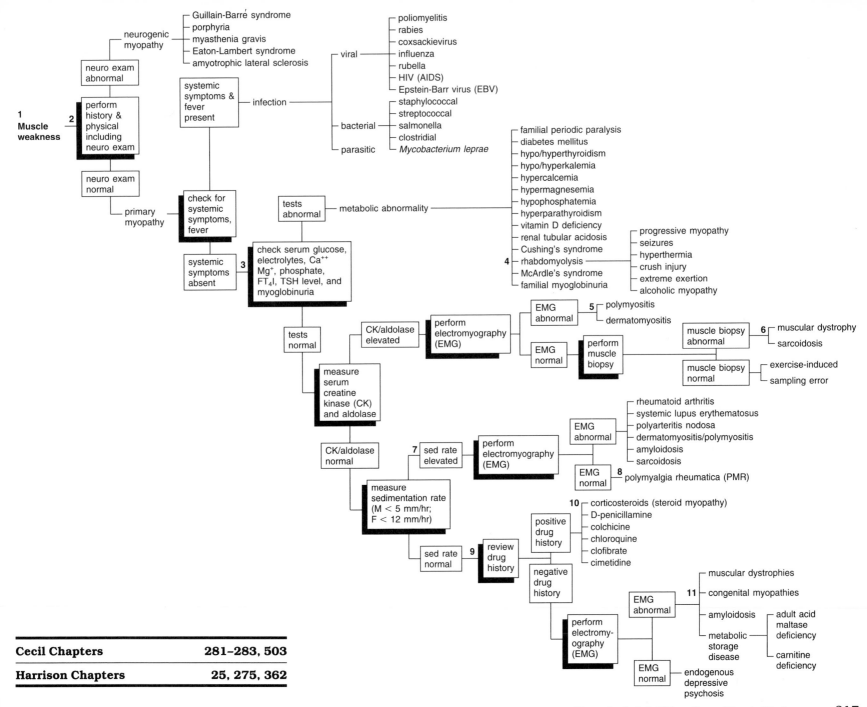

1 Muscle weakness

2 perform history & physical including neuro exam

neuro exam abnormal → neurogenic myopathy → Guillain-Barré syndrome / porphyria / myasthenia gravis / Eaton-Lambert syndrome / amyotrophic lateral sclerosis

neuro exam normal → primary myopathy

check for systemic symptoms, fever

systemic symptoms & fever present → infection:
- viral → poliomyelitis / rabies / coxsackievirus / influenza / rubella / HIV (AIDS) / Epstein-Barr virus (EBV)
- bacterial → staphylococcal / streptococcal / salmonella / clostridial
- parasitic → *Mycobacterium leprae*

3 systemic symptoms absent → check serum glucose, electrolytes, Ca^{++} Mg$^+$, phosphate, FT$_4$I, TSH level, and myoglobinuria

tests abnormal → metabolic abnormality → familial periodic paralysis / diabetes mellitus / hypo/hyperthyroidism / hypo/hyperkalemia / hypercalcemia / hypermagnesemia / hypophosphatemia / hyperparathyroidism / vitamin D deficiency / renal tubular acidosis / Cushing's syndrome / **4** rhabdomyolysis / McArdle's syndrome / familial myoglobinuria

rhabdomyolysis → progressive myopathy / seizures / hyperthermia / crush injury / extreme exertion / alcoholic myopathy

tests normal → measure serum creatine kinase (CK) and aldolase

CK/aldolase elevated → perform electromyography (EMG)
- EMG abnormal → **5** polymyositis / dermatomyositis
- EMG normal → perform muscle biopsy
  - muscle biopsy abnormal → **6** muscular dystrophy / sarcoidosis
  - muscle biopsy normal → exercise-induced / sampling error

CK/aldolase normal → measure sedimentation rate (M < 5 mm/hr; F < 12 mm/hr)

7 sed rate elevated → perform electromyography (EMG)
- EMG abnormal → rheumatoid arthritis / systemic lupus erythematosus / polyarteritis nodosa / dermatomyositis/polymyositis / amyloidosis / sarcoidosis
- EMG normal → **8** polymyalgia rheumatica (PMR)

sed rate normal → **9** review drug history
- positive drug history → **10** corticosteroids (steroid myopathy) / D-penicillamine / colchicine / chloroquine / clofibrate / cimetidine
- negative drug history → perform electromyography (EMG)
  - EMG abnormal → **11** muscular dystrophies / congenital myopathies / amyloidosis / metabolic storage disease → adult acid maltase deficiency / carnitine deficiency
  - EMG normal → endogenous depressive psychosis

Cecil Chapters	281–283, 503
Harrison Chapters	25, 275, 362

Low Back Pain

1 Low back pain is one of the most common physical complaints and is a major cause of lost work time. Most back pain is benign, and the majority of patients recover within 3 months. Less than 5 per cent of patients suffer from chronic back pain, of which only a small number have an underlying serious disease.

2 In the initial evaluation of low back pain, a complete history and physical examination should identify patients with potentially serious disease who require more extensive, immediate evaluation. The evaluation should include a complete neurologic examination. If neurologic examination uncovers muscle weakness, sensory deficits, or loss of reflexes, further prompt evaluation is indicated. In the appropriate clinical setting, the diagnosis of an abdominal aortic aneurysm should always be considered during the initial evaluation, because the mortality associated with rupture is greater than 50 per cent.

3 If neurologic findings including bowel or bladder dysfunction are present, or the physical examination is abnormal, CT or MRI should be utilized immediately.

4 Rapid onset of severe lower back pain suggests rupture or dissection of an abdominal aortic aneurysm. The diagnosis can be suspected when physical examination demonstrates a midepigastric pulsating mass. Retroperitoneal leakage of the aneurysm may result in radiation of pain to the posterior thighs. Unlike acute musculoskeletal pain in which the patient can usually find a position in which the pain is relieved, the patient with a leaking or dissecting aortic aneurysm experiences persistent pain despite position. Most abdominal aortic aneurysms are secondary to arteriosclerosis and are therefore found most often in men over 50 years old. Greater than 50 per cent of these patients have associated hypertension.

5 At times, acute lumbosacral strain can be so severe that physical examination is unable to distinguish between true weakness and weakness owing to pain. In these cases, if CT examination is normal, supportive treatment can be undertaken initially, with further evaluation if symptoms progress or pain does not resolve (see No. 6).

6 Most back pain has an acute onset, usually accompanied by a history of new, different, or vigorous physical activity. In this setting, if neurologic examination is normal and vascular rupture is unlikely, the patient can be treated supportively, with further, more extensive evaluation if the pain does not subside within several weeks. Radiographic studies are sometimes performed with the initial evaluation of back pain, but the radiographic abnormalities may not be associated with the current episode of pain.

7 Plain radiographs are relatively inexpensive and can be quite helpful in identifying a variety of abnormalities, ranging from bone lesions to kidney stones. Many of the changes that are identified by radiographs are suggestive but not diagnostic for a particular disorder, so that further study might be needed in order to confirm a diagnosis. In addition, some findings on radiography may be coincidental or contributory rather than causative of the current episode of back pain.

8 Degenerative joint disease (DJD) is probably the most common cause of chronic low back pain in persons over 50 years old. DJD is actually degenerative disc disease in which the disc has gradually collapsed with time. This alters the mechanical balance between the bony structures, including the intervertebral facet joints, resulting in pain. The patient experiences a baseline chronic low back pain with episodic occurrences of acute pain. Radiographic examination reveals disc space narrowing and marginal osteophytes along the vertebral margins.

9 Various benign and malignant pelvic disorders can be common causes for low back pain. These disorders include endometriosis, uterine fibroids, menstrual cramps, and even pregnancy. In the male, prostatic disorders, including chronic prostatitis, can result in low back pain. Some pelvic disorders, such as tumors, may be suspected on the basis of radiographs and confirmed by pelvic examination. CT or MRI may help to delineate the size and extent of pelvic tumors.

10 Based on physical findings and plain radiographs, further study may be undertaken if a diagnosis cannot be made with certainty. CT is a sensitive tool for the diagnosis of lumbar spine lesions that result in nerve root encroachment and irritation. A radionuclide bone scan can be a sensitive detector of early bone lesions when the lesions are not yet apparent on conventional radiographs.

11 Spinal infections are difficult to diagnose. Infection may involve the disc space or the bony structures of the spine. Radiographic studies may not be helpful unless a frank abscess or osteomyelitis is present, and MRI or CT may be more sensitive in detecting infection. Epidural abscess formation occurs in the setting of a history of bacteremia with the subsequent insidious development of diffuse low back pain occurring over days to weeks. Rapid progression of pain with radicular symptoms and limb weakness is an indication of the presence of an epidural abscess. Tuberculous arthritis of the spine begins in the vertebral body and ultimately leads to vertebral collapse. Acute pyelonephritis may present as low back pain, although commonly it is referred to the flank.

12 Herniated discs are not well identified on plain films but can be easily identified on CT or MRI scans. MRI may identify degenerative disc disease not visualized with CT. Disc herniations are most common at the L4-L5 or L5-S1 levels. Disc herniation at the L5 level may cause the typical pain of sciatica, with pain radiating from the back into the posterior thigh, the anterolateral leg, and the dorsolateral foot. Back pain secondary to disc disease characteristically is exacerbated by coughing or sneezing.

13 Back pain that has an onset after continuous walking is suggestive of arterial insufficiency that can result from spinal stenosis or spinal claudication. The patient complains of an aching, cramping pain in the lower back or buttocks that occurs after walking. The pain can be relieved by sitting or lying down but returns when activity is resumed. Physical examination is normal when the patient is at rest, but if the patient is examined immediately after activity, abnormalities such as weakness and reflex and sensory abnormalities will be confirmed. The CT scan is invaluable in diagnosis if the claudication-like symptoms are due to spinal stenosis.

14 PMR is a syndrome that occurs in elderly patients, most frequently as insidious shoulder pain and stiffness, associated with a markedly elevated ESR, oftentimes as high as 100 mm/hr. PMR may occur as hip girdle pain and low back pain. The significance of diagnosis of PMR is its association with temporal arteritis in 30 to 50 per cent of these patients. Temporal arteritis may lead to blindness if left undiagnosed and untreated.

15 Complaints of back pain with a paucity of abnormalities on physical exam, in the setting of secondary gain, suggest malingering. Malingering should be a diagnosis of exclusion, however, because severe lesions can, at times, be accompanied by a normal physical examination. Drug-dependent patients may complain of on-

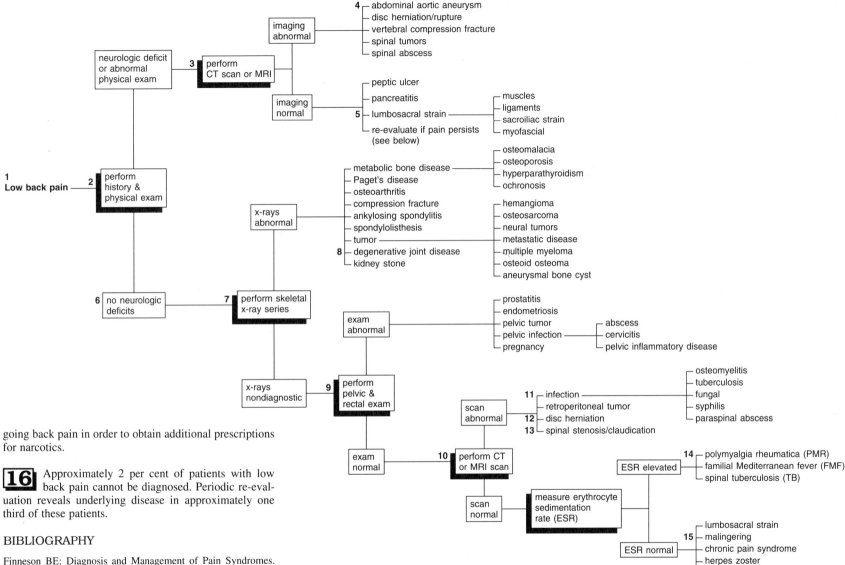

1 Low back pain

2 perform history & physical exam

neurologic deficit or abnormal physical exam

3 perform CT scan or MRI

imaging abnormal
4 — abdominal aortic aneurysm
— disc herniation/rupture
— vertebral compression fracture
— spinal tumors
— spinal abscess

imaging normal
— peptic ulcer
— pancreatitis
5 — lumbosacral strain — muscles
— ligaments
— sacroiliac strain
— myofascial
— re-evaluate if pain persists (see below)

6 no neurologic deficits

7 perform skeletal x-ray series

x-rays abnormal
— metabolic bone disease — osteomalacia
— osteoporosis
— hyperparathyroidism
— ochronosis
— Paget's disease
— osteoarthritis
— compression fracture — hemangioma
— ankylosing spondylitis — osteosarcoma
— spondylolisthesis — neural tumors
— tumor — metastatic disease
8 — degenerative joint disease — multiple myeloma
— kidney stone — osteoid osteoma
— aneurysmal bone cyst

x-rays nondiagnostic

9 perform pelvic & rectal exam

exam abnormal
— prostatitis
— endometriosis
— pelvic tumor
— pelvic infection — abscess
— cervicitis
— pregnancy — pelvic inflammatory disease

exam normal

10 perform CT or MRI scan

scan abnormal
11 — infection — osteomyelitis
— tuberculosis
— fungal
— syphilis
— paraspinal abscess
— retroperitoneal tumor
12 — disc herniation
13 — spinal stenosis/claudication

scan normal

measure erythrocyte sedimentation rate (ESR)

ESR elevated
14 — polymyalgia rheumatica (PMR)
— familial Mediterranean fever (FMF)
— spinal tuberculosis (TB)

ESR normal
— lumbosacral strain
15 — malingering
— chronic pain syndrome
— herpes zoster
16 — re-evaluate if pain persists

going back pain in order to obtain additional prescriptions for narcotics.

16 Approximately 2 per cent of patients with low back pain cannot be diagnosed. Periodic re-evaluation reveals underlying disease in approximately one third of these patients.

BIBLIOGRAPHY

Finneson BE: Diagnosis and Management of Pain Syndromes. Philadelphia, W. B. Saunders Company, 1969.
Hickling P, Golding JR: An Outline of Rheumatology. Bristol, John Wright & Sons Ltd., 1984.
Katz WA: Rheumatic Diseases: Diagnosis and Management. Philadelphia, J. B. Lippincott Company, 1977.
Kaye JJ: Arthritis: roles of radiography and other imaging techniques in evaluation. Radio *177*:601–608, 1990.
Lewis RC: Primary Care Orthopedics. New York, Churchill Livingstone, 1988.

Martinelli TA, Wiesel SW: Low back pain: the algorithmic approach. Compr Ther *17*(6):22–27, 1991.
Moskowitz RW: Clinical Rheumatology: A Problem-Oriented Approach to Diagnosis and Management. Philadelphia, Lea & Febiger, 1982.
Rothschild BM: Rheumatology: A Primary Care Approach. New York, Yorke Medical Books, 1982.
Sanchez RB, Quinn SF: MRI of inflammatory synovial processes. Magn Reson Imaging *7*:529–540, 1989.

Cecil Chapter	275
Harrison Chapter	19

Index

Note: Page numbers in *italics* refer to algorithms.

Isoimmune hemolytic disease, 126
Itching, 202, *203*
  urticaria and, 204

J

Jaundice, 64–65, *65*
  cholestatic, 64, 72
    of pregnancy, pruritus and, 202
Jodbasedow phenomenon, 188
Joint(s), degenerative disease of, 218
  inflammation of, 212, *213*, 214, *215*
Joint pain, 212, *213*, 214, *215*

K

Ketoacidosis, diabetic, 104
  generalized abdominal pain and, 56
  hyperkalemia and, 88
  hyperphosphatemia and, 98
  hypokalemia and, 86
  hypophosphatemia and, 96
  hypermagnesemia and, 102
Kidney(s). See *Renal* entries.
Kostmann's disease, 142

L

Lactic acidosis, 104
Lactic dehydrogenase, in ascitic fluid, 70
  in myocardial infarction, 24
Laparoscopy, in pelvic pain, 62
Laxatives, abuse of, causing acute diarrhea, 40
    causing chronic diarrhea, 42
    constipation and, 38
  hyperphosphatemia and, 98
Lazy leukocyte syndrome, 142
Lead colic, 58
Lead poisoning, 120
  generalized abdominal pain and, 56
Left lower quadrant abdominal pain, 60, *61*
Left upper quadrant abdominal pain, 52, *53*
Leukemia, acute myeloid, 144
  chronic myelogenous, 144
  eosinophilic, 154
  hypokalemia in, 86
  vs. aplastic anemia, 140
Leukemoid reaction, chronic, 144
Leukocytoclastic vasculitis, 206
Leukocytosis, 144
Leukoerythroblastosis, 146
Liddle's syndrome, 86, 106
Lipase, serum, abdominal pain and, 52

Lipoprotein(s), 194
Lipoprotein lipase deficiency, familial, 194
Lithium-induced hypercalcemia, 94
Liver, fatty infiltration of, 68
  inflammation of. See *Hepatitis* entries.
Liver disease, cholestatic, pruritus and, 202
  chronic, anemia of, 122
  cirrhosis as, 68
    ascites and, 70
  hepatomegaly and, 66, 68
  hypoglycemia and, 200
  impaired coagulation and, 109
Liver function tests, in jaundice, 64–65
Löffler's syndrome, 154
Low back pain, 218–219, *219*
Low-density lipoprotein, 194
Lung(s). See also *Pulmonary* entries.
  biopsy of, for cough, 12
  interstitial disease of, cough and, 12
    dyspnea and, 14
Lyme disease, 214
Lymphadenopathy, 112, *113*
Lymphedema, 30
Lymphocytic thyroiditis, subacute, 188
Lymphocytosis, 150, *151*
Lymphoma, 112
  fever of unknown origin associated with, 4
  in intrahepatic cholestasis, 64
  urticaria and, 204
Lysine hydrochloric acid, hyperkalemia and, 88

M

Macrocytic anemia, 130, *131*
Macroglobulinemia, Waldenström's, 162
  purpura and, 206
Magnesium, selective malabsorption of, 100
Magnesium sulfate, hypermagnesemia and, 102
Magnesium-containing antacids, causing diarrhea, 38, 40
Magnetic resonance imaging (MRI), of renal arteries, 32
Malabsorption, of vitamin D, 92
  selective, of magnesium, 100
Malabsorption syndrome, chronic diarrhea and, 42
Male-pattern baldness, 210
Malignancy. See *Cancer*.
Malnutrition, edema associated with, 30
  hypomagnesemia and, 100
  hypophosphatemia and, 96
  iron deficiency anemia and, 120
Mastocytosis, cutaneous, 204
Mean corpuscular hemoglobin concentration, calculation of, 118
Mean corpuscular volume, calculation of, 118
Meckel's diverticulum, 58
  bleeding in, 44
Megacolon, 38

Megaloblastic anemia, 132
Meigs' syndrome, ascites and, 70
  pleural effusion and, 20
Melanosis coli, 38
Melena, 44
MEN (multiple endocrine neoplasia syndrome), and hyperparathyroidism, 94
MEN 1 (multiple endocrine neoplasia syndrome type 1), 200
Ménière's disease, 168
Meningitis, bacterial, headache and, 166
  dementia and, 170
Menses, absence of, 180
Mental status, altered, 172, *173*, 174, *175*
Mesenteric artery occlusion, periumbilical abdominal pain in, 58
Metabolic acidosis, hyperkalemia and, 88
  hyperphosphatemia and, 98
Metabolic alkalosis, 106, *107*
Metabolism, abnormalities of, causing constipation, 38
Metastases. See also *Cancer*.
  fever of unknown origin associated with, 6
  hemoptysis associated with, 16
Methanol, acidosis and, 104
Methemoglobinemia, 138
  cyanosis associated with, 18
Microcytic anemia, 120, *121*
Micturition syncope, 28
Mid-diastolic murmur, 34
Midsystole, murmur in, 34
Migraine headache, 166–167
Miliary tuberculosis, aplastic anemia and, 128
  pancytopenia and, 140
Milk-alkali syndrome, 38
  hypercalcemia and, 95
Mitral prolapse, chest pain in, 24
Mitral regurgitation, as systolic murmur, 34
Mitral stenosis, hemoptysis associated with, 16
Monoclonal gammopathy of unknown origin, 162
Monocytosis, 148, *149*
Mononucleosis, infectious, 52, 150
''Moth-eaten'' scalp alopecia, 208
Mountain sickness, acute, alkalosis and, 106
MRI (magnetic resonance imaging), of renal arteries, 32
Mucinosis, follicular, 208
Mucosal biopsy, chronic diarrhea and, 42
Multinodular goiter(s), 186, 188
  toxic, 190
Multiple endocrine neoplasia syndrome, and hyperparathyroidism, 94
Multiple endocrine neoplasia syndrome type 1 (MEN 1), 200
Multiple myeloma, 162
  purpura and, 206
Multiple sclerosis, dementia and, 170
Murmurs, cardiac, 34, *35*
Muscle weakness, 216, *217*
Muscular dystrophy, 216
Musculoskeletal disorder(s), 212–219

U

Ulcerative colitis, arthritis and, 214
Ultrasonography, doppler, 30
   in cholecystitis, 54
   in jaundice, 64
   in oliguria, 76
Uremia, generalized abdominal pain and, 56
Ureterosigmoidoscopy, hypokalemia and, 87
Urine, sodium content of, 76
Urine dipstick, for proteinuria, 80
Urticaria, 204, *205*
Urticaria pigmentosa, 204

V

Valvular disease, cardiac, chest pain and, 24
    hypotension and, 26
Variceal bleeding, 44
Vascular disease, collagen, cardiomegaly associated with, 36
Vascular malformations, in gastrointestinal bleeding, 44
Vascular occlusion, periumbilical abdominal pain in, 58
Vasculitis, altered mental status and, 174
   leukocytoclastic, 206
   nonlupus, fever of unknown origin associated with, 6
   oliguria and, 76
Vasovagal syncope, 28

Vena cava, inferior, obstruction of, 68
Venogram, adverse reactions to, 30
Veno-occlusive disease, hepatic, 68
Ventilation-perfusion scan, for pulmonary embolus, 18
   in myocardial infarction, 24
Ventricular septal defect(s), murmur in, 34
Vertigo, 168, *169*
Very low-density lipoprotein, 196
Villous adenoma, hypokalemia and, 86–87
Viral gastroenteritis, acute diarrhea and, 40
Viral hepatitis, and hepatomegaly, 66
Viral infection(s). See also *Infection(s).*
   arthralgia and, 212
   chronic, fatigue associated with, 2
   neutropenia and, 142
   thrombocytopenia and, 158
Viral myocarditis, cardiomegaly and, 36
Virchow node, 112
Vitamin B_{12} deficiency, anemia and, 130, 132, *133*
   neutropenia and, 142
Vitamin D, and hypocalcemia, 92
   hypercalcemia and, 94
   hypophosphatemia and, 96
Vitamin D-resistant rickets, hypophosphatemia and, 96
Vitamin K-dependent factors, 108–109
Vomiting, alkalosis and, 106
   in hypokalemia, 86
Von Willebrand's disease, 110

W

Waldenström's macroglobulinemia, 162
   purpura and, 206
Washout thrombocytopenia, 160
Wegener's granulomatosis, 206
Weight gain, 10, *11*
Weight loss, 8, *9*
Wernicke's encephalopathy, 174
Western blot test, for human immunodeficiency virus, 4
Whipple's disease, arthritis and, 214
Whipple's triad, 198
Wilms' tumor, proteinuria and, 80
Wilson's disease, 80, 124

X

Xanthoma, and hyperlipidemia, 194

Z

Zenker's diverticulum, 48